MEDICINE & SOCIETY IN LATER MEDIEVAL ENGLAND

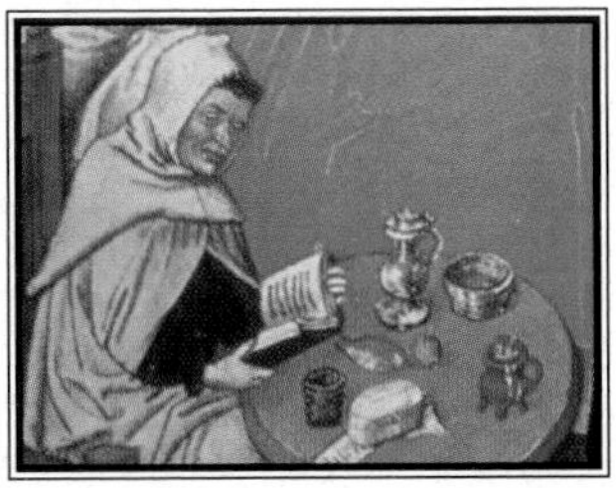

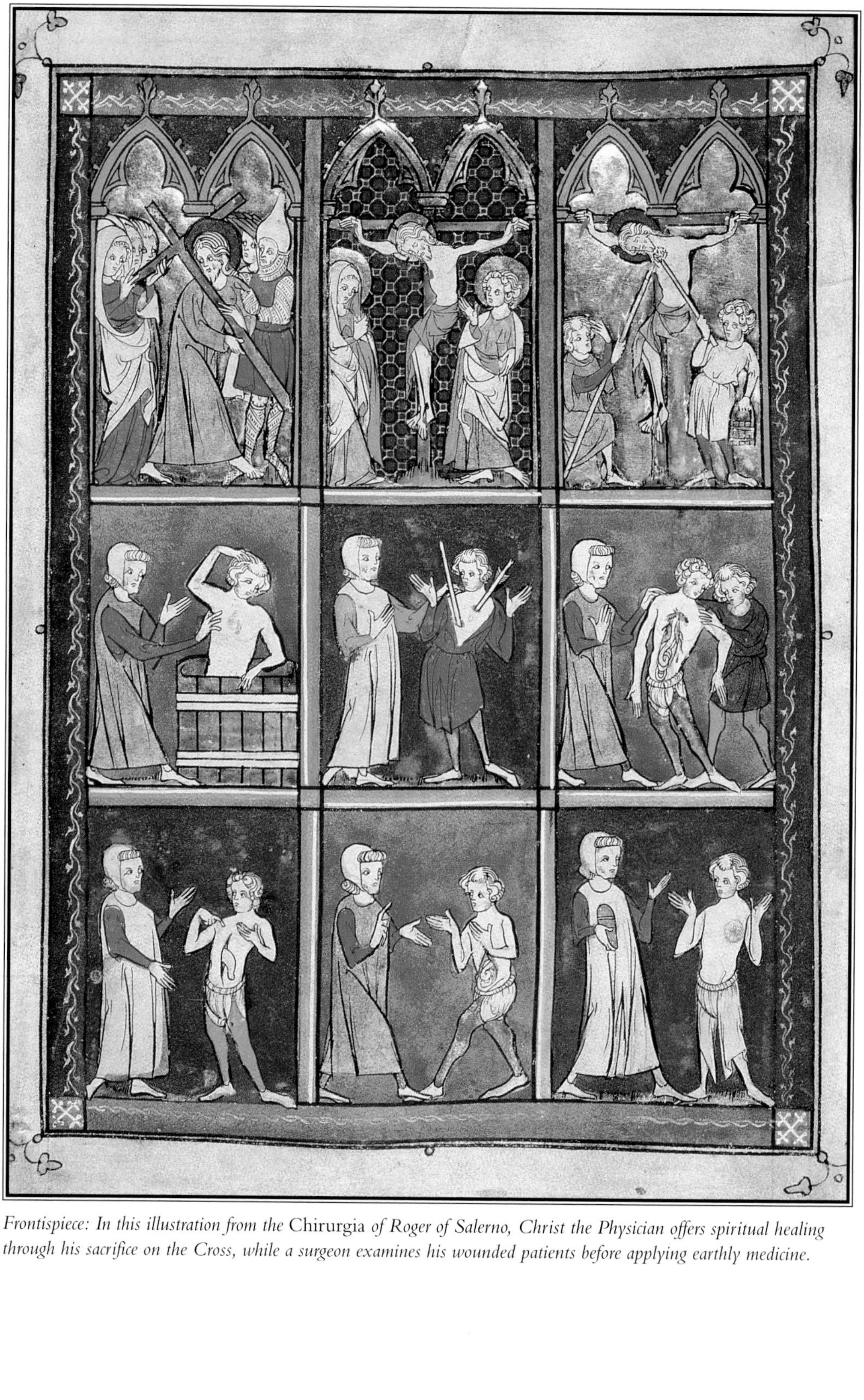

Frontispiece: In this illustration from the Chirurgia *of Roger of Salerno, Christ the Physician offers spiritual healing through his sacrifice on the Cross, while a surgeon examines his wounded patients before applying earthly medicine.*

MEDICINE & SOCIETY IN LATER MEDIEVAL ENGLAND

CAROLE RAWCLIFFE

ALAN SUTTON PUBLISHING LIMITED

First published in the United Kingdom in 1995 by
Alan Sutton Publishing Ltd · Phoenix Mill · Far Thrupp · Stroud · Gloucestershire

British Library Cataloguing in Publication Data

Rawcliffe, Carole
Medicine and Society in Later Medieval
England
I. Title
610.942

ISBN 0–86299–598–1

Library of Congress Cataloging in Publication Data applied for

Typeset in 10/13 pt Bembo.
Typesetting and origination by
Alan Sutton Publishing Limited.
Printed in Great Britain by
Butler & Tanner, Frome, Somerset.

CONTENTS

for
Peter Martin

LIST OF ILLUSTRATIONS

COLOUR PLATES

BLACK AND WHITE ILLUSTRATIONS

ACKNOWLEDGEMENTS

It is impossible in this short space to thank everyone who has helped one way or another with the writing of this book. I am indebted to the staff of the Reading Room and Manuscript Room of the British Library, of the Public Record Office, the Warburg Institute, the Norfolk Record Office, the University of East Anglia Library and of all the other institutions listed in the bibliography at the end of the volume. The unfailing courtesy and helpfulness extended over many years by the staff of the Library of the Wellcome Institute and of the Institute of Historical Research deserve especial mention. I would particularly like to express my gratitude to Miss Rosemary Taylor and Mr William Kellaway (both of whom are now retired) and Mr Donald Munro for assistance given cheerfully beyond the call of duty. Parts of this book have been read at various times at seminars run by Dr Caroline Barron, Dr Paul Brand and Mr Jim Bolton at the Institute of Historical Research, and I am grateful to those present for ideas and suggestions.

So many friends and associates have generously placed their expertise at my disposal: Miss Margaret Condon is, as always, a positively encyclopaedic source of information; Dr Anthony Gross never fails to suggest new and interesting ways of looking at the fifteenth century; and I am obliged to Professor Martha Carlin, Dr John Henderson and Dr Peter Murray Jones for supplying offprints and transcripts of documents. Dr Jones's comments on the final version of this book have been most welcome. Two dear friends and former colleagues, Miss Elizabeth Danbury and Dr Linda Clark, have not only read through and discussed the ensuing text, but have also given much-valued encouragement and support for more years than either of them probably cares to remember. So too have Miss Joan Henderson, Mrs Rochelle Haussman and Mr Alasdair Hawkyard, whose kindness is likewise recalled with gratitude.

Ironically, in view of its subject matter, the start and completion of this book coincided with the only sustained bouts of ill-health to affect me during my adult life. All medical historians should, no doubt, experience some of the physical discomfort about which they write, but a little goes a long way, and I am grateful to Dr Robert Danbury and Mr Roger Martin, heirs to the best aspects of the Hippocratic tradition, for hastening my recovery. I owe a very different debt to Professor P.M. Stell, who has made available the fruits of a long and distinguished career as a surgeon, patiently answering a host of questions and explaining the rudiments of practice with enviable lucidity.

The last chapters of this book were written after my appointment as senior research fellow at the Centre of East Anglian Studies at the University of East Anglia, a move made possible by generous funding from the Wellcome Trust for a project on the history of the Great Hospital, Norwich. The opportunity to work in such a scholarly and civilized environment is a blessing indeed: the Director, Dr Richard Wilson, has been unfailingly kind and supportive since my arrival, as have other staff and students, most notably my two colleagues, Dr Roberta Gilchrist and Miss Mavis Wesley. Thanks are also due to Dr Steven Cherry and the students who have taken part in our medical history course, and to the Women's History Group at UEA for giving me the opportunity to refine and develop many of my ideas. Dr Anthony Batty Shaw, Dr David Welch, Mr Alan Green and other members of the Norwich Medico-Chirurgical Society have also done much to make the study of medical history in East Anglia rewarding and enjoyable. It was while teaching the history of medieval medicine at Norwich that I came fully to appreciate the importance of visual aids; and most of the illustrations reproduced in this book were originally chosen to accompany these lectures.

Collaborating with the staff at Alan Sutton Publishing has, as always, been a pleasure. Mr Peter Clifford's Job-like patience in waiting years for a typescript which, when finally delivered, was twice the length first agreed, Mr Roger Thorp's exemplary skill and tact as an editor and Mrs Rosemary Prudden's help at the production stage have proved invaluable.

Although a substantial part of my academic career has been devoted to late medieval English politics, an early interest in medicine was inspired by my parents, whose constant help and encouragement can never be repaid. My mother has cast a keen eye over each and every chapter and made many suggestions: I hope she, my father and Judy enjoy the finished product, which owes such a debt to them. Finally, I must thank Peter Martin, who has invested so much time, energy and enthusiasm in this book that he could well have written it himself. Given his *métier* as a crime-writer, the plot would have been far tighter and the count of bodies even higher: as it is, the dedication goes to him.

The author and publisher wish to thank The Council of the Early English Text Society and Boydell & Brewer Ltd for their kind permission to reproduce extracts. While every effort has been made to secure permissions, we may have failed in a few cases to trace the copyright holder. We apologize for any apparent negligence.

PREFACE

My interest in the field of medieval medical history was aroused almost by accident several years ago, when I was engaged in research for an article on the settlement of lawsuits by arbitration. A case concerning a negligent physician drew my attention, not so much because of the legal aspects of the dispute, which were fairly straightforward, but chiefly on account of the fascinating insight which it provided into a new and very different side of fifteenth-century life. Having systematically investigated the political, financial and administrative affairs of their subjects, analysed their social relationships, discovered what they read and where they lived, examined their religious beliefs and determined just how litigious they may have been, historians sometimes tend to assume that little else can be learned about the men and women of late medieval England. Textbooks on the period may now concentrate more upon standards of living and mortality rates than was once the case, but on the whole they still ignore such basic questions as how the human body was believed to work, what measures might be essayed to cure or prevent illness, and who exactly assumed responsibility for healing the sick. Nor, in contrast to the prominent place occupied by the legal profession in late medieval studies, has much attention been given to the availability and cost of medical treatment or the training of practitioners. Significantly, for instance, the book of papers on *Profession, Vocation and Culture in Later Medieval England* (Liverpool, 1982), dedicated to the late A.R. Myers, does not contain a single reference to this topic.

Ideas about the nature and causes of disease are likewise rarely considered outside the pages of specialist literature. Yet, to give just one example, the belief that physical suffering in general, and leprosy and madness in particular, might be inflicted directly by God as a punishment for sin has important constitutional implications for a period in which one English king was widely rumoured to be a leper, and another endured protracted bouts of insanity. Historians have already drawn attention to the frequent use of medical metaphors in the political and religious writing of medieval England: clearly, interest in, and knowledge about, medicine extended far beyond a narrow group of university-trained practitioners. Long before the arrival of the printing press, vernacular tracts concerning the diagnosis, treatment and avoidance of disease enjoyed wide circulation among educated townspeople, the gentry and the baronage, and, in conjunction with older folk traditions, exercised a profound influence throughout society. Taken as a whole, these issues are fundamental to our understanding of the period, and I have tried to make good the lack of readily available information which hampered my own early attempts to learn more about the place of medicine in English life between the first outbreak of plague in 1348 and the early sixteenth century.

Such general surveys as C.H. Talbot's *Medicine in Medieval England* (London, 1967) and S. Rubin's *Medieval English Medicine* (New York, 1974) provide a useful background to the subject, and readers wishing to acquire an overview from Anglo-Saxon times will find both extremely helpful. Yet there is no detailed study of the fourteenth and fifteenth centuries to compare with

E.J. Kealey's *Medieval Medicus* (Johns Hopkins, 1981), which concentrates on the period 1100–54, relies heavily on primary sources and attempts to set medicine in a wider political and social context. R.S. Gottfried's *Doctors and Medicine in Medieval England 1340–1530* (Princeton, 1986) raises some interesting questions about the role and status of the emergent medical profession, but contains so many errors that it misleads rather than illuminates. (Indeed, I chose not to consult it at all when writing this book.) Many valuable articles, monographs and editions of contemporary medical texts have, however, been produced; and as my investigations progressed, I became increasingly persuaded that the fruits of this research ought to be made accessible to a far wider readership. It is important, too, that medical historians should appreciate the relevance to their work of records which are customarily the preserve of scholars active in other disciplines. Whole classes of source material, ranging from customs accounts to sermons, from political propaganda to chivalric romances, constitute a vital, but generally untapped, reservoir waiting to be used. I have drawn upon the kind of evidence which rarely appears in more traditional studies of late medieval medicine, but which will, I hope, make the subject of immediate interest to readers who are already at home in the world of the Pastons, the Stonors and the Lisles. One consequence of such an approach is that the Church (Chapter I) and women (Chapters VIII and IX) play an unusually prominent part in this study. Although women were responsible for most of the routine health care on offer in later medieval England, their contribution is often overshadowed because of the emphasis placed upon university-educated or otherwise licensed practitioners. I have also been anxious to stress the multiplicity of potential cures, including recourse to saints, magic, astrology and herbal preparations, available to the medieval patient.

Readers who wish to pursue the study of academic medicine and the dissemination of medical texts are referred to N.G. Siraisi, *Medieval and Early Renaissance Medicine* (Chicago, 1990), and to the work of F.M. Getz and L.E. Voigts listed in the bibliography. Being keenly aware of my limitations in this respect, I have concentrated here upon the social context and practical ramifications of contemporary medical theory, rather than the history of the ideas themselves, which has been admirably chronicled elsewhere. An important collection of essays on *Practical Medicine from Salerno to the Black Death*, edited by L. Garcia-Ballester and others, and M.R. McVaugh's study of medicine in medieval Aragon appeared after this book was finished. Technically speaking, neither falls within my chronological or geographical remit, but both are included in the section on further reading because they illuminate much of what I have written.

It remains to say a word about my use of source material. Quotations from Latin and French have either been translated by me into English or taken from modern, easily accessible translations. But, with a few modifications, I have cited early English texts in the original language, explaining difficult or technical words in square brackets. This, I think, provides a feeling of immediacy, and gives the past an authentic voice. My aim throughout has been to make the subject as clear and intelligible as possible, while at the same time providing detailed endnotes and a full bibliography for readers who wish to explore particular points in depth. The endnotes for individual chapters are entirely self-contained: works are cited in full on their first appearance in each chapter, and then referred to in subsequent notes by either the name of the author or, in the case of editions, a short title.

The terminology employed by fourteenth- and fifteenth-century Englishmen and women to describe medical practitioners is diverse and often perplexing. Although the style *medicus* tends, customarily, to refer to a practitioner of medicine, as opposed to surgery, this convention is not invariable. The words 'leech' and '*mire*' (from Anglo-Norman) are generally applied to dispensers of physic below the rank of graduate, but here, too, regional differences and changes of usage are common. Outside London, the royal court and the great baronial houses, surgery was mostly undertaken by barbers (whom modern historians anachronistically persist in calling barber-surgeons), while in the City itself the company of surgeons constituted a small, but influential, élite. In addition, the universities of Oxford and Cambridge produced a *cadre* of physicians, often (but not always) distinguished in the records by reference to their status as masters or doctors of medicine. To add to the confusion, leading practitioners of surgery and quite a few physicians who had never attended university were sometimes addressed as '*magister*' ('master') as well. Where possible, I have attempted to simplify matters by using a more limited vocabulary, but it is important to bear these nuances in mind. Nor should we forget that in an age before the establishment of a professional monopoly wise women, empirics and herbalists actually constituted the great majority of practitioners at work among the sick.

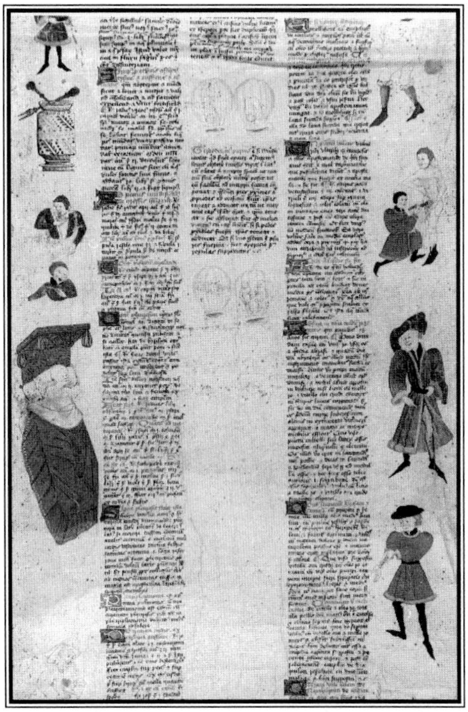

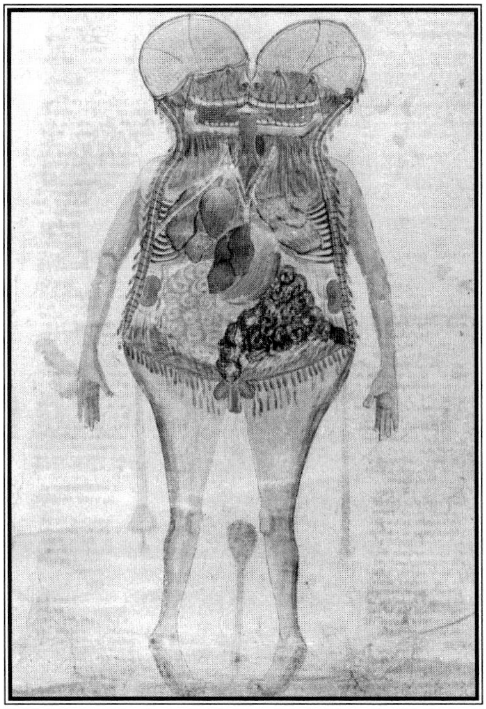

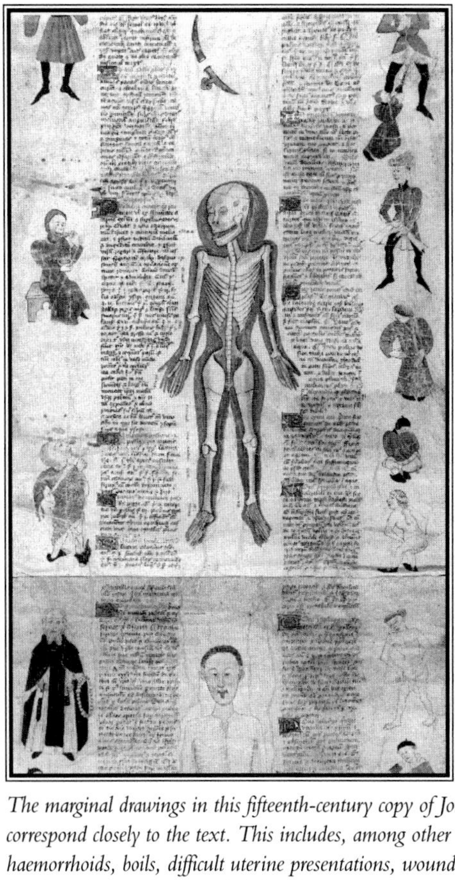

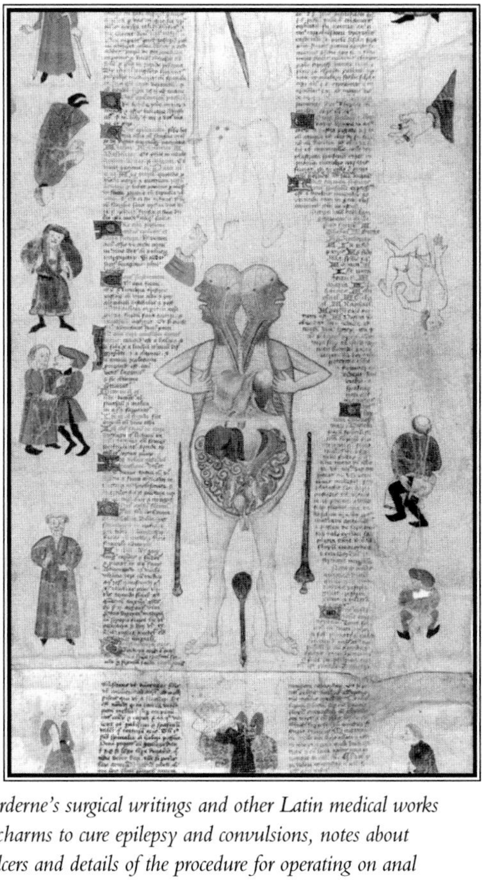

The marginal drawings in this fifteenth-century copy of John of Arderne's surgical writings and other Latin medical works correspond closely to the text. This includes, among other things, charms to cure epilepsy and convulsions, notes about haemorrhoids, boils, difficult uterine presentations, wounds and ulcers and details of the procedure for operating on anal fistulae. The artist's anatomical sketches owe more to the imagination, and provide a stark reminder of the ubiquity of Death.

CHAPTER ONE

DISEASES OF THE SOUL

God tests those he loves in the same way as the goldsmith refines gold in the furnace. The base metal vanishes completely, but the pure gold emerges truer and better than ever it was before. Sickness likewise inflicts pain and burning, but just as nothing purifies gold like fire, so nothing cleanses the soul like illness. I mean, of course, the afflictions that God sends, not other types of suffering. For many people make themselves unwell through their own foolishness or ignorance; they, not God, are thus entirely responsible. . . . Now, the remedy against sickness visited by God is fortitude: be patient, and thank God for his favour in selecting and testing you in this way. And as regards ill-health caused by immoderation or folly, beg his mercy and forgiveness because you have through your own stupidity so damaged your body that you may no longer serve him as you ought. . . . Thus sickness brings spiritual healing, and cures the wounds of the soul, and prevents it from sustaining further damage, as it surely would had God not intervened. Sickness helps man to understand what he really is, and to know himself. He is a good master indeed who beats into man the knowledge of his own frailty, compared with the might of God, and teaches him the nature of this wretched world. Sickness is your goldsmith, who, in the bliss of heaven adds gilding to your crown. The more intense your suffering, so the more elaborate the goldsmith's work becomes: and the longer it lasts, the brighter shines the gold in the dusk when the martyrs gather in heaven, because of the pain you have endured on earth with a good will. Surely, there can be no greater sign of grace to you, who have deserved and earned the pains of hell, world without end, than to pass through a brief moment of woe here, today?

The English Text of the Ancrene Riwle

A recent article on terminal disease, written by one of the many medical correspondents now contributing to the popular press, noted that today an appreciable number of Englishmen and -women reach middle age before experiencing the loss of a close friend or relative.[1] 'Coming to terms' with death, he concluded, has become a serious problem for those of us fortunate enough to lead comfortable lives in the West, not least because polite society finds the subject as embarrassing and distasteful as the public discussion of sexual matters was to our Victorian forebears. Such scruples are, of course, only possible when a range of social, political, economic and medical factors combine to ensure that a relatively large sector of the population will survive in reasonable health to enjoy its allotted three score years and ten, finally departing this world from the isolation of a hospital bed or of an institution devoted to the care of the elderly. However much they may have wished to avoid the unpalatable facts of mortality, sickness and pain, our ancestors had no choice but to look Death repeatedly and squarely in the face, and in so doing devise very different strategies for dealing with physical suffering and bereavement. Whether, as Philippe Aries believed, the fascination with the macabre characteristic of much late medieval western art and literature was in fact 'the sign of a passionate love for this world and a painful awareness of the failure to which each human life is condemned', rather than an

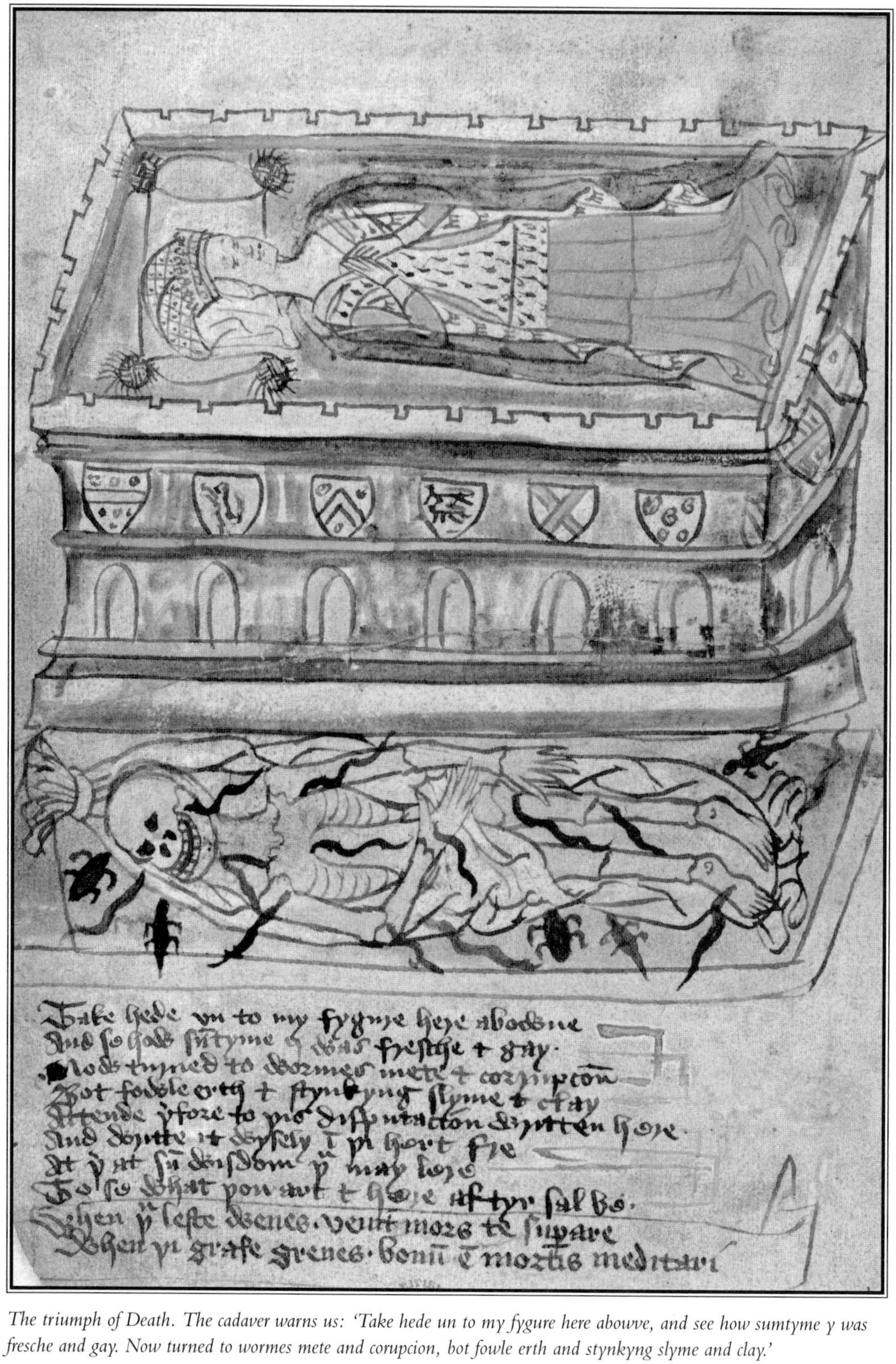

The triumph of Death. The cadaver warns us: 'Take hede un to my fygure here abouve, and see how sumtyme y was fresche and gay. Now turned to wormes mete and corupcion, bot fowle erth and stynkyng slyme and clay.'

unhealthy obsession with corruption and decay, the spectacle of cadavers, skeletons and open graves loses none of its power to disturb.[2]

It is impossible for modern readers truly to comprehend the shock and terror generated across Europe by the plague of 1348–9. Nor can we assume that subsequent epidemics caused any less panic and despair: a further twelve occurred throughout England between then and 1485, as well as numerous regional outbreaks which, cumulatively, did far more to hasten demographic decline.[3] Intestinal and pulmonary infections, typhus, measles and sickness arising from malnutrition were all endemic, often hitting local communities in waves, one after another. Thus, for example, a Scottish chronicler laconically recounted how, within a few months in 1439, spiralling grain prices were first followed by famine, then an unusually violent outbreak of dysentery with the highest death rate yet known in the country, and lastly a visitation of plague so virulent that all its victims died within twenty-four hours.[4] In this context, William Langland's famous depiction of the unassailable forces of Death, Nature and Old Age, unleashed upon the world as a warning to the ungodly, seems far more than a literary conceit:

> Elde the hore was in the vaunt-warde,
> And bar the baner by-fore Deth: by right he hit claymede.
> Kynde [Nature] cam after hym with menye kynne sores,
> As pockes and pestilences, and muche people shente;
> So Kynde thorgh corupcions culde full menye.
> Deth cam dryvyng after, and al to douste paschte [dashed]
> Kynges and knyghtes, caysers [emperors] and popes;
> Lered ne lewide [learned or ignorant], he lefte no man stande;
> That he hitte evene sterede nevere after.
> Many a lovely lady and here lemmanes [lovers] knyghtes
> Sounede and swelte for sorwe of Dethes dyntes.[5]

Epidemics and famines apart, medieval life was beset by constant threats to health arising from poor diet (at both ends of the social spectrum), low levels of hygiene, high rates of infant mortality, the risks of childbirth and repeated pregnancies, accidents and injuries. An examination of the skeletal remains of Sir Hugh Hastyngs, a Norfolk landowner who died in 1347 aged less than forty, reveals that he suffered from osteoarthritis, probably caused by continuous practice with a broad-sword or other heavy weapon, and compounded by the physical wear and tear of military campaigns in France. Although he was the son of a nobleman and had spent time at Court, he evidently consumed coarse bread containing particles of grit (of the sort eaten by the peasantry), which had caused progressive dental deterioration. A blow to the mouth had, moreover, deprived him of at least five or six front teeth, so that by the time of his death he must have found eating very difficult indeed.[6]

Facial disfigurements were by no means uncommon during this period: the heroes of one of the most popular chivalric romances of the fifteenth century, *Le Morte d'Arthur*, regularly identify each other by their most recent wounds; and in this respect, at least, the author (who must have sustained quite a few cuts and bruises during the course of his own turbulent career) seems to have been drawing on personal experience. We know that in 1374 about a quarter of recruits serving in the Provençal army were badly scarred on the hands or face; and that many English soldiers mutilated in the wars with France returned home in a parlous condition to beg.[7] Even allowing for the exaggeration common in such cases, one cannot but marvel at the powers of survival mustered by one Thomas Hostell, whose misfortunes had begun in 1415 at the siege of Harfleur. There he had been

> smyten with a springolt through the hede, lesing his oon ye, and his cheke boon broken; also at the bataille of Agingcourt, and after at the takyng of the carrakes on the see, there with a gadde of yren his plates smyten in sondre, and sore hurt, maymed and wounded; by meane wherof he being sore febeled and debrused, now falle to great age and poverty, gretly endetted, and may not helpe himself.[8]

Soldiers could hardly expect to avoid danger, but even the home (where a significant proportion of accidents still occur today) was beset by constant hazards. The children of the labouring poor, whose energy was consumed by the struggle to survive, often remained unsupervised for long periods. The juxtaposition in dark, cramped surroundings of open hearths, straw bedding, rush-covered floors and naked flames posed a continuous threat to curious infants, as did wells, ponds, agricultural or industrial implements, stacks of timber, unattended boats and loaded waggons, all of which appear with depressing frequency in coroners' reports as causes of death among the young.[9] Besides the obvious risk to health presented by the close proximity of domestic animals, which either shared their owners' quarters or wandered in off the streets, the very real possibility that one would maim or kill a child increased the odds against survival even more. In 1322, for example, Bernard de Irlaunde's baby daughter died just a few hours after being bitten on the head by a sow which had roamed into her father's shop in London. Citizens who wished to keep pigs were under strict orders to shut them up at home, but this can hardly have improved conditions for any children living on the premises.[10]

Evidence from Florence in the late 1420s suggests that the average expectation of life among the laity may have been twenty-nine-and-a-half years from birth for women and about one year fewer for men. Although these conclusions are tentative, they correspond roughly with statistics for the life expectancy of monks at Westminster Abbey during the same period, when a young man of twenty could hope, again on average, to survive for another decade. During the last quarter of the fifteenth century the mortality rate in this monastic community rose sharply as boys still in their teens, who lived communally in conditions likely to foster the spread of disease, stepped in to take the place of dead cloister monks, and themselves fell victim to epidemics. A similar picture emerges at Christ Church, Canterbury, where, between 1395 and 1505, an average of one year in every four witnessed some crisis in mortality. This meant that up to one monk in three died of a contagious disease, and any who lived beyond their early twenties could consider themselves fortunate.[11] Both of these houses were, however, situated in centres of high population density and thus risked exposure to infections, such as certain strains of tuberculosis, against which youngsters from the countryside had few defences. It may be that more isolated monasteries fared better, at least to the extent of avoiding the hazards of urban life.

So far as women of moderate or comfortable means were concerned, the contemporary belief that females lived longer than males may well have been founded in fact. If she could survive the diseases and accidents of infancy and the dangers of childbirth she would be spared a life of heavy manual labour, and with luck escape the brawls and other violent confrontations which so often claimed the lives of men in an age before antisepsis, blood transfusion and anaesthetics gave major surgery a viable chance of success. But the death rate among young and early middle-aged women of all classes remained high, partly because of epidemics but largely on account of the perils of pregnancy, parturition and post-natal infections. At least 1,992 of the Members returned to the English House of Commons between 1386 and 1421 are known to have been married, and of these a bare minimum of 397 (20 per cent) lost one wife and took another, while seventy-six had two wives or more. Only one of them was divorced. Since a substantial proportion of the rest are relatively obscure figures, about whom little is known, we can be reasonably confident that the incidence of mortality among MPs' spouses was, in fact, much higher. It is, however, worth noting that 536 (27 per cent) of the married MPs were themselves the second, third, fourth or even fifth husbands of women who had already been widowed, which supports the presumption that, after a certain point, females from the middle and upper classes probably stood a better chance of reaching old age.[12]

As medieval correspondents so often remind us, Death came unannounced, without warning, returning time and again to claim his unsuspecting victims. In 1453, for example, Margaret Paston informed her husband that

> as for tydyngys, Phylyppe Berney is passyd to God on Monday last past, wyt the grettes peyn that evyr I sey man. And on Tuysday Sere John Henyngham gede to hys chyrche and herd iij massys, and cam hom agayn nevyr meryer, and seyd to hese wyf that he wuld go sey a lytyll devocion in hese gardeyn and than he wuld dyne; and forth-wyth he felt a feyntyng in hese legge and syyd doun. Thys was at ix of the clok, and he was ded or none.[13]

The circumstances of Henyngham's death, after he had looked upon the Host with its promise of spiritual healing and eternal life, would have seemed enviable to contemporaries, although unless he had also been able to confess and repent his sins, receive absolution and take the viaticum, his immortal soul might still have been condemned to centuries of torment in purgatory or even the unending pains of hell. Fear of *mors improvisa*, the sudden and unexpected death which struck while its prey was unshriven and in a state of mortal sin, gave rise to a genre of devotional literature designed to inspire good works and foster an appropriate sense of contrition in the reader.[14]

Contemplation of the four last things (death, judgement, heaven and hell) was encouraged by the Church as a means of concentrating the mind upon the ordeal to come (colour plate 1). An unhealthy soul, troubled with nagging sores, unhealed injuries and the pernicious infection of sin would find the journey to heavenly bliss difficult, if not impossible. But spiritual medication was always at hand; and although the patient might be reluctant to take it, and 'make a sowre face', a few moments reflection on the fleeting, vulnerable nature of life on earth provided a powerful inducement:

> thou seeste, I saye, thy selfe yf thou dye no worse death, yet at the least lying in thy bedde, thy hed shooting, thy backe akyng, thy vaynes beating, thine heart panting, thy throte ratelyng, thy fleshe trembling, thy mouth gaping, thy nose sharping, thy legges coling, thy fingers fimbling, thy breath shorting, all thy strength fainting, thy lyfe vanishing, and thy death drawyng on. If thou couldeste nowe call to thy remembraunce some of those sicknes that have most grieved thee and tormented thee in thy dayes, as everi man hath felt some . . . as parcase the stone or the strangurye [intensely painful and difficult excretion of urine] have put thee, to thine own minde, to ne lesse torment than thou shouldest have felt if one

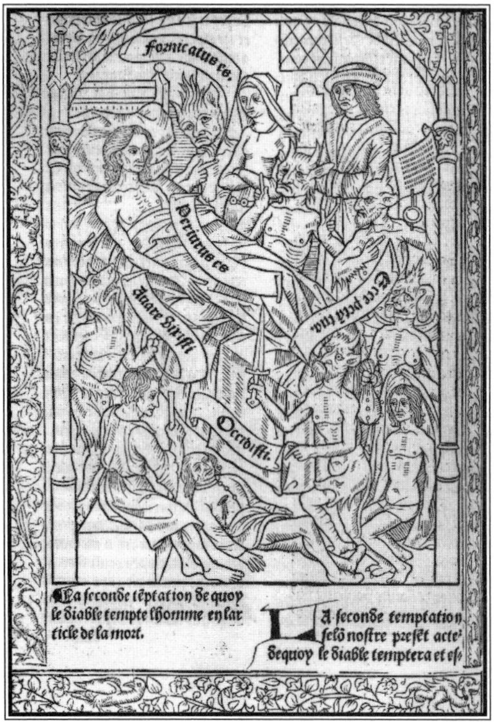

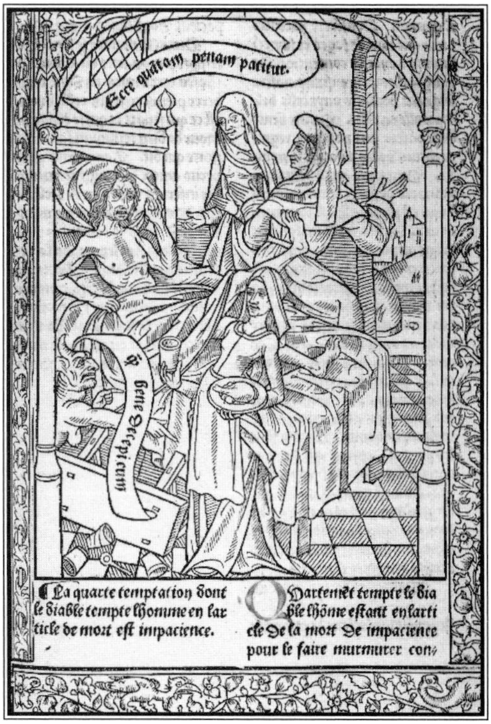
Ecce quātam penam patitur.
q̄ bene decepi eum
La quarte temptation dont le diable tempte lhomme en lar ticle de mort est impacience.

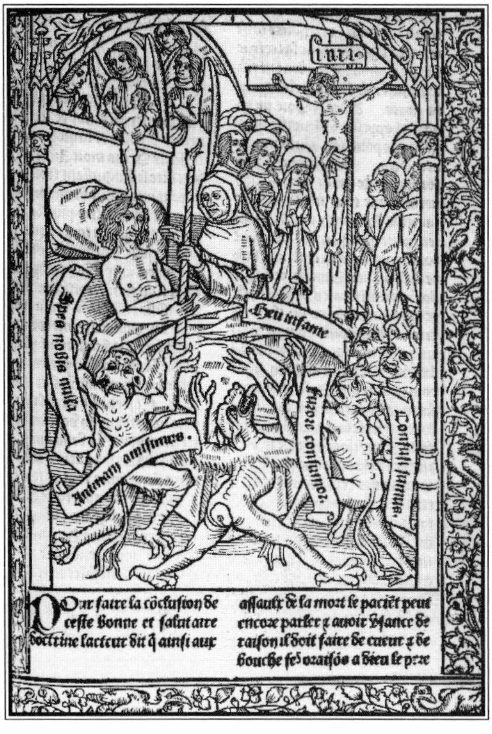

Pages from the Ars Moriendi, *or* Art of Death, *advise the reader on how to overcome the various temptations which may beset him or her at the end. With the help of Christ and the saints, the devil will be defeated, and the soul of the departed rise to heaven.*

> had put up a knife into the same place, and wouldest, as thee then seemed, have bene content with such a chaunge, think what it wil be than, whan thou shalt fele so many such paines in every part of thy bodi, breaking thy vaines and thy life stringes, with like pain and grief, as though as many knives as thy body might receive shold everiwhere enter and mete in the middes.[15]

Works such as this, devoted to the *ars moriendi*, or art of making a 'good death', dwell repeatedly upon the need to endure, even welcome physical pain in order to obtain spiritual redemption. Nor was this emphasis upon stoicism in the face of suffering restricted to an individual's last moments on earth: as the quotation at the start of this chapter reveals, illness was commonly regarded as either a gift from God, intended to add gilding to the martyr's crown, or else, more commonly, a punishment for irresponsibility or sin to be borne with a good grace.[16]

The invention of the microscope by Anthonie van Leeuwenhoek (d.1723) eventually made it possible to understand how diseases are spread by organisms invisible to the human eye, but during the Middle Ages and early modern period other, very different explanations offered a logical and theologically orthodox solution to the problem. Two main lines of thought, which derived, respectively, from the ancient Greeks (discussed in Chapter II) and the Fathers of the Christian Church, dictated how the human body and its disorders were perceived. While accepting without question the classical idea that the immediate, physical cause of most illnesses could be traced to an imbalance of the four humours, for which the sufferer himself was often to blame, medieval ecclesiastical and medical authorities alike believed that, in the long term, illness

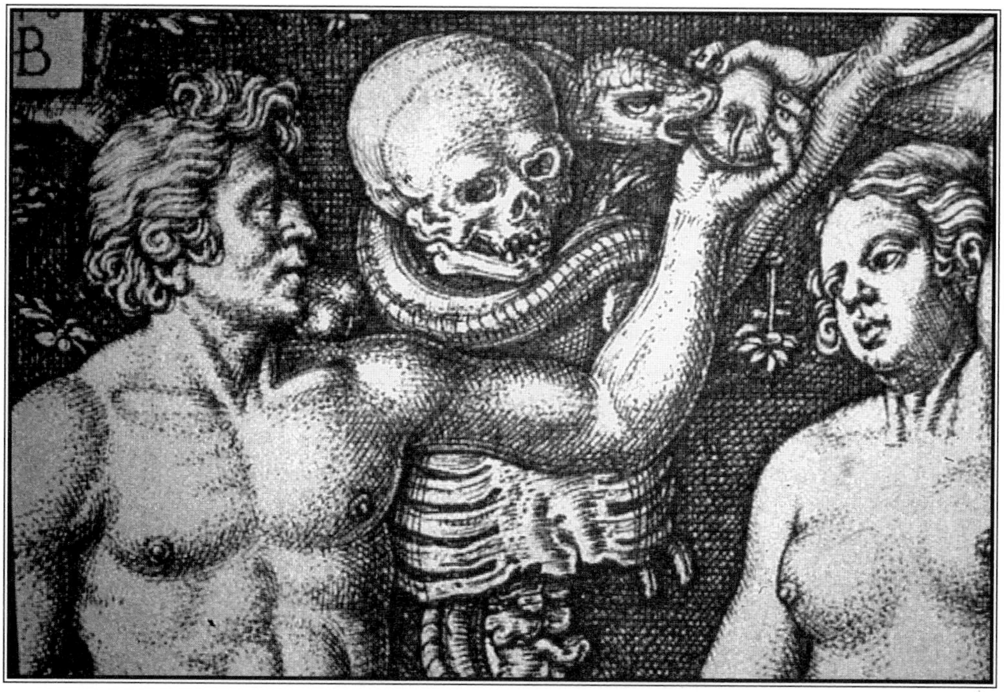

In this graphic depiction of the consequences of Original Sin, the Tree of Knowledge, whose fruit Eve tempts Adam to eat, is transformed into a skeleton. Thus illness and Death enter into Paradise.

and death were visited upon man by God. From the very moment of conception, as St Augustine of Hippo (d.430) maintained, every single human embryo was contaminated by the Original Sin of its first parents, Adam and Eve. Thus 'shackled by the bond of death' to the guilty pair, who had defied their maker and eaten of the forbidden fruit, all men and women became reluctant heirs to a legacy of suffering and mortality.[17] The consequences of Eve's fatal 'inabstinence' were described centuries later by John Milton (d.1674) in Book XI of *Paradise Lost*, at the stage where Adam is made to realize the full implications of her insubordination and his weakness. These lines, reminiscent of the passage from Langland given above, reflect assumptions about the cause and inevitability of disease current throughout the medieval period and beyond:

> . . . . Immediately a place
> Before his eyes appear'd, sad, noisome, dark,
> A Lazar-house it seem'd, wherein were laid
> Numbers of all diseas'd, all maladies
> Of ghastly Spasm, or racking torture, qualms
> Of heart-sick Agony, all feaverous kinds,
> Convulsions, Epilepsies, fierce Catarrhs,
> Intestine Stone and Ulcer, Colic pangs,
> Deamoniac Phrenzy, moping Melancholy
> And Moon-struck madness, pining Atrophy,
> Marasmus, and wide-wasting Pestilence,
> Dropsies, and Asthmas, and Joint-racking Rheums.
> Dire was the tossing, deep the groans, despair
> Tended the sick busiest from Couch to Couch;
> And over them triumphant Death his Dart
> Shook, but delay'd to strike, though oft invok't
> With vows, as thir chief good, and final hope.[18]

Added to the burden of original sin carried by all men and women, irrespective of their own personal conduct, was the private load shouldered by each individual as a result of his or her failure to behave as a good Christian should. To the author of *Dives and Pauper*, a tract on the virtues of holy poverty and obedience, some people were more 'enclynyd to synne' than others, and thus liable to be chastised with diseases which they had brought upon themselves through overindulgence. Punishment for the wickedness of parents was, moreover, frequently inflicted by God upon their children, notably in the case of sexual incontinence (even by married couples) or excessive displays of affection towards the young. 'Also God smytyght hem wyt sekenesse and myschef sumtyme for the fadrys synne and the modrys', he warned, 'for they lovyn hem to mechil [much] and welyn goon to hell to makyn hem riche and grete in this world.'[19]

Because they appeared to question, or even openly rebel against, the divine will, unrestrained displays of grief on the death of children were heavily criticized by such writers. Mothers, in particular, came under attack for their unseemly tears and intemperate words when, as so often happened, their offspring died young. The once fashionable idea that parental love flowered only after the heightening of middle-class sensibilities during the eighteenth century has, rightly, been exploded by historians over the last decade.[20] However much they might inveigh against 'thys women that wepe so sorowfully whan that hyr chyldryn dey them froo', preachers found it hard to subdue maternal instincts. John Wycliffe's complaint about the 'riche wifis' who 'wepen, grucchen and crien ayenst God, as God schulde not do ayenst her wille, and axen God whi he takith rathere here children fro hem than pore mennis, sith thei may betre fynde [support] here children than may pore men' speaks for itself.[21]

Yet good Christians still tried hard to accept pain and bereavement with humility, on the assumption that they would thus be spared a far worse ordeal in purgatory. Perhaps the Church's teachings about the expiatory nature of physical suffering offered some form of spiritual anaesthesia, a real opium of the people, as the sick or wretched consoled themselves with thoughts of celestial joy to come:

> Ther-fore, man, behold the goodness of God, how that he forgeveth the this grett longe peyne in chaunchynge the gret peyn of purgatorie in-to temperall peyn; that is, sekenes of bodie, lose of catell [goods], pursewynge of thin enmye. For thoo thou had all maner of sekenes of bodye all thi liffe tyme that all men myghte have, and thoo that thow lyveste an hundreth wyntere, yitt it were not so grevous as one daye in purgatorie. And yitt on [one] daye in this worlde of peyne is more helpynge to the towarde the blisse of heven than xxti [twenty] in the peyn of purgatorye, yiff that thow take it mekeliche.[22]

Although sleeping draughts, in the form of soporific drinks liberally laced with alcohol, were widely employed in the Middle Ages, the means of deadening pain were at best rudimentary and unpredictable. Discomfort caused by such chronic conditions as gout, hernias, intestinal parasites, rotten teeth and gums, ulcerated limbs and untreated gynaecological problems was, moreover, common. It would be naive to assume that these trials were invariably borne with resignation (Sir John Mandeville, for one, railed against 'the gowtes artetykes that me distreynen . . . agenst my will'); but for some the promise of a speedier passage through purgatory must have brought partial relief. Despite the agonies of arthritis, which often left her crying with pain, Henry VII's mother, the Lady Margaret Beaufort, remained a model of piety, throwing herself upon the will of God, and actually exacerbating her condition by spending hours on her knees every day in prayer.[23] Others may have found it harder to make sense of the divine purpose, yet there is plenty of evidence to suggest that pious men and women did their best to count the positive blessings of illness.

In the early 1420s, for example, the poet Thomas Hoccleve, who had apparently experienced a serious bout of mental collapse some five years before, explained what he considered to be the dual purpose of his ordeal. He, too, employs the conventional image of disease as a refiner's fire, melting away base impurities:

> Gold purgyd is, thou seyst, in the furneis,
> For the fyner and clenner it shall be;
> Of thy disease, the weyght and the peis [heaviness]
> Bere lyghtly, for God, to prove the,
> Scorgyd the hath with sharpe adversitie;
> Not gruche and sey 'Why susteyn I this?'
> For yf thow do, thow takest amis.
> But thus thow shuldest thinke in thyn herte,

And sey, 'To the, Lorde God, I have a-gylte
So sore: I moot for myn offensis smerte,
As I am worthy. O Lorde, I am spilt,
But [unless] thow to me thy mercy grante wilt.'[24]

Hoccleve's misery, as his 'witt were a pilgrime and went fer fro home', seems to have intensified after his recovery, for although he was duly grateful to God, 'the curtese leche [physician] moste sovereyne', for restoring him to his senses, his sickness had by then lost him many friends.

Except in rare cases, where apparent madness could, in fact, be seen as an attribute of sanctity, the insane aroused particular fear and unease because (in theory, at least) their sins seemed so terrible and their punishment so extreme. 'Natural' forms of insanity (as opposed to daemonic possession, which came, like a thunderbolt, directly from God) were often held by the Church to reflect a pernicious enthralment to one or more of the seven deadly sins, leading, in turn, to humoral disorders sufficiently violent to upset the brain. Wrath, gluttony or sexual vice would, for example, produce an intense level of heat and thus give rise to frenzy, while a corresponding degree of coldness was generated by sloth or the anguish experienced by disappointed lovers or the bereaved parents described above. This caused listlessness, the inability to concentrate and sometimes even stupor. Alternatively, the mentally ill might have succumbed to malign planetary influences, especially those of the moon, which gave its Latin name to lunacy and predisposed those men and women born under its sway towards irrational behaviour.[25] Yet even in the face of blind astrological forces, the good Christian was expected to put up a fight and keep his emotions under control. In short, whatever his particular brand of depravity or weakness, the madman seemed wilfully to have alienated himself from God by destroying his own reason: the one characteristic which distinguished him from brute animals and brought him closer to his Maker. This was, indeed, a fearsome thing to do.[26]

Extreme cases of dementia were customarily explained in terms of possession by demons, who could only enter a human body if the soul had already been weakened by sin or if God had instructed them to act on his behalf. He might wish to warn the proud or complacent of the folly of their ways before it was too late, giving them a sharp taste of the fire and brimstone to come. This was certainly how Margery Kempe (b.*c.* 1373) came to regard the eight months of puerperal insanity which she describes in some detail at the start of her spiritual autobiography. She had, in her own words, gone 'owt of hir mende' after a near-fatal confinement because of fear and desperation following her failure to make a full confession of some 'thyng in conscyens whech sche had nevyr schewyd be-forn'. Under constant restraint because of her repeated attempts at self-mutilation, she believed herself to be possessed by a pack of devils from whom she was eventually rescued by a vision of Christ, 'syttyng up-on hir beddys syde', like a caring physician.[27] Margery remained painfully aware that her devotional zeal, which found expression in bouts of uncontrollable weeping and religious ecstasy, might be mistaken for 'natural' madness, daemonic possession or the falling sickness. Her fears were more than justified, for many of the men and women who encountered her in this state were convinced that she must be an epileptic, and thus without question prey to diabolic forces. 'Than folke spitted at hir for horrour of the sekenes', she recounts, 'and sum scornyd hir and seyd that sche howlyd as it had ben a dogge, and bannyd hir and cursyd hir, and seyd that sche dede meche harm a-mong the pepyl.'[28]

Margery Kempe was fortunate in enjoying the support of a devoted husband and some powerful friends, who saved her from persecution and enabled her to enjoy a remarkable degree of freedom. Others, lacking such protection, were either forcibly detained, because they posed a threat to themselves and their neighbours, or expelled from the community to cause a nuisance elsewhere. The biographer of St Hugh, Bishop of Lincoln (d.1200), records how, on a ride through Cheshunt, Hertfordshire, they encountered a lunatic 'possessed by a terrible demon' who was lying bound with his head, hands and feet chained to posts. Even under restraint, he presented such a terrifying prospect that his own bishop had galloped past not long before 'as if pursued by the Furies', although Hugh felt no such fear in the presence of evil and soon restored him to his senses. The demon had apparently entered his victim's body while he lay asleep and defenceless on board a ship, near London; and the young man had been brought home in shackles to be kept safe by the villagers, who realized that only supernatural help would cure him.[29]

The connection between violent, antisocial behaviour and the powers of darkness continued to be made for centuries to come: in 1541, for example, the mayor and aldermen of Norwich issued orders for the expulsion of one Ralph Chamberlain, 'beyng vexid wyth a dyvyll and beyng lunytick', from the city under pain of imprisonment; and a few years earlier Sir Thomas More had advocated the use of 'betynge and correccyon' in the treatment of a man possessed by 'frantike heresyes'. As we shall see, heretics were more commonly described as spiritual lepers, but it is interesting to note that insanity, too, with its connotations of sin, figures in the vocabulary of abuse.[30] The idea that a devil might be flogged or starved out of the body of its demented host remained current throughout the Middle Ages, and likewise reflects an essentially 'moral' approach to mental illness. Clearly, the patient was in no state to make a full confession of sins, as, from 1215 onwards, the Church required all persons seeking either medical or surgical help to do; but at least he or she could be obliged to mortify the flesh in penance.[31]

Yet the confused or otherwise mentally disturbed did not always meet with hostility and rejection, nor were they invariably held responsible for their plight. Birth, wealth and connections usually guaranteed a degree of acceptance, as did a fairly general belief that some lunatics, at least, were unfortunate rather than evil. The jurors who returned a verdict of misadventure on the death of one of the brothers at a hospital in Beverley, Yorkshire, in 1285, seem not only to have been moved by the tragic circumstances involved, but also anxious to establish that the homicide could not be blamed for killing his dearest friend. While agreeing that he had acted at 'the instigation of the devil', they maintained that a previous *illness* had rendered him 'frantic and mad' and thus susceptible to the wiles of Satan. At no point was his sickness equated with sin.[32]

As they became more widely assimilated throughout society, medical theories concerning the cause and treatment of 'natural' madness (which are explored in subsequent chapters) led people to think in terms of diet, lifestyle and temperament. And although it was perfectly compatible with the Church's pronouncements about divine retribution, this emphasis on the management of disease clearly encouraged a more sympathetic approach. The tone of a letter sent, in about 1503, by the Earl of Oxford to Sir John Paston certainly reflects a very different attitude to that described above:

> And where as your broder, William, my servaunte, ys so troubelid with sekenes and crasid in his myndes that I may not kepe hym aboute me, wherfor I am right sory, and at this tyme sende hym to you; preying especially that he may be kepte surely and tendirly with you to suche tyme as God fortune hym to be bettyr assurid of hym-selfe and his myndes more sadly [wisely] disposid, whiche I pray God may be in shorte tyme.[33]

William, who was then entering his sixteenth year in the earl's service, had been 'sore dysesyd' at least once before, in 1492, when his infirmity had prevented him from joining an expedition to France. Noblemen were usually liberal over the provision of medical help for staff and retainers, although even the most compassionate would have found it difficult to tolerate eccentric behaviour in their households.

The problem of looking after those who were too deranged to be left untended was by no means confined to the upper ranks of society. During her long bout of puerperal psychosis, Margery Kempe was 'bowndyn and kept wyth strength bothe day and nyght', as also was another victim of the disease whom she encountered in the course of her travels. Both women had loving husbands who may have believed in diabolic possession but were certainly not disposed to abandon them to the devil, choosing rather to provide reliable keepers and pray for a speedy recovery.[34] A government enquiry of 1402 into the management of the London hospital of St Mary Bethlehem, the only institution in medieval England known to specialize in the care of the insane, revealed a catalogue of abuses caused by absenteeism and corruption. Some of the revenues embezzled by the warden had been collected from the friends and relatives of patients who paid for long periods to have them kept (as they believed) in reputedly secure and comfortable accommodation with the constant solace of religion available in the hospital chapel. The neighbours of Agnes Coteneys had, for instance, collected alms for eighteen months so that she could make a full recovery in the hospital, where she evidently remained, at their expense, after regaining her reason. Quite large sums of money also came from charitable donors all over England, who expected to improve the health of their own souls by helping men and women afflicted with madness: since Christ himself had cast out devils, it could be argued that the possessed, however sinful, deserved no less help and compassion than the hungry, sick or homeless.[35] Even after the implementation of sweeping reforms, conditions in St Mary Bethlehem (which owned stocks, manacles and chains for the restraint of violent inmates) probably left much to be desired, but it was generally perceived as performing a valuable, positive social function. As one London chronicler noted:

> Yn that place ben founde many men that ben fallyn owte of hyr wytte. And fulle honestely they ben kepte . . . and sum ben restoryde unto hyr wytte and helthe a-gayne. And sum ben a-bydyng there yn for evyr, for they ben falle soo moche owte of hem selfe that hyt ys uncrerabylle unto man. And unto that place is grauntyde moche pardon, more thanne they of the place knowe.[36]

So far as the propertied classes were concerned, the obligation to provide a reasonable level of support for the mentally ill and exercise responsible stewardship over their estates was enshrined in English law. There can be little doubt that many such 'idiots' were victimized by unscrupulous relatives, although in theory a sophisticated set of legal procedures existed for establishing whether or not a person was, indeed, insane, appointing guardians to manage his or her affairs and ensuring that they rendered proper accounts. The case of Emma Beston of Bishop's Lynn shows that in some instances, at least, the law could not only provide protection for vulnerable men and women, but also be applied with considerable sensitivity. Emma was initially examined in November 1382 by the escheator of Norfolk, who found that she had been suddenly deprived of her senses 'by the snares of evil spirits' some four years earlier, pronounced her incapable of managing her own affairs and placed her in the custody of a kinsman. Various appeals, ostensibly in her own name as well as on behalf of the municipal authorities, who resented the escheator's intervention, challenged this decision, claiming that she was perfectly sane and accusing her new guardian of fraud. But Emma had been abducted with the mayor's connivance, and it was only after the issue of successive royal writs that she was finally produced, in the following July, for interrogation at Lincoln. Four lawyers then embarked upon a systematic line of questioning:

> The said Emma . . . was asked whence she came and said that she did not know. Being asked in what town she was, she said that she was at Ely. Being asked what day that Friday was, she said she did not know. Being asked how many days there were in a week, she said seven, but could not name them. Being asked how many husbands she had had in her time she said three, giving the name of one only and not knowing the names of the others. Being asked whether she had ever had issue by them, she said that she had had a husband with a son, but did not know his name. Being asked how many shillings there were in forty pence, she said she did not know. . . . They examined her in all other ways which they thought best and found that she was not of sound mind, having neither sense nor memory, nor sufficient intelligence to manage herself, her lands or her goods. As appeared by inspection, she had the face and countenance of an idiot.[37]

Emma was duly returned to the care of her relative, although as a further safeguard her estates were entrusted to three other men, on the understanding that they would support her out of the proceeds and restore any additional profits if she recovered.[38] It is, of course, now impossible to tell how she actually fared, but the law had at least adopted a pragmatic approach to her problem, leaving the evil spirits to the Church.

No such protection was available for the disturbed or half-witted poor, who were forced to rely upon public charity and often took to the roads as beggars. The poet William Langland wrote movingly of their plight, reminding his readers of the moral obligation to help such 'murye-mouthed men, mynstrales of hevene and Godes boyes':

> The whiche aren lunatik lollers and leperes a-boute,
> And mad as the mone sitt, more other lasse.
> Thei caren for no cold, ne counteth of no hete,
> And arn meuvynge after the mone. Moneyles thei walke,
> With a good wil, witlees, meny wyde contreys,
> Right as Peter dude, and Paul, save that thei preche nat,
> Ne myracles maken. Ac meny tymes hem happeth
> To prophecien to the puple, pleyinge, as hit were;
> And to oure sight, as hit semeth, suthe [since] God hath the myghte
> To yeven eche a wyght wit, welthe and his hele,
> And suffreth such so gon, hit semeth to myn inwitt [knowledge]
> Hit arn as hus aposteles, suche puple, other as his privye
> disciples.[39]

In certain quarters, however, the stigma of sin remained sufficiently potent for otherwise charitable and pious individuals to shun the mentally disturbed and actually deny them help. John Baret, a prominent native of Bury St Edmunds, whose preoccupation with the next world was, even by contemporary standards, unusually obsessive, gave voice to this prejudice in the 1460s, when drawing up his last testament. 'I will that in no wyse noon ydiot nor fool occupye the seid goods', he instructed his executors with regard to a major bequest, 'but refuse hym and take anothir that is next, that the seid name of Baret may contynwe goodly as longe as God wochesaffe.'[40]

Because of their special commitment to assist the passage of the souls of founders and benefactors through purgatory, some hospitals went so far as deliberately to exclude anyone who threatened to disrupt the regimented hours of private prayer and liturgy devoted to this purpose. More to the point, the undesirables in question, who generally comprised lunatics, epileptics, lepers and pregnant women, seemed impure as well as disconcerting to the ecclesiastical authorities who ran these institutions, and therefore likely to render any devotions ineffective.[41] The insane thus found themselves in a highly equivocal position, although they were probably less exposed to extreme, often contradictory ideas about sickness than lepers, who also fell victim to the belief that their fate must, of necessity, have come as chastisement from God.

With certain notable exceptions, medieval theologians took a harsh view of leprosy (and all the other conditions with which it was often confused), sometimes portraying the disease as a symbol of deep-seated moral decay or as a real, physical manifestation of wickedness on the part of the sufferer or his parents. Orders issued by the third Lateran Council of 1179 for the isolation of lepers and subsequent attempts by ecclesiastical and lay authorities throughout Europe to restrict their movements have been seen by historians as part of a wider crusade against heretics, Jews, homosexuals and anyone else whose conduct or beliefs gave rise to suspicion.[42] Significantly, in this context, the heretic was frequently described in medical terms as a spiritual leper, infected by a poisonous contagion from which his soul was unlikely to recover, expelled from the community of the faithful and driven by uncontrollable sexual urges to contaminate those who fell into his clutches.[43] The horrific effects of lepromatous leprosy and the fear it inspired made it seem an especially appropriate punishment for the two sins of concupiscence and pride, which, in turn, were invariably represented as leprosy or cancer of the soul. 'For just as leprosy makes the body ugly, loathsome and monstrous,' ran one medieval homily, 'so the filth of lechery makes the soul very loathsome spiritually, and the swelling of secret pride is leprosy, that no man may hide':

> For man quaim sinne mad unhale,
> Hafd noht ben bette of his bale,
> Bot yef Crist haved til him comen,
> And his seknes opon him nomen,
> And clensed him of leper of sinne,
> That alle mankind was fallen in.
> For riht als leper mas bodi
> Ugli, and lathe, and unherly,
> Sua mas the filth of licheri
> The sawel ful lath, gastelye,
> And the bolning [swelling] of prive pride
> Es leper, that na man mai hide.[44]

By the start of the period considered here, leprosy seems already to have been in retreat, and many lazar houses were being closed or converted to other purposes. But the disease still claimed a regular quota of victims and lost none of its popularity with moralists, who used it as a kind of literary shorthand when describing the consequences of pride, the worst and most dangerous of the seven deadly sins. The widespread rumour, put about by his many enemies, that Henry IV had turned leprous after ordering the execution of Archbishop Scrope, in 1405, served to reinforce the image of an arrogant usurper, brought low by the wrath of God. Whatever his real, physical symptoms (which suggest heart disease), Henry's conduct marked him out as a moral and political leper. Medieval congregations were, after all, familiar with the biblical story of King Uzziah, who had contracted leprosy after merely presuming to serve as a priest in the Temple; nor was there any need to elucidate the battery of cautionary tales on the theme of beautiful women deformed beyond recognition because of their vanity.[45] Another type of homily, concerning the priest or visionary permitted by God to see and diagnose the spiritual ailments of parishioners taking communion, was likewise intended to shock by invoking an image of decay and corruption past redemption.[46] With varying degrees of sophistication, poets and storytellers further elaborated the theme of leprosy as a punishment for crime or depravity, especially of a sexual nature. It is, for example, interesting to note that all the lecherous conspirators in Hoccleve's tale of Jereslaus's wife are struck down by incapacitating diseases, the most evil of them all being turned into a 'foul leepre'; and that only after making a full confession of their sins are they cured by the heroine herself.[47]

Since both the Church and the medical profession maintained that carnal relations between a man and a menstruating woman (which were strictly forbidden by canon law) might well result in leprous offspring, and also regarded leprosy as a sexually transmitted disease, the association with lechery is easy to understand. Lepers were, moreover, believed to be especially libidinous: a fact which explains both the draconian measures for mortifying the flesh with prayer and fasting adopted by many lazar houses and the appearance in chivalric romances of marauding packs of lepers with voracious sexual appetites.[48] How appropriate that the lovely Cresseid, who is not only vain, blasphemous and proud but also little more than a harlot with 'wantoun blude', should be condemned to end her days in the dirt and penury of a 'spittail-hous':

My cleir voice and my courtlie carrolling,
Quhair I was wont with ladyis for to sing,
Is rawk as ruik, full hiddeous, hoir and hace;
My plesand port all utheris precelling,
Of lustines I was held maist conding;
Now is deformit the figour of my face;
To luik on it na leid now lyking hes.
Sowpit in syte, I say with sair siching
Ludgeit amang the lipper-leid allace.
O Ladyis fair of Troy and Grece, attend
My miserie, quhilk nane may comprehend,
My frivoll fortoun, my infelicitie,
My greit mischief quhilk na man can amend.
Be war in tyme, approchis neir the end,
And in your mynd ane mirrour mak of me.[49]

[My clear voice and melodious singing,
when I used to perform with the ladies,
is hoarse as a rook, truly hideous, feeble and rasping;
my pleasing gait, which excelled all others
(for I was held to be the liveliest of all);
now the shape of my face is deformed,
and no man wants to look at it.
Drowned in sorrow, I cry with great sighing,
lying among the leper-folk, alas!
O, fair ladies of Troy and Greece, pay heed
to my misery, which none can measure,
my fickle fortune, my unhappiness,
my terrible disease, which nobody can cure.
Learn your lesson before it is too late; the end is nigh,
so see in me a reflection of yourselves.]

It might be supposed, in view of the judgement passed against him, that the medieval leper had little choice but to hide away in some isolated spot far from his persecutors. But other, very different ideas about his social worth and spiritual status confused the issue: like the mentally sick, who aroused conflicting emotions and provoked a variety of responses, he could also be seen as one of the elect, permitted by God to endure purgatory on earth and thus pass directly to heaven. To Hugh of Lincoln, whose sympathy for the insane has already been noted, lepers were 'the flowers of paradise and the lucent pearls in the crown of the eternal king'; the more deformed their bodies, the brighter shone their souls; and the greater their suffering, the more certain they were of salvation.[50] His desire to wash the feet of lepers, embrace them and kiss their sores was by no means unusual: many devout Englishmen and -women, including Margery Kempe, sought to do likewise, partly as an act of Christian humility, partly out of sympathy for the afflicted and also because of their respect for those whom God had marked as his own. So great was their longing to identify with the crucified Christ, some female mystics even prayed that they might themselves contract the disease and thus experience similar extremes of pain and rejection. They hoped, too, that their sacrifice would ease the punishment endured in purgatory by other sinners, just as Christ had redeemed mankind through his ordeal on the cross.[51]

If the majority of benefactors could not quite overcome their fear of contagion to follow Hugh's example, let alone offer themselves as victims, they were at least generous in the matter of endowing and maintaining lazar houses and providing alms for the inmates of such institutions. These customarily stood at the very gates and walls of English towns and cities, reflecting the ambivalent, liminal position of the leper. Having actually been obliged to undergo a symbolic funeral on admission, he was, in the eyes of the Church, neither dead nor alive, neither in heaven nor on earth, neither an outcast nor a full member of the community. But he remained a common sight, with his staff, begging bowl and clapper; and, so far as we can tell from surviving municipal records, attempts at segregation were often half-hearted and ineffective.[52] Tolerance may have increased as the disease began to retreat, but long before then individual writers had stressed the need for charity and compassion. At the opposite extreme from the homiletic literature threatening leprosy as a punishment for sin may be found another genre, extolling the merits of those who showed kindness to lepers and reaped their due reward, either in heaven or more immediately on earth. One story tells how a woman cared secretly for 'lepre folk' against her husband's wishes and risked death by smuggling a particularly sad case into her own room. Wild panic followed the knight's unexpected return, at which point the chamber was miraculously filled with perfume and he himself 'wex als meke as a lambe', devoting the rest of his life to God and good works.[53]

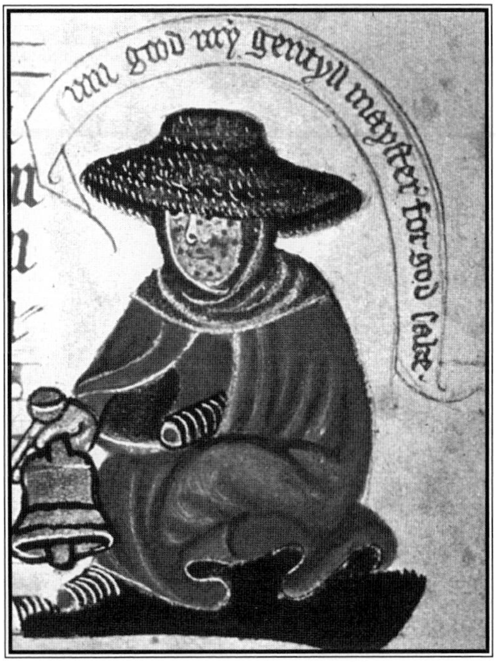

A female leper, in an advanced state of the disease, warns passers-by of her presence by ringing a bell, which also serves to attract alms. So does her cry: 'Sum good my gentyll mayster for God sake.'

Just as 'natural' madness could be attributed to humoral imbalance, astrological forces or changes in the sufferer's circumstances or environment, similar factors (as well as contagion and heredity) figured prominently in the aetiology of leprosy. But whereas the Church tended to blame lunatics and lepers for the sin, self-indulgence or weakness which had caused them to destroy their own health, the medical profession adopted a rather less judgemental approach. By concentrating upon the need for a careful diagnosis, and attempting to understand the nature of the disease, physicians and surgeons grew disinclined to moralize. They still accepted (or at least did not deny) that leprosy might well have been inflicted as an act of divine retribution, but at the same time recognized the psychological damage likely to result from too much sermonizing:

> Firste, in clepynge Goddes help, he schall conforte ham and saie that this passioun [suffering] or sekenesse is salvacioun of the soule and noght to say the trouthe, for if leprouse men were reproved, it were a purgatorie to the soule. And if the world have hem in hate, neverthelatter God have hem not in hate. Ye, but he loved Lazer [Lazarus], the leprouse man, more than other men. If soche men forsothe be noght reprovede, thai schal stande in pees.[54]

The evidence of Christ's healing miracles (the Lazarus whom he loved was 'sick', however, not leprous: John 9: 1) did much to counter the prejudice felt at all levels of society towards the lepers, epileptics, lunatics and outcasts whose condition marked them out as wastrels or sinners. On a more general level, it helped to reconcile the Church to the practice of earthly medicine, which appeared, on the face of things, to defy the will of God by alleviating pain and prolonging life.[55] Another potent influence stemmed from the idea of *Christus Medicus*, Christ the physician of diseased souls, a concept which drew heavily upon contemporary medical theory, and bestowed implicit approval upon the work of mortal practitioners. The latter were, of course, seen to be fallible, since unlike God they were not dealing with men and women whom they

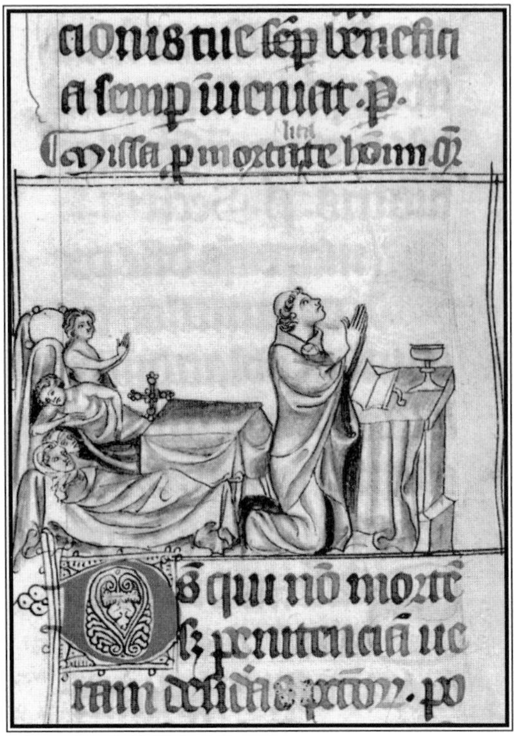

During times of pestilence, special masses were said to protect the faithful from contagion. No earthly medicine can save the patients on the left, although the Eucharist provides balm for troubled souls, and offers a promise of salvation.

themselves had created; but in other respects the comparison made much of their skill and sensitivity, not to mention the range and ingenuity of the treatment at their disposal. The writings of St Augustine contain numerous passages on the theme of Christ's devotion to his spiritual patients, however difficult and fearful they might be. His ordeal on the cross is, for example, compared to the reassurance offered by a physician who agrees to taste unpleasant medicine first:

> Drink, O sick one, of the bitter cup in order to become well, you, whose internal organs are diseased without exception. Do not fear to drink. For to dispel your fear the Physician drank first, that is, the Lord drank first the bitterness of the passion. He had no sin, he had nothing to be cured; yet he drank. Drink until the bitterness of this age passes away, until there comes a time when there will be no scandal, no anger, no wasting disease, no bitterness, no fever, no deceit, no enmities, no old age, no strife.[56]

Augustine and successive generations of theologians further maintained that the holy panacea itself derived from Christ's body and blood (as revealed to the faithful during the mass) and could heal the most ulcerated and festering soul if properly administered. This was a widespread belief, reflected in popular devotional literature: one of the much-loved prayers of St Bridget of Sweden (d.1373), who experienced many visions of the Passion, invoked Jesus, the 'hevenly leche', and his tormented body as sure protection against the contagion of sin; while for St Catherine of Siena (d.1380) the 'fire of love' which had led God to sacrifice his only son might prove a painful cure, but alone offered the certain hope of salvation. 'When we realize how sweet and dear a medicine we have within us', she wrote, 'we must . . . stretch out our hands in the self-contempt the sick person has, who hates to be sick and loves the medicine the doctor gives.'[57]

In view of these assumptions about Christ's role as a heavenly physician, it is easy to see how the sacrament of the Eucharist came to be accorded miraculous powers, even to the extent of combating earthly disease.

> The blode, sum tyme of geete [goat], or ellis of calff,
> Was sprente on the people, to leche ther sore;
> But now the blode of Crist, by doble halff
> Lechith the people, and clensith well more,
> Which dayly at the auter, his prist beffore

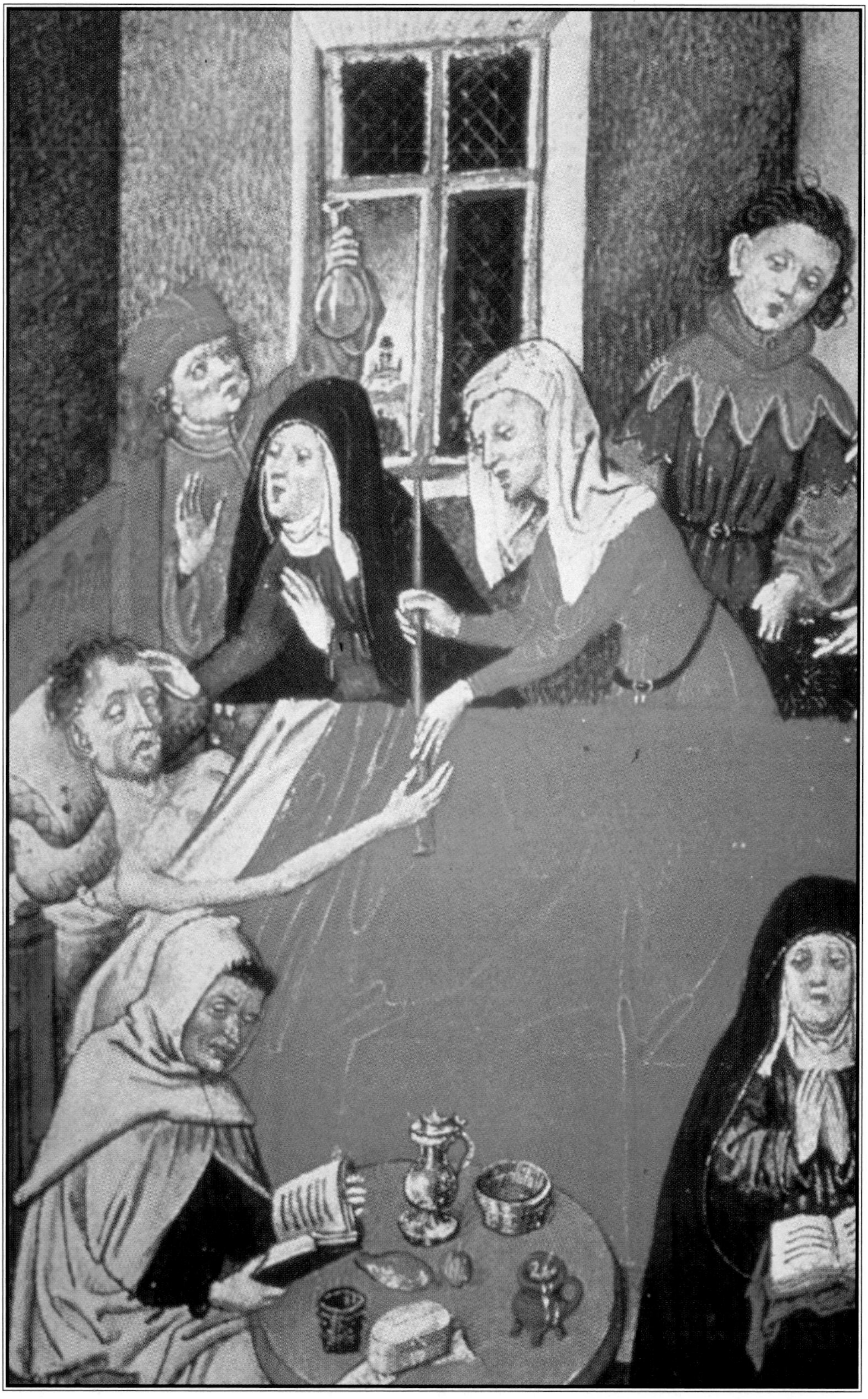

Plate 1: Religion takes precedence over medicine at the deathbed. A physician scrutinizes his patient's urine in the background, but the scene is dominated by praying figures, vessels for the administration of Extreme Unction and a lighted candle to ease the passage of the dying man's soul through purgatory.

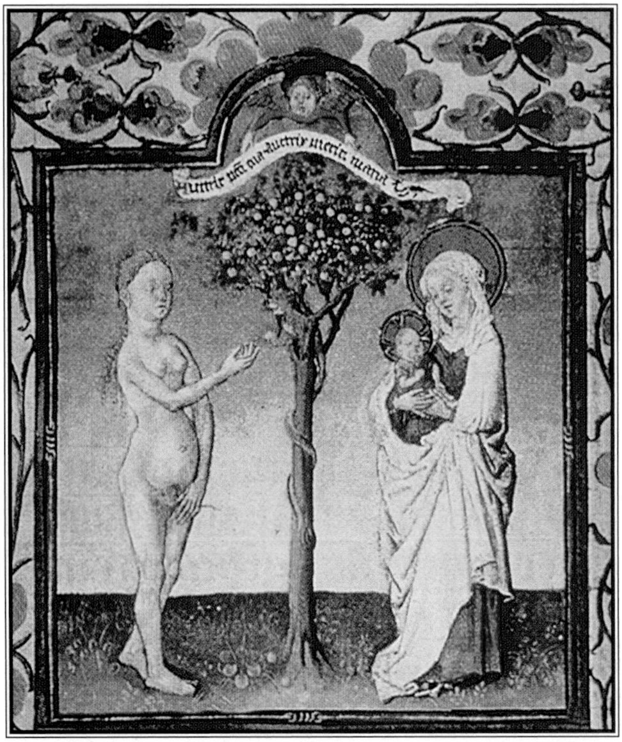

Plate 2: Eve, 'authoress of sin' and thus of death, suffering and disease, stands at the opposite side of the Tree of Knowledge from the Virgin Mary, 'authoress of merit'. Her nakedness and the Virgin's heavy clothing underscore the contrast between them.

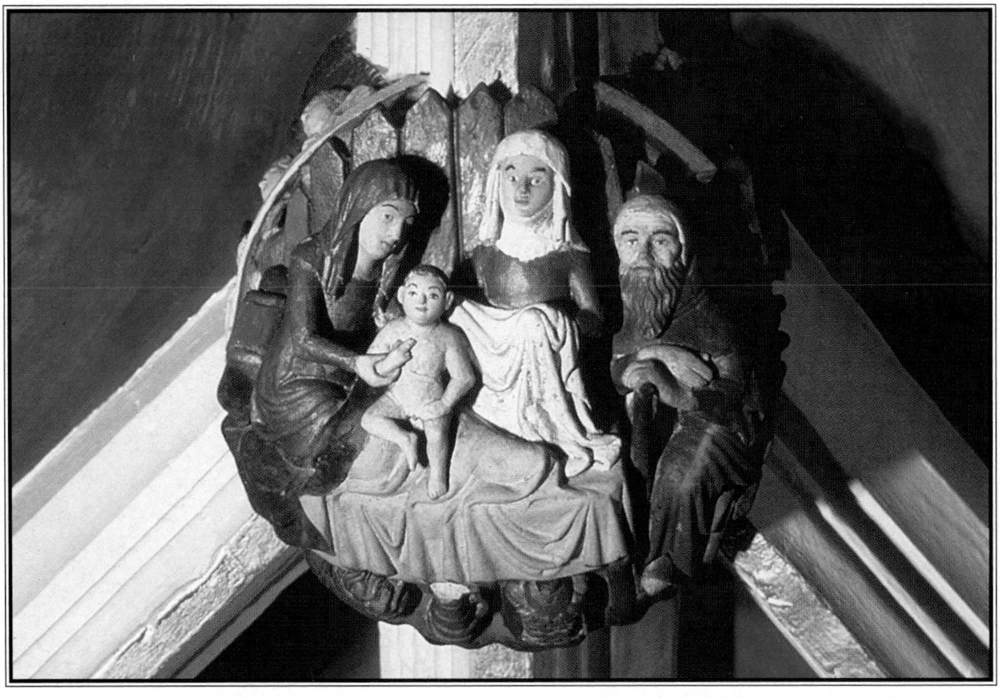

Plate 3: Although they were taught that the Virgin Mary was herself the product of an immaculate conception, fifteenth-century men and women still saw her mother, St Anne, in a homely, domestic light. This attractive depiction of the Holy Family reflects, and helps to explain, the popularity of her cult.

Consecrate with worde and mynde of entent,
Wher God, in fowrm of bred, his body doth present.[58]

For this reason the 'Sainte Hostie' bearing the image and blood of Christ given by Pope Eugenius IV to Philip the Good of Burgundy in 1433 (as a reward for distinctly secular endeavours on his behalf) became the focus of a healing cult at Dijon. It was credited with saving the life of Louis XII of France, who gave his coronation crown to the shrine as an ex-voto offering for deliverance from a serious illness.[59] Even at a humble parochial level, regular attendance at Holy Communion was believed to promote physical as well as spiritual well-being, although it was for the latter purpose that most English hospitals of any size accommodated their patients in churches or chapels. The infirm poor who entered these institutions were effectively guaranteed an immediate improvement in the health of their souls, if not their bodies, as the provisions of the fourth Lateran Council with regard to the confession of sins by the sick were naturally enforced there, along with similar regulations promulgated nearer home by English bishops.[60] Cynics might argue that the authorities showed less thought for the spiritual welfare of the inmates than the need to improve the 'quality' of their prayers on behalf of wealthy patrons; but the exercise clearly brought peace and calm to troubled minds:

My dedly woundis are derne [dire] and depe,
I have no place to represse them aryght,
And smertynge wyll nott suffer me to slepe
Tyll a leche with dewte have them dyght [treated].
Hitt most be a curate, a crownyd [tonsured] wyght,
Thatt knew the querely off bene and pese
[That knows how to read the mass-book];
And els thes medicynys have no myght
To geve us lycense to lyve in ese.[61]

Confession may even have imparted some physical benefits, at least if the penitent was convinced that his or her sufferings came as a punishment from on high. By teaching that the administration of 'goostliche medicyne' freed the soul from sin and enabled the good Christian once again to 'resceyve God, dwellynge in parfait charite', the Church offered repentant wrongdoers the hope that they would either make a speedy recovery or else accrue 'muche merit in blisse after this lyf'.[62] The indigent poor, however, had no choice but to swallow their dose of spiritual linctus. Before gaining admittance to the hospital of St Mary in the Newarke, Leicester, for instance, paupers incapable of fending for themselves were obliged to confess and receive absolution from the warden, who was also a priest. The hospital had been founded by Henry, Earl of Lancaster, in the 1330s, and reorganized on impressive lines by his son and namesake, the first duke, in 1356. Duke Henry's new regulations contained the specific provision that all the patients lying in the nave of the hospital church should be able 'devoutly to behold the elevation of the Body of Christ' during the mass, which was to be celebrated before them twice a day, at dawn and nine in the morning.[63] He, of all men, was well aware of the therapeutic effects of the Eucharist upon souls consumed with sin, having just completed his *Livre de Seyntz Medicines* (*Book of Sacred Medicines*), a long meditation on the subject of Christ the Physician.

The work begins with a desperate appeal for medical help, in which the duke compares

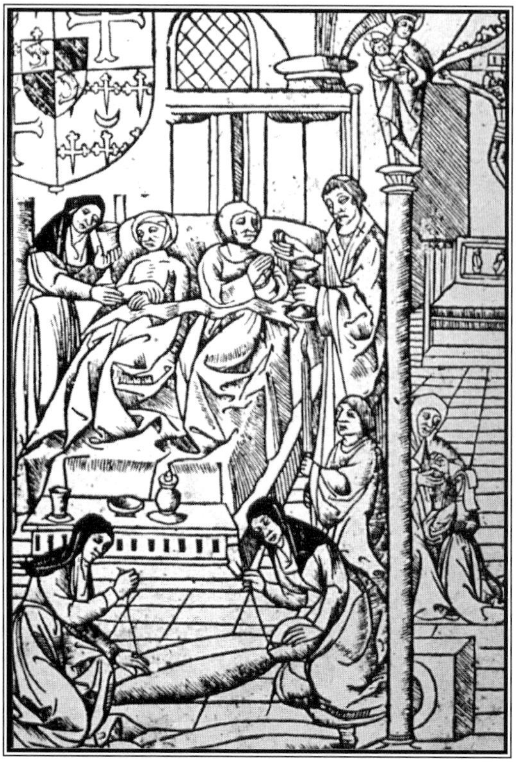

Lying within view of the high altar, a patient at the Hotel Dieu in Paris receives the last rites. A statue of the Virgin Mary, who was sometimes described as a nurse in the service of her son, Christ the Physician, stands on the right, while the sisters themselves tend the sick and sew up bodies in shrouds.

himself, in spiritual terms, to one of the bruised, battered and terminally sick patients in his own hospital:

> Ah! Gentle Lord Jesus Christ, I am the one, poor and bereft of goods, who is so badly injured with seven such putrefying and dangerous wounds [the seven deadly sins] that I can only wait for death – see what an evil death! – if I do not immediately receive the comfort and aid of the good master. That is you, blessed Lord God, who is the leech and the physician, and who shelters all those who believe in you with a good heart. And since, Lord, I have so little and my wounds are so deadly, so horrible, so full of poison through the rottenness of vile, stinking filth, it is too shameful for me to speak of them, or examine them or even think about them. Ah! Gentle Lord God, how can I possibly be so bold as to show them to you?[64]

From start to finish, the reader is presented with a dazzling array of medical metaphors, for although Duke Henry's sole preoccupation lies with the fate of his immortal soul, he describes the quest for salvation in terms of a protracted (and sometimes extremely painful) course of treatment, with the Virgin Mary as his solicitous, forgiving nurse. His vivid use of terms drawn from the specialist vocabulary of the university-trained physician illustrates (as do many other works cited in the course of this book) the extent to which scientific ideas had been absorbed into the discourse of well-educated laymen. The analogy between Christ and a surgeon presiding over the dissection of corpses at Montpellier may have raised some clerical eyebrows, but there can be no denying the effectiveness of such an image:

> Most Gentle Lord, I beg that it will please you to have me cut up and opened before you, my Lord and my Master, in the same way as certain bodies are dissected before the surgeons in the schools at Montpellier and elsewhere. For when a man has been condemned to death he is given to them to open, to see and to recognize how and in what manner the veins, the nerves and the other bodily parts are to be found in man. Gentle Lord, observe how I am opened up before you, so that you can see quite clearly how my flesh and my veins and all my members are replete with sin. . . . And also since I am a man condemned to death for my wickedness, you can with good reason cut up and open my body rather than anyone

> else's and make an example out of me to others, of the tumours that they can see and identify in me.[65]

Yet however sick their souls might be, and however rank the sores of wrongdoing, good Christians were taught to believe that, if they showed sufficient humility and contrition, the heavenly leech would always save them with the ointment of his blood. A wide variety of medication was in fact available, ranging from the harsh extremes of penance and self-denial (which ranked as the spiritual equivalent of major surgery) to prophylactic measures for avoiding infection in the first place.[66] One of the medieval physician's principal tasks was to provide his patients with advice about the best means of preserving their health; and Christ, too, had explained to man how he could protect himself against sin:

> The most sovereyn leche nought only taughte hym how he shulde moun lyvyn withouten ende, but overmore he warnyd hym to what sekenesse he was most dysposyd, wherby he myghte lesyn that lyf and deyin wytouten ende; and taughte hym medecynys agens thoo sekenessis whanne he bad hym nought sleen [kill], doon noo leccherye, noo thefte, beryn noo fals wygtnesse, wurshepyn fadyr and modyr, and in his reulyng lovyn his neyghebore as hymself. . . .[67]

Since immorality and selfishness caused disease, it followed logically that righteous living would not only be good for the immortal soul but also likely to offer immunity against earthly pestilence. As San Bernardino urged his Italian congregations in the early fifteenth century, charity rather than physic should be their first resort during epidemics; there could be no better preventative medicine than almsgiving, which pleased God and disposed him, in turn, to show compassion.[68] But knowing from personal experience that generosity alone could not guarantee survival, or erase the spots and stains of sin, medieval men and women also sought to safeguard their physical, as well as spiritual health, through prayer and pilgrimage.

The use of healing prayers and incantations is explored at length in Chapter IV, along with the Church's persistent, but often unsuccessful, attempts to prevent laymen and -women from straying off the narrow path of religious orthodoxy by employing them out of context as part of some pagan or magical rite. It is, however, important to remember that the ecclesiastical authorities actively encouraged pious Christians to invoke the help of God and his saints, placing their chief trust in heavenly medication should they fall ill or run the risk of catching the plague. By the close of the Middle Ages printed books of hours contained scores of prayers for the sick or fearful: not surprisingly, appeals for protection against the pestilence and the horror of *mors improvisa* were by far the most common, although pregnant women, epileptics and even those who were about to be phlebotomized could find devotions appropriate to their needs.[69] The rich might choose to pay for special masses to be said during epidemics; or secure for themselves the promise of a year free from the malign effects of 'want, emptiness, loss of cattle, fumes and evil vapours, cramps, dropsy, cancer, leprosy, asthma, unclean spirits, shame, bad luck . . . water, fire, lightning, tempest, plague and sudden death' simply by fasting on bread and water and having a mass of St Anthony celebrated on their behalf.[70]

For many, pilgrimage to the tomb of a holy man or woman noted for his or her healing powers or to the site of a wonder-working relic, such as the piece of the true cross at Bromholm in Norfolk, which was credited with the power to raise the dead and cure lepers, promised a

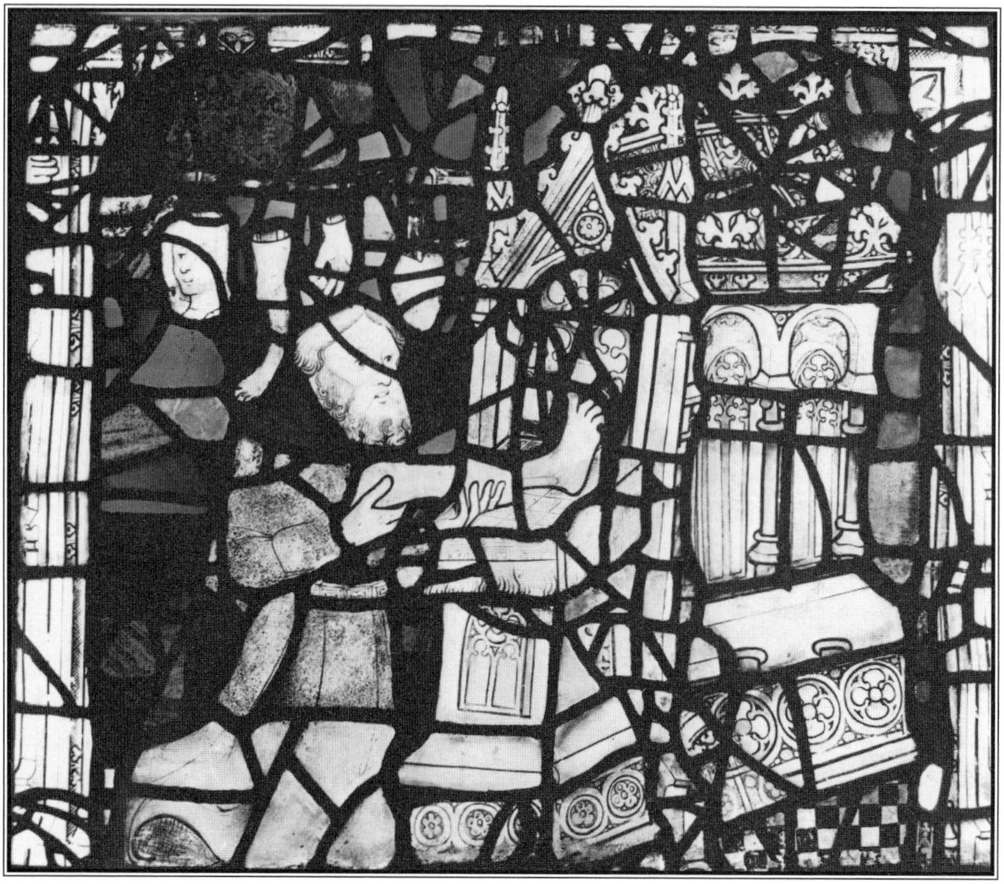

A pilgrim presents a wax model of a leg at the shrine of St William in York Minster, either hoping for a cure or in gratitude for one already bestowed through the intercession of the saint. Other ex voto *offerings, including a head, hand and heart, hang on the left.*

more certain insurance against illness or hope of recovery.[71] Constant preoccupation with the joys or torments awaiting them after death did not prevent thousands of Englishmen and -women from undertaking long and sometimes dangerous journeys all over Europe in the hope that they might be spared further misery on earth through the intercession of a patron saint. Medieval shrines were covered with wax or metal images of arms, legs, hearts and other diseased bodily parts (not to mention models of sick animals) presented by those who hoped for, or believed they had already received, a miraculous cure. The tomb of Archbishop Scrope in York Minster, for example, was surrounded by rods from which hung hundreds of such offerings, often made of precious metal, while costly jewels and cups given by devotees of the local 'saint and martyr' (he was never actually canonized) were displayed separately on rich pieces of cloth. The vendors of these 'ymages' posed a problem to the civic authorities, who fined a group of chandlers in 1475–6 for setting up stalls illegally in the street and peddling their wares along the major approaches to the minster.[72] That rich pickings were to be had from this lugubrious trade is evident from a report made by papal commissioners sent to inspect the shrine of Thomas Cantilupe at Hereford Cathedral in August 1307, during the course of inquiries leading to his

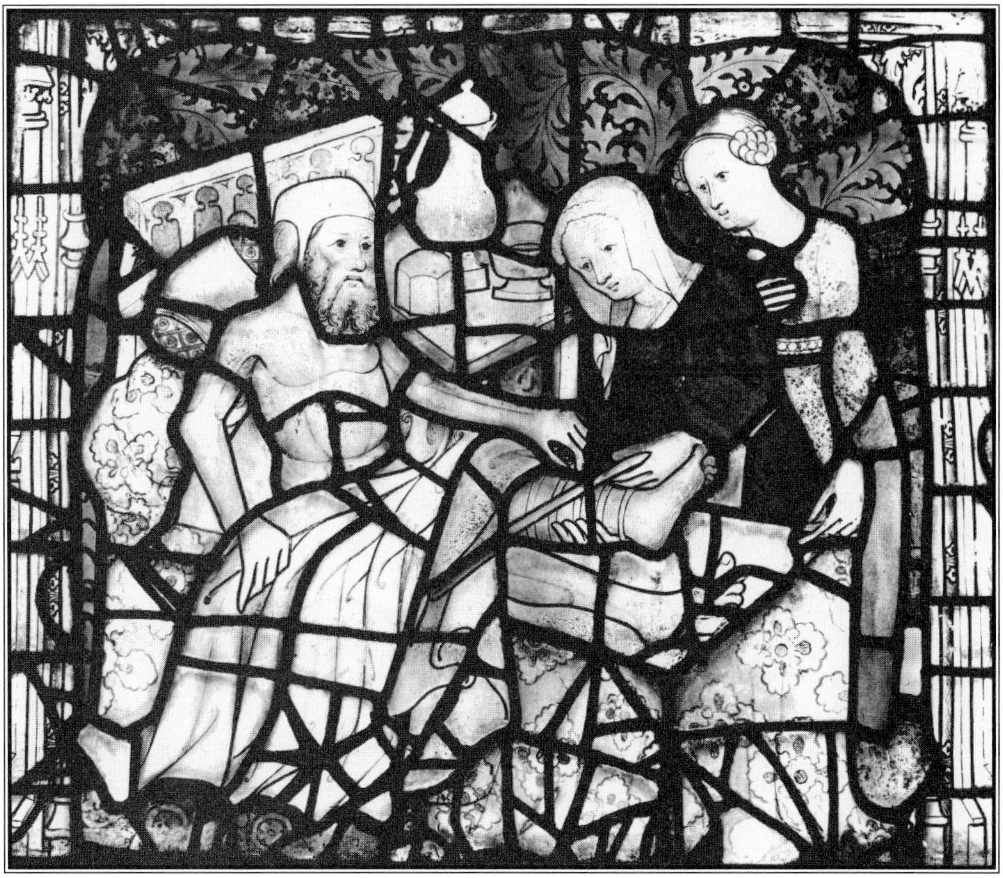

Measuring the patient's leg so that a candle of the appropriate length may be burnt at St William's shrine. Conventional medicine, in the form of salves and potions at the bedside, has so far proved ineffective.

canonization. They noted almost 2,000 models of whole bodies or recognizable human limbs fashioned in silver or wax, 108 discarded walking-sticks and crutches, 95 children's shifts and 'an uncountable quantity of eyes, breasts, teeth and ears'. On returning a few months later, they found that nearly a hundred more items had been deposited by new visitors.[73]

Candles, too, burnt in profusion around these shrines, often corresponding in height to the stature of the donor, or else containing a wick which, when fully extended, had been made according to specific measurements taken while a sick or injured person lay *in extremis*. Sir Thomas More's tale of the custom at St Valery's shrine near Abbeville, where men piously measured their 'prevy membres at the aulters ende' and offered up candles of the appropriate size in order to avoid bladder stones, cannot be taken too seriously (even from the pen of one who was himself destined to become a saint), but the practice of dedicating a representative 'light' in cases of illness was ubiquitous.[74] The 174 'more evident and more famous' miracles posthumously attributed to King Henry VI contained a lengthy description of one such case, which, in common with hundreds of others recorded throughout the medieval period, also dwelt upon the powerlessness of the medical profession. In 1487 the infant son of one of the Archbishop of Canterbury's servants contracted a painful and debilitating illness:

> And so, his disease seeming now past bearing and past comfort, physicians were called in from all sides, that his parents might not let the care of him seem vain and idle: moreover the most skilled surgeons of London were consulted, and those also who were in attendance on the archbishop himself, men of learning and repute, made diligent search and enquiry into the boy's condition, yet nothing could they find in him but the presages of impending death. Some said he was suffering this discomfort and these incurable pains from gout, or from some paralytic trouble: others that . . . his weakness came from the contagious venom of some evil spirit. But all alike, deeming that he could not be healed by any man or any natural treatment, refused to bestow their pains upon him further. . . . Seeing her labours all in vain, and all the remedies they had sought at such cost unavailing, so that all human help had now failed her, [his mother] knelt on the ground, like the devout soul she was, over her son's body, and called upon heaven for succour. And anon, taking a measure, which was that of a wax candle, such as those which are wont to be made rolled together after the manner of a *rotula* [a coiled-up taper], she began to measure the child's body. And having great faith in the most blessed King Henry, she commended her child in Christ's name to his prayers only, making mention of no other saints at all.[75]

At the sound of Henry's name, the child immediately gained strength, sat upright and began to walk: a supernatural cure rendered all the more dramatic in view of the manifest inadequacy of the secular medical experts.

This apparent antagonism towards the healing profession may, in part, have resulted from a genuine concern about the merits of any treatment which did not come directly from God, although less creditable financial and political considerations were clearly at stake. The clergy responsible for recording miracles were usually involved in campaigns for the canonization of the individuals whose relics lay in their possession, so they had a vested interest in stressing the impotence, incompetence or venality of physicians and surgeons. There was, furthermore, an understandable desire to attract as many visitors as possible in order to boost the reputation and revenues of newly established shrines. Competition was fierce: all but the most famous saints tended to lose their appeal and go out of fashion after an initial burst of carefully orchestrated publicity.[76]

Criticism of the overt commercialism of some priests, who shamelessly exploited the fears and hopes of vulnerable pilgrims, was voiced long before the Reformation, although recourse to the saints and their relics remained one of the first avenues to be explored by the sick right up to the mid-sixteenth century and beyond. The seasonal nature of many ailments, caused by lack of vitamins in the medieval winter diet, meant that many people did, indeed, recover from temporary disabilities when pilgrimages started up in springtime, while others, troubled by psychosomatic disorders or simply in need of a rest and change of scene, began to improve once they left home.[77] Such 'cures', no doubt greatly embellished in the telling, were enough to fuel the hope of ordinary men and women who desperately needed to believe that something could be done to ease their pain. Clearly, if God had visited them with sickness in the first place, an appeal to him, through the agency of his saints, offered the best prospect of help.

In certain cases, notably with regard to scrofula (tuberculosis adenitis), the touch of God's anointed on earth might in itself prove sufficient to dispel the disease. In England the ritual of 'touching' placed great emphasis upon the sacerdotal role of the monarch, who not only laid his hand upon the swollen or ulcerated glands of the sufferer, but also blessed him or her with the

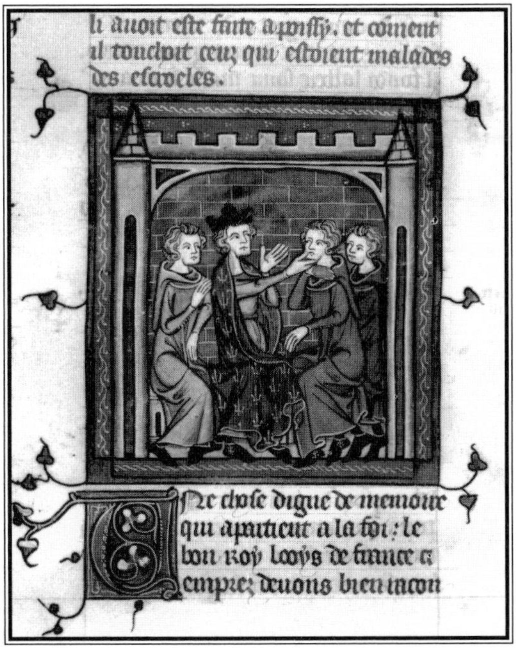

A scene from a fourteenth-century French chronicle shows supplicants suffering from scrofula being cured of the disease by the annointed hand of St Louis (d.1270), King of France.

sign of the cross and in the name of Christ. The idea that the chrism, or holy oil, used to anoint the king's hands at his coronation bestowed supernatural healing powers, also found expression (from the fifteenth century onwards) in a ceremony performed on Good Friday for the production of 'cramp' rings. These were worn to protect against muscular pain or epilepsy, the close connection with the Passion, and the monarch's ritual obeisance to the cross, being considered especially potent in the face of daemonic possession. Not surprisingly, the king's ability to channel 'divine grace' through his hands into the bodies of the sick proved a formidable weapon in the armoury of royal propaganda; and it is worth noting that opponents of the Yorkist regime maintained that neither Edward IV nor Richard III, as usurpers, could possibly have received the gift from God.[78]

Medical opinion in both England and France accepted without question that an anointed ruler would usually be able to cure scrofula, although individual writers disagreed over the best time to employ such an awesome remedy. Some felt that it should be a last resort, to be essayed after medication and even surgery had failed, while others preferred to try it first.[79] The fact that patients would seek a combination of spiritual and physical cures, invoking God and the practitioner at more or less the same time, was taken for granted: if, as the Church required, treatment actually began with confession, the two medicines would of necessity be administered together, not least because most university-trained physicians had themselves taken holy orders. However much they may have dwelt upon the need for passive acceptance of earthly trials, late medieval theologians knew well enough that frail, frightened human beings would try all the means at their disposal to avoid pain and postpone death. In most cases this involved a combination of religious and medical practices which recognized the intimate connexion between body and soul. The idea of separating the two, of treating physical symptoms without addressing the spiritual malaise of the sufferer, would have seemed both profane and pointless. Historians of medieval medicine can hardly avoid making such an anachronistic distinction, and in concentrating almost exclusively upon the treatment of the body the rest of this book illuminates just one corner of a far broader canvas.

NOTES

1. The *Independent on Sunday*, 9 January 1994, *Sunday Review*, p. 45.
2. P. Aries, *The Hour of Our Death*, trans. H. Weaver (pbk, London, 1987), pp. 128–32. Aries challenges here the far gloomier interpretation advanced by J. Huizinga in Chapter XI of his classic work, *The Waning of the Middle Ages*, trans. F. Hopman (pbk, London, 1976), which was first published in 1924.

3. J. Bolton, *The Medieval English Economy 1150–1500* (pbk, London, 1980), pp. 62–3.
4. *Ane Addicioun of Scottis Croniklis and Deidis*, ed. T. Thomson (Edinburgh, 1819), p. 34.
5. William Langland, *Piers the Plowman*, ed. W.W. Skeat (2 vols, Oxford, third impression, 1961), vol. I, p. 585 (C passus XXIII, vv. 95–105). For a discussion of the surprisingly limited response of late medieval English writers to the plague, see S. Wenzel, 'Pestilence and Middle English Literature: Friar John Grimestone's Poems on Death', in *The Black Death: The Impact of the Fourteenth-Century Plague*, ed. D. Williman (New York, 1982), pp. 131–59.
6. B. Hooper, S. Rickett, A. Rogerson and S. Yaxley, 'The Grave of Sir Hugh de Hastyngs, Elsing', *Norfolk Archaeology*, XXXIX (1984), pp. 88–99. Riding accidents constituted a routine hazard of medieval life, not just on military campaigns: in 1448, for example, the wife of Nicholas Radford, an eminent West Country lawyer, was said to be 'a full sike woman hardely, for she hadd sore falle of hire horse' (*Letters and Papers of John Shillingford*, ed. S.A. Moore (Camden Soc., new series, II, 1871), p. 64).
7. Thomas Malory, *Le Morte d'Arthur*, ed. J. Cowen (pbk, 2 vols, London, 1986), vol. II, pp. 398, 405; M. Hebert, 'L'Armée Provençale en 1374', *Annales du Midi*, XCI (1979), pp. 5–27.
8. *Original Letters Illustrative of English History*, ed. H. Ellis (3 series in 11 vols, London, 1824–46), second series, vol. IV, pp. 95–6.
9. B.A. Hanawalt, 'Childrearing among the Lower Classes in Late Medieval England', *Journal of Interdisciplinary History*, VIII (1977–8), pp. 1–22. It is interesting to note that, of the miracles attributed to King Henry VI, a total of 55 out of the 138 recorded in sufficient detail to make analysis possible concern young people under twenty, many of whom were the victims of accidents, notably by drowning or concussion (*The Miracles of King Henry VI*, ed. R. Knox and S. Leslie (London, 1923), *passim*).
10. *Calendar of the Coroners' Rolls of the City of London 1300–1378*, ed. R.R. Sharpe (London, 1913), pp. 56–7; *Calendar of the Letter Books of the City of London, A*, p. 220; *C*, p. 5; *D*, p. 251.
11. D. Herlihy, 'Life Expectancies for Women in Medieval Society', in *The Role of Women in the Middle Ages*, ed. R.T. Morewedge (London, 1975), p. 13; B. Harvey, *Living and Dying in England 1100–1540: The Monastic Experience* (Oxford, 1993), Chapter IV, *passim*; J. Hatcher, 'Mortality in the Fifteenth Century: Some New Evidence', *Economic History Review*, second series, XXXIX (1986), pp. 19–38.
12. *The History of Parliament: The House of Commons 1386–1421*, ed. J.S. Roskell, L. Clark and C. Rawcliffe (4 vols, Stroud, 1993), vols II–IV, *passim*.
13. *Paston Letters and Papers of the Fifteenth Century*, ed. N. Davis (2 vols, Oxford, 1971–6), vol. I, p. 39.
14. E. Duffy, *The Stripping of the Altars: Traditional Religion in England* c. *1400*–c. *1580* (Yale, 1992), pp. 309–15.
15. *The Workes of Sir Thomas More, Knyght* (London, 1557), p. 75. See also p. 72, where More contrasts the 'short medicine' God prescribes for the soul 'conteinyng onely foure herbes, comen and well knowen, that is to wit: deth, dome, pain and ioy' with the esoteric, expensive and often useless drugs employed by earthly physicians and apothecaries to dose their patients' bodies.
16. *The English Text of the Ancrene Riwle*, ed. A. Zettersten (Early English Text Soc., CCLXXIV, 1976), pp. 79–80.
17. E. Pagels, *Adam, Eve and the Serpent* (pbk, London, 1990), p. 109. For Eve's particular responsibility, see below, pp. 171–2, 174. Among the desperate consequences of Original Sin, as listed by St Augustine, 'are the evils that arise from the body, in the shape of diseases; and there are so many of them that all the books of the physicians cannot contain them all. And . . . in almost all of them, the treatment and the medicines are themselves instruments of torture.' (St Augustine, *Concerning the City of God against the Pagans*, trans. H. Bettenson (pbk, London, 1984), p. 1067).
18. John Milton, *Paradise Lost*, ed. M.Y. Hughes (New York, 1935), p. 372 (Book XI, vv. 477–93).
19. *Dives and Pauper*, ed. P. Heath Barnum (Early English Text Soc., CCLXXV, 1976, and CCLXXX, 1980), vol. I, p. 129.
20. As, for example, R.A. Houlbrooke in *The English Family 1450–1700* (pbk, London, 1984), pp. 134–40.
21. *A Common-Place Book of the Fifteenth Century*, ed. L.T. Smith (London, 1886), p. 69; *Select English Works of John Wyclif*, ed. T. Arnold (3 vols, Oxford, 1869–71), vol. III, p. 199.
22. *Middle English Sermons*, ed. W.O. Ross (Early English Text Soc., CCIX, 1940, reprinted 1960), pp. 41–2. The idea that 'sekenesse of body, meekliche suffrid maketh helthe of sowle, and soule-helthe is not but oonliche of God' is common to much late medieval religious writing. See, for example, *Yorkshire Writers: Richard Rolle of Hampole*, ed. C. Horstman (2 vols, London, 1895–6), vol. II, pp. 450–1.
23. John Mandeville, *Mandeville's Travels*, ed. P. Hamelius (Early English Text Soc., CLIII, 1919), p. 210; *English Works of John Fisher*, ed. J.E. Mayor (Early English Text Soc., extra series, XXVII, 1876), p. 300. Margaret Beaufort's health may also have been damaged by an unusually early confinement, when she was just thirteen, see M.K. Jones and M.G. Underwood, *The King's Mother* (Cambridge, 1992), pp. 40, 96. For the use of anaesthesia in the medieval period, see below, p. 77.
24. Thomas Hoccleve, *Hoccleve's Works: The Minor Poems*, ed. F.J. Furnivall and I. Gollancz (Early English Text Soc., extra series, LXI, 1892, LXXIII, 1925, reprinted in one vol. 1970), p. 108.
25. See Chapter IV below.

26. P.B.R. Doob, *Nebuchadnezzar's Children: Conventions of Madness in Middle English Literature* (Yale, 1974), pp. 10–32.
27. *The Book of Margery Kempe*, ed. S.B. Meeche (Early English Text Soc., CCXII, 1940), pp. 6–9 (a modern English edition of this work has been produced by W. Butler-Bowdon (Oxford, 1954), and the corresponding passage is on pp. 9–11). Margery's experience is considered by R. Porter, *A Social History of Madness* (pbk, London, 1989), pp. 105–13, who rightly cautions against the 'psychodynamic post mortems' undertaken on her by 'psychoanalytical sleuths'.
28. *The Book of Margery Kempe*, ed. Meeche, p. 105; ed. Butler-Bowdon, p. 137.
29. *The Life of St Hugh of Lincoln*, ed. D.L. Douie and H. Farmer (2 vols, London, 1961–2), vol. II, pp. 125–6.
30. *Records of the City of Norwich*, ed. W. Hudson and J.C. Tingey (2 vols, Norwich, 1906–19), vol. II, pp. 168–9; Thomas More, *The Apology*, ed. J.B. Trapp (*The Complete Works of St Thomas More*, New Haven, IX, 1979), p. 118.
31. Doob, op. cit., pp. 37–41; J.R. Guy, 'The Episcopal Licensing of Physicians, Surgeons and Midwives', *Bulletin of the History of Medicine*, LVI (1982), p. 531.
32. *Calendar of Inquisitions Miscellaneous*, vol. I, no. 2279. Although, in the eyes of the Church, the insane were ultimately responsible for any crimes committed while they were mad because they had brought the affliction on themselves through sin, the law accepted that a person who had been demonstrably possessed by madness for any significant time (*furia continuce detinebatur*) could not be held culpable for their actions (see, for example, PRO, C260/20/9, 25/2).
33. *Paston Letters and Papers*, op. cit., vol. II, p. 486.
34. *The Book of Margery Kempe*, ed. Meeche, pp. 6–9, 177–9; ed. Butler-Bowdon, pp. 10–11, 233–5.
35. PRO, C270/22.
36. *The Historical Collections of a Citizen of London*, ed. J. Gairdner (Camden Soc., new series, XVII, 1876), p. ix.
37. *Calendar of Inquisitions Miscellaneous*, vol. IV, no. 227; *Calendar of Patent Rolls, 1381–85*, pp. 212, 351.
38. *Calendar of Patent Rolls, 1381–85*, p. 471.
39. Langland, op. cit., vol. I, p. 235 (C passus X, vv. 107–18).
40. *Wills and Inventories from the Registers of the Commissary of Bury St Edmunds*, ed. S. Tymms (Camden Soc., XLIX, 1850), p. 25.
41. M. Carlin, 'Medieval English Hospitals', in *The Hospital in History*, ed. L. Granshaw and R. Porter (pbk, London, 1990), p. 25.
42. R.I. Moore, *The Formation of a Persecuting Society* (Oxford, 1987), pp. 11, 47–80.
43. *Idem*, 'Heresy as Disease', in *The Concept of Heresy in the Middle Ages*, ed. W. Lourdaux and V. Verhelst (*Mediaevalia Louaniensia*, series one, IV, 1976), pp. 1–11; S.N. Brody, *The Disease of the Soul: Leprosy in Medieval Literature* (Cornell, 1974), pp. 125–7.
44. *English Metrical Homilies*, ed. J. Small (Edinburgh, 1862), pp. 129–30. Part of this poem is cited by Brody in a modern English version, op. cit., p. 138.
45. P. McNiven, 'The Problem of Henry IV's Health, 1405–1413', *English Historical Review*, C (1985), pp. 747–72; *Middle English Sermons*, op. cit., p. 211; *The Book of the Knight of la Tour-Landry*, ed. T. Wright (Early English Text Soc., XXXIII, 1868), pp. 69, 90. See also, *An Alphabet of Tales, A–H*, ed. M.M. Banks (Early English Text Soc., CXXVI, 1904), pp. 170–1, for the case of a woman 'so smytyn with canker and seknes that sho rotid so . . . that no creatur mot fele the stynk of hur' as a punishment for unduly fastidious behaviour.
46. M. Rubin, *Corpus Christi: The Eucharist in Late Medieval Culture* (pbk, Cambridge, 1992), pp. 148, 220.
47. *Hoccleve's Works: The Minor Poems*, op. cit., pp. 140–78. Another version of this popular tale may be found in *The Early English Versions of the Gesta Romanorum*, ed. S.J.H. Heritage (Early English Text Soc., extra series, XXXIII, 1879), pp. 311–19.
48. *The Book of Vices and Virtues*, ed. W.N. Francis (Early English Text Soc., CCXVII, 1942, reprinted 1968), p. 249; Brody, op. cit., pp. 179–86. For the sexual transmission of leprosy, see below, p. 175.
49. *The Poems and Fables of Robert Henryson*, ed. H.H. Wood (Edinburgh, 1958), pp. 120–1.
50. *The Life of St Hugh of Lincoln*, op. cit., vol. II, pp. 12–14.
51. *The Book of Margery Kempe*, ed. Butler-Bowdon, pp. 232–3. C.W. Bynum, *Holy Feast and Holy Fast: The Religious Significance of Food to Medieval Women* (University of California Press, 1987), pp. 121, 200, 209, 234, 248.
52. R. Gilchrist, 'Christian Bodies and Souls: The Archaeology of Life and Death in Medieval Hospitals', in *Death in Towns: Urban Responses to the Dying and the Dead, 100–1600*, ed. S. Bassett (Leicester, 1992), pp. 113–15; M.B. Honeybourne, 'The Leper Hospitals of the London Area', *Transactions of the London and Middlesex Archaeological Soc.*, XXI (1967), pp. 5–8.
53. *An Alphabet of Tales, A–H*, op. cit., pp. 117–18.
54. *The Cyrurgie of Guy de Chauliac*, ed. M.S. Ogden (Early English Text Soc., CCLXV, 1971), p. 381. L. Demaitre, 'The Description and Diagnosis of Leprosy by Fourteenth-Century Physicians', *Bulletin of the History of Medicine*, LIX (1985), pp. 327–44, stresses the 'natural' attitude to leprosy adopted by continental physicians. For a diagnosis by English practitioners, see below, p. 114.
55. The 'tension, even if only latent, between secular medicine and theology, between the cure of the soul and the cure of the body' is explored in D.W. Amundsen and G.B. Ferngren, 'Philanthropy in Medicine: Some Historical

Perspectives', in *Beneficence and Health Care*, ed. E.E. Shelp (*Philosophy and Medicine*, XI, 1982), pp. 1–31. See also below, pp. 84–85.

56. Cited by R. Arbesmann, 'The Concept of *Christus Medicus* in St Augustine', *Traditio*, X (1954), p. 15.

57. *The Prymer off Salysburye Use* (John Growle, London, 1533), the third of the fifteen 'Oes' of St Bridget; *The Letters of St Catherine of Siena*, ed. S. Noffke (4 vols in progress, Medieval and Renaissance Texts and Studies, Binghampton, New York, 1988 onwards), vol. I, p. 258.

58. *Songs, Carols and Other Miscellaneous Poems*, ed. R. Dyboski (Early English Text Soc., extra series, CI, 1907), p. 69.

59. J.P. Lecat, *Le Siècle de la Toison d'Or* (Paris, 1986), p. 58. The 'Sainte Hostie' was displayed in an elaborate gold monstrance, surmounted with Louis's crown, a depiction of which, dated 1674, may be seen in the Musée des Beaux Arts, Dijon.

60. *Councils and Synods, 1205–1313*, ed. F.M. Powicke and C.R. Cheney (2 vols, Oxford, 1964), vol. I, pp. 173, 371, 444; vol. II, p. 993.

61. *Religious Lyrics of the Fifteenth Century*, ed. C. Brown (Oxford, 1962), p. 273. This poem, on the theme of medicines to cure the deadly sins, lists appropriate 'herbal' remedies: humility, love, charity, almsgiving, the 'dowbyll flour' of prayer and watchfulness, abstinence and chastity, mixed with contrition 'that wasshith the woundis as doith a well', confession 'that wyll nott suffyr no ded flessh dwell' and good works 'that soverayn sanatyfe'. See below, pp. 58–9, for medical analogies.

62. *Yorkshire Writers*, op. cit., vol. II, p. 450.

63. A.H. Thompson, *The History of the Hospital and the New College of the Annunciation of St Mary in the Newarke, Leicester* (Leicestershire Archaeological Soc., 1937), pp. 18, 47.

64. Henry of Lancaster, *Le Livre de Seyntz Médicines*, ed. E.J. Arnould (Oxford, 1940), p. 7. In his *Etude sur le Livre de Saintes Medecines du Duc Henri de Lancastre* (Paris, 1948), Arnould devotes one chapter (pp. lxxix–cviii) to the duke's sources, but dwells only briefly on his use of medical symbolism.

65. Ibid., p. 86. As in so many other areas, the Church maintained an ambivalent attitude towards dissection; see below, pp. 127–8.

66. See below, p. 58.

67. *Dives and Pauper*, op. cit., vol. I, p. 68.

68. R. Palmer, 'The Church, Leprosy and Plague in Medieval and Early Modern Europe', *Studies in Church History*, XIX (1982), pp. 86–9.

69. An interesting selection of prayers may, for example, be found in *Horae Beatae Mariae Virginis*, ed. E. Hoskins (London, 1901), pp. 111, 117–18, 120, 122, 129, 145, 149, 151, 165.

70. *Missale ad Usum Insignis Ecclesiae Eboracensis*, ed. W.G. Henderson (Surtees Soc., LXIX and LX, 1872), vol. II, pp. 233–4; Duffy, op. cit., pp. 293–4. It is worth noting that, in 1496, Pierre Picot, a royal physician, arranged for the mystery play of St Sebastian to be mounted at Chalon-sur-Saone in order to bring to an end an outbreak of plague. Along with St Roch, St Sebastian was frequently invoked during pestilences (E. Wickersheimer, *Dictionnaire Biographique des Médecins en France au Moyen Age* (Paris, 1936), p. 655).

71. F. Wormald, 'The Rood of Bromholm', *Journal of the Warburg Institute*, I (1937–8), pp. 31–45. The subject of medieval pilgrimage is explored more fully in Duffy, op. cit., pp. 183–205; and R.C. Finucane, *Miracles and Pilgrims: Popular Beliefs in Medieval England* (London, 1977), *passim*.

72. *Fabric Rolls of York Minster*, ed. J. Raine (Surtees Soc., XXXV, 1858), pp. 225–6; *York City Chamberlains' Account Rolls 1396–1500*, ed. R.B. Dobson (Surtees Soc., CXCII, 1978–9), p. 145. For similar examples from the tomb of Bishop Edmund Lacey (d.1455), see U.M. Radford, 'The Wax Images Found in Exeter Cathedral', *Antiquaries Journal*, XXIX (1949), pp. 164–8.

73. Finucane, op. cit., p. 98. The offering of wax images was heavily satirized during the Reformation. A classic jibe may be found in *Acts and Monuments of John Foxe*, ed. G. Townsend and S.R. Cattley (8 vols, London, 1837–41), vol. V, p. 405.

74. Thomas More, *A Dialogue Concerning Heresies*, ed. T.M.C. Lawler and others (*The Complete Works of St Thomas More*, New Haven, VI, 1981), pp. 228–9, 667–8.

75. *The Miracles of King Henry VI*, op. cit., pp. 173–6.

76. Repeated but unsuccessful attempts by the monks of Norwich Cathedral to establish a lasting cult, even to the extent of indiscriminately buying up relics, are described by J.R. Shinners, 'The Veneration of Saints at Norwich Cathedral in the Fourteenth Century', *Norfolk Archaeology*, XL (1987), pp. 134–41.

77. Finucane, op. cit., pp. 79, 107.

78. M. Bloch, *The Royal Touch: Sacred Monarchy and Scrofula in England and France*, trans. J.E. Anderson (London, 1973), pp. 54–9, 66–9, 92–3, 97–8, 103–5, 310, 313, 331–2; *The Miracles of King Henry VI*, op. cit., pp. 109–10.

79. Bloch, op. cit., pp. 67–9.

CHAPTER TWO

IDEAS ABOUT THE BODY

Sanguineus:
Of yiftes large, in love hath grete delite,
Iocunde and gladde, ay of laughyng chiere,
Of ruddy colour meynt somdel with white;
Disposed by kynde to be a champioun
Hardy i-nough, manly, and bold of chiere.
Of the sangwyne also it is a signe,
To be demure, rigth curteys, and benynge.

Colericus:
The coleryk: froward and of disceyte,
Irous in hert, prodigal in expence,
Hardy also, and worchith ay by sleyght.
Sklendre and smalle, ful light in existence,
Right drye of nature for the grete fervence
Of heete; and the coleryk hath this signe,
He is comunely of colour cytryne.

Fleumaticus:
The flewmatyk is sompnelent and slowe,
With humours grosse, replete, ay habundaunt,
To spitte invenons the flewmatik is knowe,
By dulle conceyte and voyde, unsufficiaunt
The sutill art to complice or haunt;
Fat of kynde, the flewmous, men may trace,
And know hym best by whitnes of his face.

Malencolicus:
The malencolicus thus men espie:
He is thought and sette in covetise,
Replenysshith full of fretyng envye;
His hert servith hym to spende in no wise,
Trayterous frawde full wele can he devise;
Coward of kynde when he shuld be a man,
Thow shalt hym knowe by visage pale and wan.

Secular Lyrics of the Fourteenth and Fifteenth Centuries

The classical tradition loomed large in all aspects of late medieval learning, and nowhere more so than in the study of medicine. Not only was the curriculum followed by medical students based largely upon the work of Greek physicians active well over a thousand years before the emergence of the oldest European universities in the twelfth and thirteenth centuries, but more widespread ideas about the human body, common throughout the middling and upper ranks of society, derived from the same source. Laymen with a smattering of formal education shared with clerks and scholars a profound veneration for Hippocrates and Galen, the two greatest stars in the medical firmament, whose names alone seemed to guarantee a successful cure. Often in association with Socrates (an approximate contemporary of the historical, as opposed to the legendary Hippocrates), they were regularly invoked in fulsome language of the kind more usually employed by hagiographers:

> Thus seith Ypocras the goode surgean,
> And Socrates and Galean,
> That wore ffilosophers alle thre
> That tyme the best in any cuntre,
> In this world were noon hure peere
> As fer as any man myght here,
> And practisedem medycyns be Godus grace
> To save mannus lyf in dyvers place.
> Cryst that made bothe est and west
> Leve here soules have good reste,
> Evere-more in ioye to be
> In heven with God in trinite.[1]

The formidable reputation posthumously acquired by Hippocrates of Cos (b.*c.* 460 BC) had little factual basis. He may, as a successful physician, perhaps have composed a small part of the miscellaneous corpus of writings which bears his name, but this is by no means certain. Quite probably, the collection was compiled from a variety of sources by scholars working in Alexandria during the third century BC; the fact that it became associated with a man singled out for praise by Plato and Aristotle because of his fame as a doctor encouraged others to accept and elaborate the legend of authorship. Not all Greek medical experts were uncritical in their approach to these treatises, but the attention and praise lavished upon them by Galen, a towering figure in the medieval medical pantheon, bestowed a lasting imprimatur.[2]

We are on safer historical ground when describing the career of this remarkable man. Born in about 129 AD and trained as both a surgeon (his experience at a school for gladiators in his native Pergamum must have proved invaluable) and physician, he was celebrated in his own lifetime as a practitioner, experimental scientist and medical theorist. Such was his fame that he worked for some years in Rome as personal physician to the emperor, Marcus Aurelius, although he still managed to produce an impressive *oeuvre*, including lengthy commentaries on nineteen so-called Hippocratic texts.[3] While noting certain omissions and even errors in Hippocrates' work, Galen none the less hailed him as a master 'whose views on medical and biological matters were to be adopted wherever possible', most notably with respect to the theory of the humours first adumbrated in that part of the corpus known as *The Nature of Man*.[4]

Ironically, given Galen's mistrust of practitioners who learned their skills from books, his work

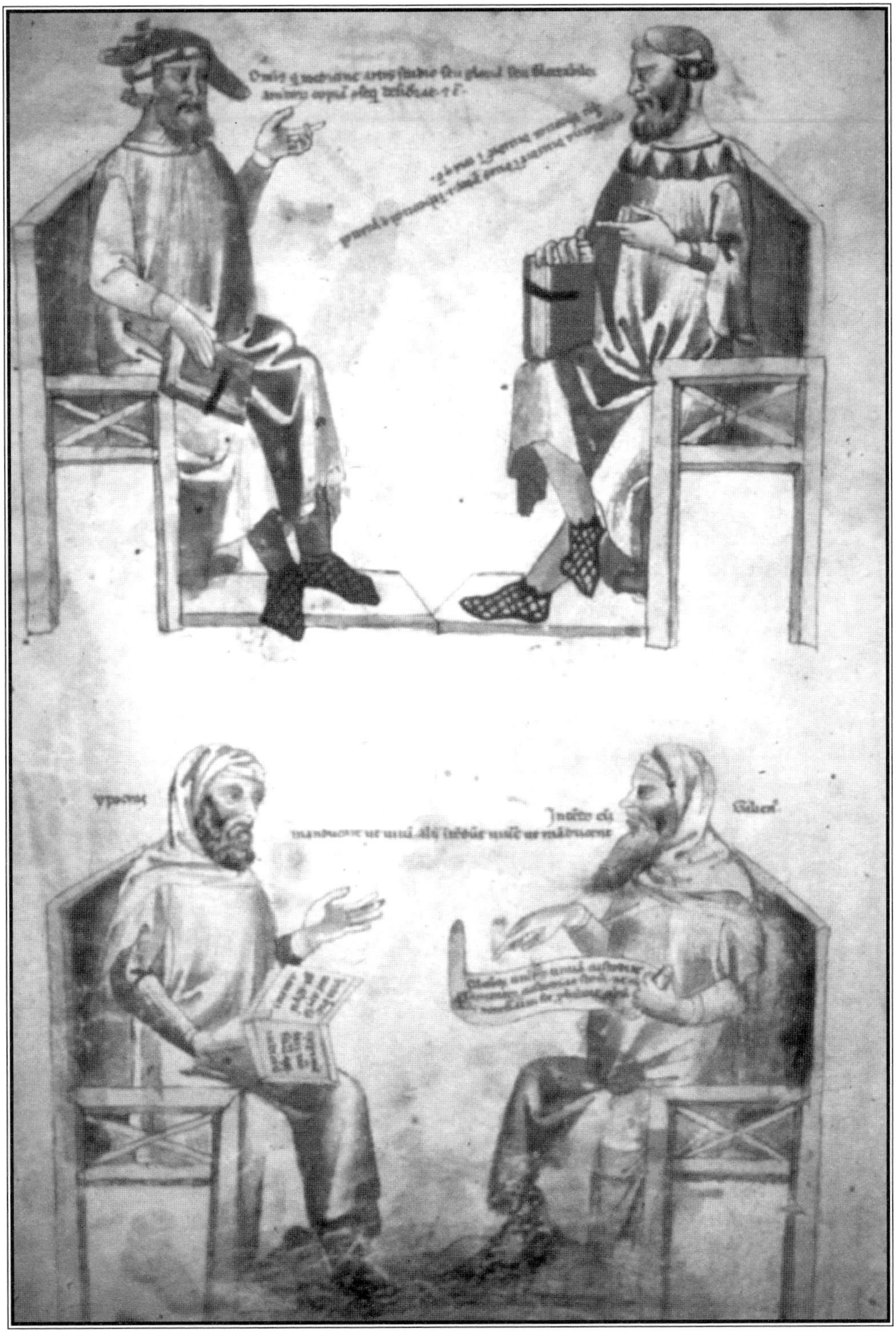

Homage to the work of Constantine the African (d.1087). This illuminated page from a fourteenth-century French herbal shows scholars consulting the translations of Galen and Hippocrates made by him from Arabic into Latin.

cast a long, inhibiting shadow upon medical education until the sixteenth century. Commentaries, digests, summaries and encyclopaedias, designed to preserve his own teachings like a fly in amber, supplanted empirical studies based on clinical observation of the sort he himself had recommended to students. An analysis of the works of Bernard Gordon (b.1258), who taught and practised at Montpellier for over thirty years, has revealed no fewer than 600 direct references to 'God's servant', Galen (colour plate 13). Indeed, this 'prince of physicians' is actually cited almost as often as all the other medical authorities used by Gordon put together, which is understandable in view of the superhuman skill and intelligence generally attributed to him.[5] At first, however, it seemed that the West would preserve only a small, unrepresentative fragment of Greek medical literature: the division of the Roman Empire and the survival in the western part of no more than a handful of texts translated into Latin brought an abrupt halt to intellectual speculation, and even in Italy, where some Galenic and Hippocratic writings were readily available, the emphasis inevitably shifted away from theory to the acquisition of basic workaday skills.[6]

The balance was more than redressed by the spread of Greek learning throughout the Arab world. Translations of most important philosophical and scientific works, including those by leading medical authorities, were made and augmented by Muslim and Jewish scholars, many of whom regarded themselves as natural heirs to the Hippocratic tradition. From the eleventh century onwards, as the centres of Islamic scholarship in Spain, Sicily and the Near East became more accessible to Christians, the writings of Rhazes (d.925), Isaac Judaeus (d.*c.* 932), Avicenna (d.1037), his near contemporary Albucasis, Averroes (d.1198) and other eminent commentators began to circulate in the West, along with new translations of the Greek masters. An initial trickle of exciting discoveries became a veritable flood, thanks to such enthusiasts as Gerard of Cremona (d.1187), whose output included translations from Arabic into Latin of nine treatises by Galen, three by Rhazes and Avicenna's encyclopaedic exposition of Galen's work, the *Canon of Medicine*.[7]

The teaching of medicine in the West underwent a dramatic transformation as a result of this scientific renaissance. New universities grew up throughout Europe with schools and faculties for the training of physicians, who were expected to have first obtained a thorough grounding in the liberal arts. In principle, this meant that they were already familiar, through the newly available works of Aristotle, with Greek ideas about natural philosophy; they then proceeded to consolidate their knowledge by studying a prescribed group of classical texts and commentaries. The *Articella*, or *Ars Medicinae*, which comprised a selection of works by Galen and Hippocrates, provided the basis of the syllabus; to it was added Avicenna's *Canon* (where the student learnt that 'the immutable principles of philosophy' could never be disproved by fallible human experience), as well as works by Averroes and Rhazes.[8]

The university-trained practitioner prided himself upon his formidable academic and largely classical training; but, as we have already seen, he was not alone in his reverence for the past. As the Middle Ages drew to a close, the underlying principles of Hippocratic and Galenic medicine had become common currency at all levels of the profession, and were assimilated, albeit with varying degrees of understanding, across a broad spectrum of society. What made these ideas so popular?

In order to make sense of disease and illness with the limited scientific knowledge at their disposal, the Greeks had evolved an all-embracing, and eminently coherent, explanation of the workings of the human body. This derived from the concept that each and every individual, being a microcosm of the universe, functioned in exactly the same way as did the universe itself, sharing the same components and responding with great sensitivity to environmental and planetary influences. Such a theory was readily absorbed into the mainstream of Christian tradition, where it assumed an important place alongside the biblical account of the Creation. In the words of the German mystic, Hildegard of Bingen (d.1179): 'O man, look to man. For man has the heavens and earth and other created things within him. He is one, and all things are hidden within him.'[9]

Just as the universe was made up of the four basic elements of fire (hot and dry), water (cold and wet), earth (cold and dry) and air (hot and wet), so too the body depended for its existence upon four corresponding humours: choler or yellow bile, phlegm or mucus, black bile, and blood. Galen's unreserved admiration for Hippocrates hinged largely upon his genius in being the very first to demonstrate these 'interacting qualities, through the agency of which everything comes to be and passes away'.[10] Although good health could only be achieved by maintaining a careful balance between them, and ensuring that none grew either too powerful or too weak, a combination of heredity, age and circumstances usually conspired to make one or two of the humours somewhat stronger than the others. This gave each individual his or her 'complexion'; and so pervasive was the medical vocabulary used to describe the appearance and behaviour of the humoral types, that it is still widely employed today.

fire	hot and dry	choler or yellow bile	choleric
water	cold and wet	phlegm or mucus	phlegmatic
earth	cold and dry	black bile	melancholic
air	hot and wet	blood	sanguine

A modern reader has no difficulty in picturing Chaucer's Franklin, whose ruddy, 'sangwyn' colouring accords well with his jovial manner and lavish hospitality, or in creating a mental picture of the 'sclendre colerik' Reeve, made gaunt and irritable through an excess of yellow bile.[11] Women, being colder and moister than men, were generally held to be heavy, slow and phlegmatic, but they, too, might tend towards a sanguine, choleric or, worst of all, melancholic disposition. Melancholia arose from the spleen's failure to absorb black bile, which was 'ane odious humour to nature and to al membris of the body for his yvel qualitez', and thus, not surprisingly, the most potentially dangerous of them all.[12] In extreme cases, the retention of 'melancoliouse filthes' could corrupt the whole body, producing the 'greyny flesche and horrible' of leprosy; a less dramatic superfluity of black bile engendered covetousness, guile, cowardice and an unhealthy pallor.[13]

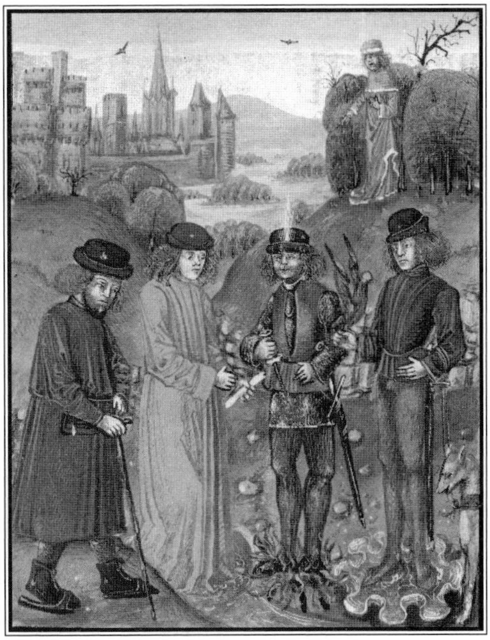

The four humoral types or complexions depicted with their corresponding attributes: a melancholy clerk stands on the earth, a phlegmatic merchant (with a model ship) on water, a choleric knight in the fire and a sanguine nobleman (carrying a hawk on his wrist) in the air.

Medieval writers derived great intellectual satisfaction from devising numerical categories into which they placed everything from the sorrows of the Virgin to prohibited degrees of kinship within marriage. Humoral theory lent itself particularly well to a series of analogies based upon the number four, which might include the ages of man, the seasons of the year, the points of the compass or, as in this fifteenth-century verse, times of day:

God made all mankynd that lyves on the erthe
Of iiij elementys, als we in bokys rede:
Of fyre and of ayre, of watir and of erthe,
That gendirs in us humors, als Arystotille us lers [teaches].
Blod raynes in man at mydnyght, fleume in the mornyng,
Colericus comys at none, melancole in the evyng:
And of thir iiij homers comys qualites sere,
After that thai have myght in man and powere.
Sanguine is the fyrst, the ij fleumatyk;
the iij is melancole, the iiij coleryk.
Of these iiij humors ilk man is made,
Bot all is noght in lyke of qualite and state.[14]

Nor was all 'in lyke of qualite and state' within the body, for each particular organ had its own 'complexion' or humoral composition, as well as occupying a specific place in the hierarchy of physical parts. Medical authorities disagreed to a certain extent over the relative dryness of the heart, 'the firste organyk membre' of the body, although all believed it to be hot. The kidneys were manifestly 'fleschy and sanguine', while the brain (which could only be observed after death, thus bearing out the humoral stereotype) seemed cold and moist, albeit with areas of warmer matter.[15] Some organs actually served to house reserves of blood, phlegm or bile, which, in a healthy person, would remain where nature intended:

The splen is to Malencolie
Assigned for herbergerie:
The moiste Flweme with his cold
Hath in the lunges for his hold
Ordeined him a propre stede,
To duelle ther as he is bede;
To the Sanguin complexion
Nature of hire inspeccion
A propre hous hath in the livere
For his duellinge mad delivere;
The dreie Colre with his hete
Be weie of kinde his propre sete
Hath in the galle [bladder], wher he duelleth,
So as the Philosophre telleth.[16]

Ideally, any superfluous and potentially harmful humours would be excreted in the sweat, tears, urine and faeces. In addition, sneezing was seen as a valuable way of clearing impurities

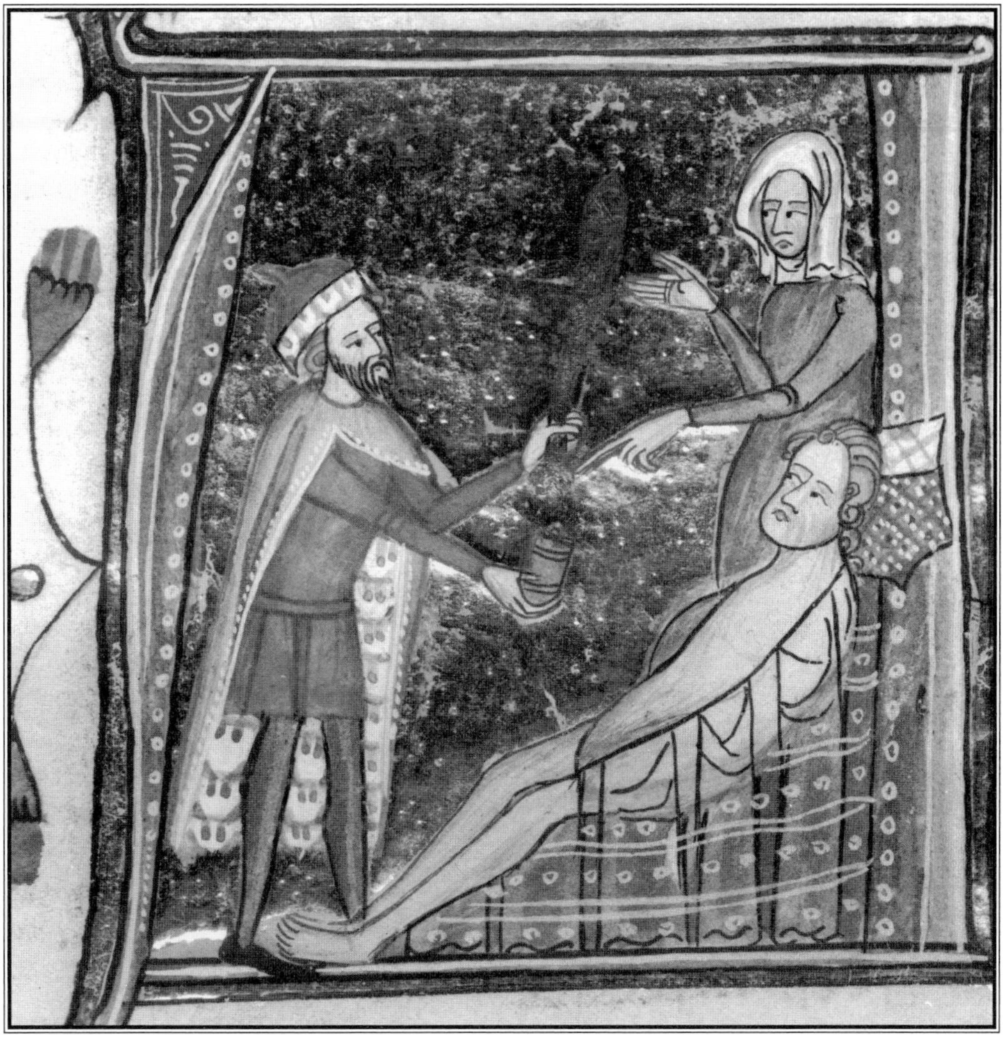

According to this fourteenth-century English encyclopaedia, 'A' stands for apostume, or swelling, which the practitioner must reduce by applying medication to disperse the concentration of humours beneath the skin.

from the head: 'For manse brayn is more moyste then the brayne of odur bestes, ther fore humours be ther gederit, and be put out with nesyng.' Once, however, the body's natural mechanism for waste disposal began to break down or proved in any way inadequate, the delicate humoral balance itself came under threat, with painful, if not fatal, consequences. In certain circumstances, for example, an excess of choler 'made lyghte with hete of hit selfe' would be drawn inexorably upwards 'in fumosite and smoke' to the moist atmosphere of the brain, causing frenzy and delirium, while the descent of cold, thick humours to the feet and ankles was likely to result in painfully swollen joints.[17]

Tumours, ulcers and other afflictions accompanied by suppuration, swelling or discoloration of the flesh were generally blamed upon the inability of that part of the body to absorb the healthy matter provided for nourishment, perhaps because of trauma or exposure to the cold. Not only did writers such as the French surgeon, Henri de Mondeville (d.*c.* 1320), believe that failure to expel 'evil humidity' through sweating might lead to an unpleasant catalogue of skin diseases: they also shared a conviction that either fleas or lice (depending on the degree of heat on the skin's surface) might be generated as a result.[18] The cause of external eruptions, or 'apostumes' as they were commonly called, was relatively easy to determine because of the coloration and relative sensitivity of the affected area. It might appear red, throbbing and sore (sanguine), yellowish and acutely painful (choleric), pale and soft (phlegmatic) or hard and dark (melancholic), depending upon the humour or combination of humours trapped beneath the skin.

The physician faced a harder task when attempting to diagnose internal apostumes. Most diseases of the liver, kidneys, spleen and other vital organs were attributed to blockages or local disruptions of this kind, which, given the current understanding of human physiology and the absence of effective techniques for surgical exploration, provided a convenient solution for some knotty medical problems. It is worth noting, for example, that the English physician, John of Gaddesden (d.1361), described pleurisy as an apostume of the ribs or midriff, pneumonia as an apostume of the lungs and both frenzy and lethargy as apostumes of the brain.[19]

Since almost any illness or bodily dysfunction could be convincingly and authoritatively ascribed to a humoral imbalance, it is hardly surprising that medical practitioners, who were by nature conservative, continued for the best part of two thousand years to describe, diagnose and treat the sick within these terms of reference. Having been called upon to perform an autopsy on the son of an influential Florentine official in the hope that his findings might be used to safeguard the health of the boy's surviving siblings, the physician Bernard Tornius (d.1497) reached some predictable conclusions. Dissection revealed several abscesses of the liver (probably caused by septicaemia), which Bernard explained in terms of an abundance of phlegm, accentuated by the child's 'humid age'. The retention of putrid matter and noxious fumes around the body's 'principal members' had provoked 'a withdrawal of heat to the inner parts', but not in sufficient quantities to counteract and expel the fatal poison. He thus urged the official to take particular care of his other children until their 'natural heat' had become strong enough to drive out 'superfluities and humidity', and especially to avoid the production of heavy vapours which might well prove fatal. To this end, he devised a course of medical treatment designed to keep the youngsters fit until they reached the warmer climes of puberty.[20]

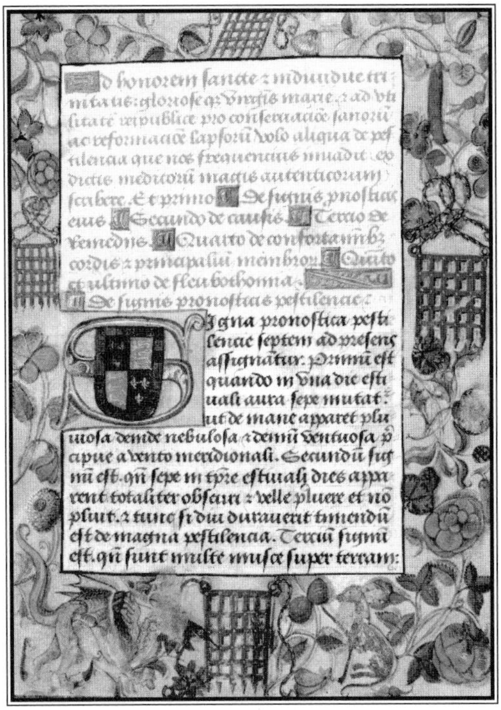

Advice literature on avoiding pestilence followed a standard format, but was more carefully produced and embellished for high-born readers. Lady Margaret Beaufort's personal copy of one such Latin treatise is easily recognized by her heraldic devices.

As in classical times, great importance was placed upon the need to preserve health. At best an uncertain gamble, the business of curing people once they fell ill was fraught with dangers and difficulties for doctor and patient alike, so it made sense to concentrate upon preventative medicine. From the twelfth century onwards theologians with an interest in natural science emphasized the positive contribution to be made by practitioners in keeping disease at bay, with the result that medical writers began to explore the possibilities of didactic literature composed specifically for an educated lay readership. Even before the outbreak of the Black Death the *regimen sanitatis*, or guide to healthy living, was a growing genre; and successive epidemics generated a huge popular market, avid for information.[21] Ideally, the physician was supposed to provide each patient with a *regimen* tailored to his or her individual 'complexion' and lifestyle, but the time and labour involved meant that only the very rich could afford such a personal, customized service.

In 1424, for example, the distinguished Oxford *medicus*, Gilbert Kymer, composed a *Dietariam de Sanitatis Custodia* for his patron, Humphrey, Duke of Gloucester, containing a great deal of advice, meticulously set out in twenty-six chapters, about diet, digestion, exercise and (appropriately, given the duke's rather tortuous marital history) the dangers of sexual excess.[22] Much of what he wrote had, however, already become available to a wider, albeit less tutored, readership as shorter, more accessible works written in the vernacular began to circulate among the gentry and merchant classes. Some, such as John Lydgate's 'Dietary and Doctrine for Pestilence', were ostensibly intended to advise people about avoiding infection, although their insistence upon a light, nourishing diet, fresh air and gentle exercise drew upon over a thousand years of medical tradition:

For helthe of body keep fro cold thyn hed,
Ete no rawe mete, take good heed herto,
Drynk holsom wyn, feede the on lyht bred,
With an appetite ryse from thi mete also,
With women aged flesshly have na a do,
Upon thy sleep drynk nevyr of thi cuppe,
Glad toward bedde and at morwe, bothe too,
And use nevir late for to suppe.

Temperat diet kyndly digestioun,
The golden sleep braidyng upon pryme,
Naturall appetite abydyng his sesoun,
Foode accordyng to the complexioun,
Stondyng on iiij, flewme or malencolie,
Sanguey, colre, so conveid bi resoun,
Voidyng al trouble of froward maladie.[23]

From their study of the *Articella*, medieval physicians learnt to distinguish between three basic classes of phenomena which together determined the health or sickness of their patients. The first were naturals, such as the humours, elements and qualities, which made up the human body; the second, contra-naturals, or pathological conditions hostile to survival; and the third, non-naturals. The latter comprised agents necessary to life, loosely grouped under the categories of environment, motion, nourishment, sleep, evacuation and mental equilibrium. Each of these was capable of either harming or strengthening the individual according to the way he or she chose

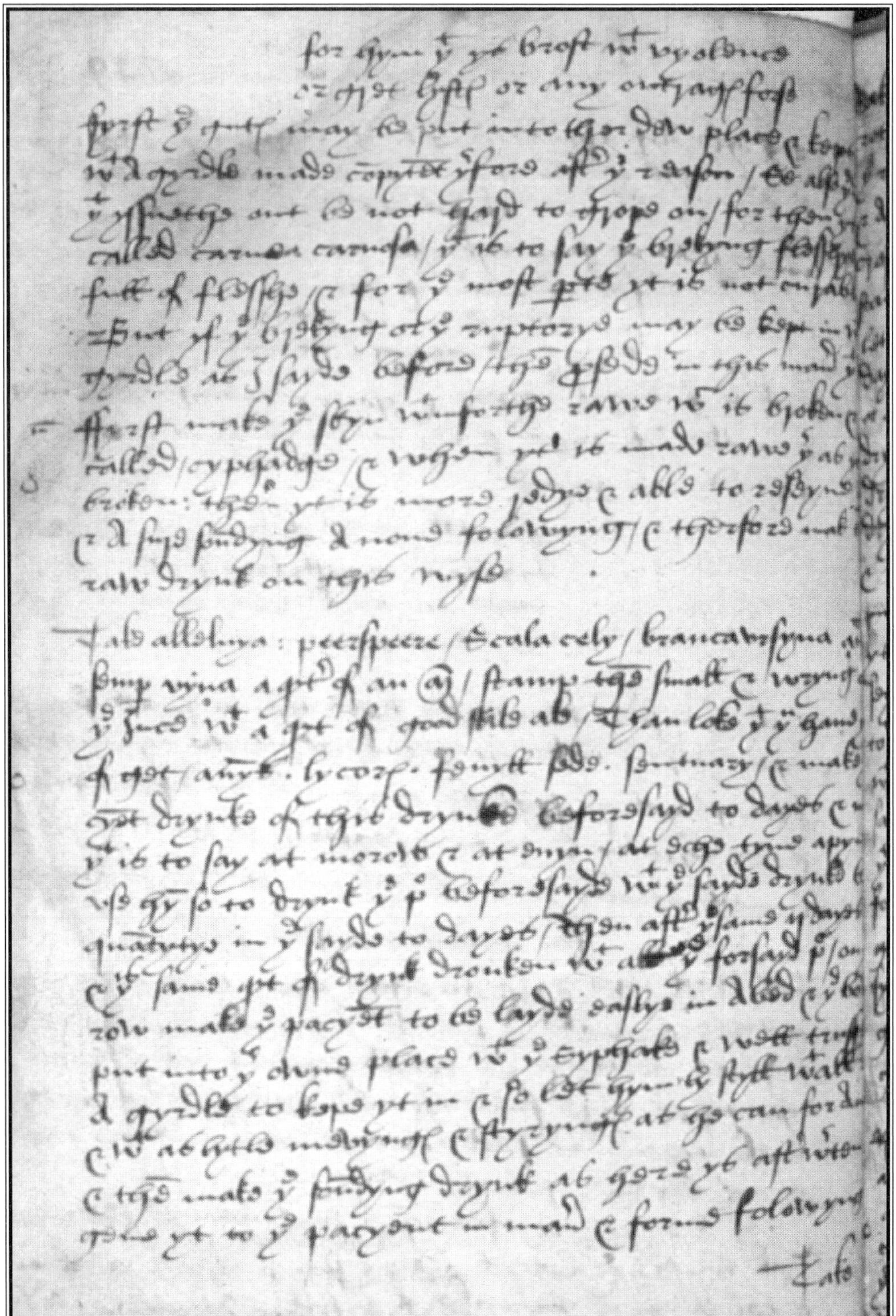

The workmanlike text of Jean de Bourgoyne's extremely popular plague tract, translated and abridged for the benefit of an anonymous English owner in the early fifteenth century.

to live: sensibly managed, in keeping with each person's 'complexion' or humoral make-up, non-naturals could become a positive source of well-being and fitness; but abuses, either as a result of excess or deprivation, spelt disaster.[24]

By explaining how best to achieve the golden mean the *regimen sanitatis* encouraged a holistic approach to medicine with which modern readers can easily identify: the repeated emphasis upon sensible eating habits, relaxation, the avoidance of stress and keeping on good terms with colleagues and neighbours has about it a timeless, pragmatic quality, which (unlike certain other aspects of medieval therapeutics) ought to have proved remarkably successful. Having read what his 'master', Galen, had to say on the subject, Bernard Gordon wrote perceptively about the harmful effects of noise and the many other disagreeable nuisances of contemporary urban life. He was critical of colleagues who preferred 'the lucrative treatment of diseases' to 'the preventative application of a good *regimen*' (which made less money); and he advised his students to examine the patient's living quarters as well as his body, checking to see if he was 'disturbed by an adjoining shop occupied by a carpenter, hammerer, tanner of hides, melter of tallow or by any persons who work with sulphur and the like'. Barking dogs, drunks and, more alarmingly, bandits were rightly identified as causes of anxiety and therefore of disease, although it is hard to see how Bernard's less affluent patients could have avoided such hazards.[25]

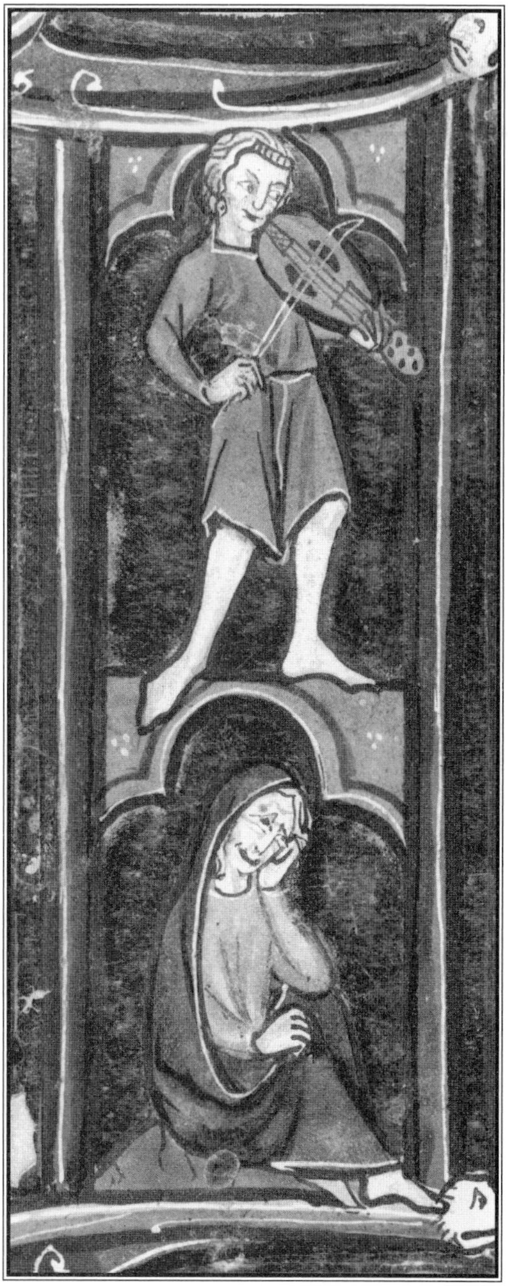

This illuminated capital from a late thirteenth-century copy of Aldobrandino of Siena's Li Livres dou Sante (Books of Health) *depicts the power of music to overcome melancholy and restore the spirits. The artist draws upon the well-known Biblical story of David, the musician, and King Saul.*

Overindulgence at mealtimes was discouraged on the ground that it would disrupt the process of 'coction' or digestion, producing unhealthy quantities of one particular humour or dangerous fumes likely to generate disease. Just as a dish could easily be ruined by too much or too little cooking, so too the measured conversion of food into phlegm, bile and blood required a steady temperature and level of moisture. Chaucer's physician in *The Canterbury Tales* clearly practised as he preached, adopting a 'mesurable' diet 'of no superfluitee, but of greet norissyng and digestible', exactly as he would have prescribed for his patients.[26] All foodstuffs could, like the human complexion itself, be categorized by their intrinsic heat, dryness, cold or moisture, and were either recommended or prohibited by the practitioner according to his patient's special circumstances. The French physician who attended Honor, Lady Lisle, when she was suffering from a phantom pregnancy in the late 1530s blamed 'the many and diverse cold and slemysh humours', which lay at the root of the problem, upon her undisciplined eating habits. Having prescribed purges and potions to cleanse her body of the noxious residue, he proceeded to lecture her about the need for moderation, not least with regard to pastries and late-night snacks:

> Madame, furthermore, ye must, if it pleaseth you, have regard that at your meat ye do nothing that may be contrary to your disease and that might increase or augment the same. Ye must above all things keep from indigestion, for of the same proceedeth all evil corruption and all diseases and infirmities to man's body, and thereby is engendered an humour which is the food and nourishing of your disease. Wherefore, it shall be good and requisite that there be a great space between your dinners and suppers, and that ye eat but twice a day. . . . Ye shall not use cold meats, as powdered beef that is cold, or cold veal. Ye shall not eat of gross meats, beef, of all venison flesh, except of pheasants, nor of mutton, but seldom and little, for it engendreth slymysh humours. . . . Ye shall not eat any raw fruit nor raw herbs, whatsoever they be, nor roasted, boiled or parboiled. . . . All manner of pastry is contrary for you, as tarts, pies, cakes and other pastry which the cooks or bakers thereof do accustom to ordain. As far as shall be to your possibility, ye shall eat nothing after supper; that if ye be constrained to the same (which I would not gladly that it should so chance with you), ye shall then eat a little marmalade for to comfort your stomach.[27]

Warm and moist foods, such as chicken and almonds (the principal ingredients of *blanc mangier*, a dish commonly served to medieval invalids), were considered the most 'temperate' or closely akin to the ideal humoral state. For this reason Lady Lisle was urged to eat stewed capon, broth from the bones and other types of poultry. On the other hand, because they lived in water, fish naturally seemed phlegmatic and hard to digest unless the cook took pains to dry them out, while too much red meat could produce a harmful superfluity of 'grosse blode' in those of a sanguine disposition.[28] An invalid's refusal to forgo potentially dangerous meals, or to follow the diet recommended by his physician, seemed tantamount to a rejection of professional help, and could in fact be presented as such by the defence in cases of alleged malpractice. When accused of negligence in 1433, the York leech, Matthew Rillesford, countered by asserting that his patient's wilful consumption of 'unwholesome food', against all advice, had not merely nullified the effect of whatever medicines he might have been given, but had actually caused them to be eliminated from his body.[29]

During outbreaks of plague or sweating sickness strict dietary measures assumed particular importance as a means of keeping the pores closed to 'infectabyl ayer', so hot spices, leeks, garlic, 'suttel wynes' and anything else likely to raise the body temperature were immediately banned from the kitchen.[30] Although alcohol was often used medicinally (not least because of the almost supernatural resemblance between red wine and blood), writers stressed the need for moderation.

'Be cleyn in your sowle and in your body, swere no gret othis, let not your drynke be your master', ran one set of maxims, adding, somewhat tendentiously, that 'chef medycen is abstynence'.[31] Besides causing such chronic pathological conditions as gout, flatulence and haemorrhoids, 'froward drounkenesse' could do spectacular damage to the snoring inebriate if the attendant fumes had no means of escape. Dedicated topers (most notably those encountered in Germany by the Elizabethan traveller, Fynes Moryson) took appropriate precautions for self-ventilation:

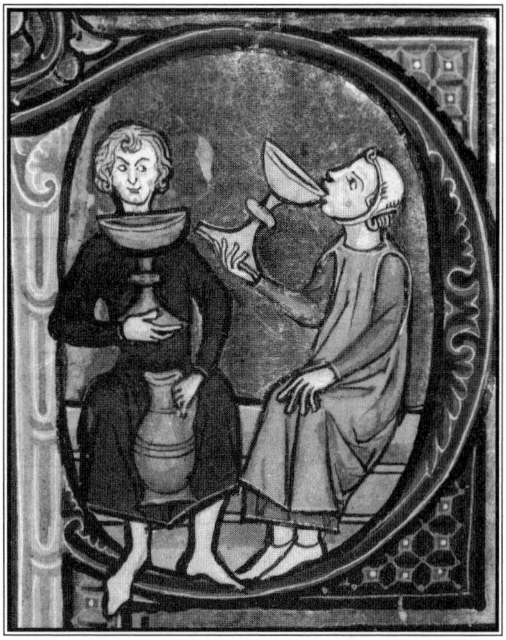

While recognizing that alcohol had many therapeutic qualities, writers on the regimen of health, such as Aldobrandino, stressed the need for moderation. Drinking on an empty stomach, or consuming too much young wine was not encouraged.

> They seldome or never drinke with their hats on, for sitting in a warme stove bare-headed, they find their heads more speedily eased of the vapours that arise from drinking. Many of [them] going to sleepe, doe by the advice of the Physitian, put little stones into their mouthes, to keepe them open: for as a boyling pot better seethes the meat if the fier be coverid, so the fier be moderate: but if it be extraordinarilie great and hot, the pot lid must be taken off, lest it boyle over; so it is good to helpe a man's concoction, if he sleepe with his mouth shut, so his diet be sparing or moderate: but in such excesse as the Germans use, not onely the mouth, but (if it might be) the very brest is to bee opened, that the heate of the inward parts may have vent.[32]

During his continental travels, Moryson made frequent allusion to the effects of environment upon the humoral make-up of the people he visited. He believed, for instance, that the striking numerical preponderance of women over men in the Netherlands was due largely to the 'flegmaticke humors' bred by the 'watery Provinces'. The cold, wet climate (together with alcohol abuse of almost Germanic proportions) made it harder for the men 'to beget males', since boys naturally inclined towards a sanguine temperament.[33] In this he was reiterating ancient ideas about the part played by the weather at the time of conception: the pure, invigorating north wind, which seemed to cleanse the air of unhealthy vapours and 'stimulate natural energy', was, not surprisingly, equated with the positive qualities of masculinity, while the humid south wind, a carrier of rain, and not infrequently sickness, created conditions more favourable to the generation of females.[34]

Medieval writers gave considerable thought to the proper location of houses and gardens so that they could derive maximum benefit and minimum danger from the prevailing winds. When describing the health-giving properties of a well-ordered pleasure garden, Albertus Magnus (d.1280) was quite specific on this score:

> Let the garden stand open to the North and East, since these winds bring health and cleanliness; to the opposite winds of the South and West it should be closed, on account of their turbulence bringing dirt and disease; for although the north wind may delay the fruit, yet it maintains the spirit and protects the health.[35]

Along with the common assumption that meteorological conditions had a direct effect upon the human body ('such as is the Aire, such be our spirits, and as our spirits, such are our humours'), went an even stronger belief in the transmission of epidemics by corrupt air.[36] Once again, the 'naturelly infectyf' south wind was regarded as the principal culprit, to be avoided at all costs, especially during outbreaks of plague:

> Also, it is gode to a pacient every daye for to chaunge his chaumbre and often times to have the wyndowes opene ayenst the north and east, and to spere the wyndowes ayenst the south. For the south wynde hath ij causes of putrifaction: the first is it maketh a man beyng hole or seke feble in their bodyes; the seconde cause is, as it is writon in the iij of *Amphorismys* [the third book of *Aphorisms* in the Hippocratic corpus, number five], the south wynde grevyth the heeryng and hurteth the herte by cause it openeth the poores of man and entreth the herte. Wherfore it is gode to an hole man in tyme of pestilence when the wynde is in the south to bee within the hous al daye.[37]

The idea that infectious diseases were spread by airborne vapours and absorbed through the open pores of the body had, like humoral theory, a long classical pedigree; and it, too, continued to find advocates until the eighteenth and nineteenth centuries.[38] Hallowed by tradition, and apparently supported by empirical observation, it gave rise to measures for public health which may well have proved quite effective, albeit for entirely different reasons. Local authorities sought to eliminate such obvious sources of miasmic contagion as 'stynken caryn cast on the water nye the cytees or townes', 'the corrupcon of privys' and 'the castyng of stynkyng waters and many other foule thinges in the stretes', secure in the knowledge that they were not only making urban life less disagreeable but also, and of far more importance, cleansing the air of potentially lethal fumes.[39] Complaints made in 1415 about the state of a public latrine near 'the Moor' outside the walls of London, for example, drew attention to the 'many sicknesses and other intolerable maladies arising from the horrible, corrupt and infected atmosphere proceeding from the latrine aforesaid'. As a result, the offending structure was demolished and rebuilt over the waters of the Walbrook, comparable regulations being promulgated with regard to the disposal of domestic waste in the area.[40]

The same theory lay behind the desire to isolate lepers, whose polluted breath was believed to contaminate the surrounding atmosphere, and thus infect anyone to whom they spoke. For this reason they were warned not to engage in outdoor conversation with healthy individuals until the latter had placed themselves upwind some distance away, and were naturally banned from frequenting narrow lanes or confined spaces where such precautions could not be taken. Rabies was likewise attributed by some authorities to noisome 'exhalations' from unburied corpses.[41] The enormous popularity of scented clothes and pomanders, as well as powders, incense and perfumes for use in the homes of wealthy men and women, was thus (as almost all the surviving plague treatises attest) not simply a means of camouflaging unpleasant smells but an important prophylactic measure, intended to combat infection.[42]

Medical practitioners, who could not, of course, honourably follow the advice given in these manuals and stay well away from plague victims (although Galen had beaten a hasty retreat from Rome when pestilence struck in AD 166), took careful precautions to wear 'many scented things', have rose-water sprinkled throughout the sickroom and press a sponge soaked in vinegar to their noses when visiting the afflicted. Needless to say, a dangerous build-up of contagious fumes around the patient was to be prevented by proper ventilation, and any urine sample or other 'voided matter' removed for examination was to be covered with a heavy cloth to prevent the escape of noxious air.[43]

Erasmus of Rotterdam, an obsessive hypochondriac who spent much of his life either fleeing from or worrying about epidemics, felt that the English had only themselves to blame for successive outbreaks of sweating sickness and other contagious diseases. Not only were they generally indifferent to the direction of the prevailing winds and the need to air their houses properly, but also, as he complained to Cardinal Wolsey's physician in 1524, their domestic habits left much to be desired. This picture of unremitting squalor should not be taken too literally (we know from surviving accounts that floors in baronial households and large institutions, at least, were covered with matting and kept fairly clean), although Erasmus' views on the subject of hygiene proved extremely influential with civic reformers:

> To begin with, they do not consider which quarter of the sky their windows or doors will face, and then their rooms are as a rule so planned as to make a through draught impossible, which Galen especially recommends. Then a great part of the walls consists of transparent glass panes which admit light in such a way as to exclude air, and yet admit through chinks what they call filtered air, which is considerably more unhealthy and stands there motionless for long periods. The floors too are generally spread with clay and then with rushes from some marsh, which are renewed from time to time but so as to leave a basic layer, sometimes for twenty years, under which fester spittle, vomit, dogs' urine and men's too, dregs of beer and cast-off bits of fish, and other unspeakable kinds of filth. As the weather changes, this exhales a sort of miasma which in my opinion is far from conducive to bodily health.[44]

It is easy to see why the medieval layman, haunted by the omnipresence of death, and perhaps even more terrified of a long, incapacitating and painful illness, constantly strove to avoid infection and restrain his warring humours, even if he could boast little more than a smattering of medical knowledge. And we may certainly assume that the more affluent, book-owning classes were quite well informed about the way their bodies worked (or were believed to work), not least because of the pervasiveness of ideas and terminology which went far beyond the pages of the *regimen sanitatis*. The equation of health with humoral balance, and physical fitness with moderation was not lost on political commentators, who readily drew comparisons between the human body and society as a whole.

Thomas Brinton, Bishop of Rochester (d.1389), followed a long-established tradition in identifying different bodily parts with specific social or economic groups, starting with the prince at the head and ending, predictably enough, with farmworkers and labourers at the feet.[45] Others embarked on more detailed anatomical conceits, involving, for example, judges (the neck or the eyes), priests (the chest or the ears), noblemen (the spine), knights (the arms), squires (the hands), yeomen (the fingers), men of law (the ribs), merchants (the thighs), artisans (the legs), ploughmen (the feet) and domestic servants (the toes). Whatever their choice of similes, most thought in hierarchical terms. For the Oxford humanist Thomas Starkey (d.1538) the problem of maintaining a stable balance of power in society was as subtle as that of keeping his own humours under control: a preponderance of phlegm, black bile or choler might well prove manageable, just as an oligarchy or even a democracy might function adequately, but the ideal lay elsewhere:

> How be hyt, as of physycyonys the sanguyn complexyon ys gugyd of ther chefe and best for the mayntenance of helthe of the body, so the state of a prynce, where as he ys chosen by fre electyon most worthy to rule, ys, among the other, chefe and pryncypal jugyd of wyse men for the mayntenance and long contynuance of thys commyn wele. . . .[46]

In an urban context, particularly after the upheavals of the Peasants' Revolt and other civic disturbances of the late fourteenth and early fifteenth centuries, mayors, aldermen and local dignitaries fought hard to defend their position at the head of a 'corps politike', utilizing the ritual of plays and festivals to reinforce this image and remind their social inferiors of the distance between neck and feet.[47] If a man fell sick because one bodily part or humour had usurped the others, so by analogy neither the state nor the city could tolerate the disease of political disaffection:

> I likne a kyngdom in good astate
> To stalworthe man, myghty in hele.
> He is myghty, with a-nother to dele.
> Yif eche of his lymes with other debate,
> He waxeth syk, for flesch is frele.
> His enemys wayte erly and late,
> In his feblenesse, on hym to stele.[48]

Medical theory further inspired these writers to envisage the 'body politic' in terms of class and rank because it also recognized certain 'noble', 'principal' and 'spiritual' organs, whose exalted function placed them in a position of authority over the rest. Such a tripartite system of classification is itself reminiscent of the conventional division of Christian society into those who fought, those who laboured and those who prayed; and some parts of the anatomy were similarly evaluated.[49] A combination of sensitivity and position determined the relative 'nobility' of each organ: the eyes or ears, for example, were demonstrably high-ranking members of the corporeal aristocracy when compared with the lowly knees or feet, not least because of their vulnerability to pain or infection. It goes without saying, that, although their vital importance was acknowledged, the digestive tract and reproductive organs lacked the social cachet of the denizens of the upper thorax, and were indeed separated from them by the diaphragm, just as a great landowner might seek to isolate himself from the vulgar herd (upon whose labour he depended) by walling off his grounds.[50]

Another scale of values, defined by a recent historian as 'economic' rather than 'feudal', ordered bodily parts in terms of their relative usefulness. However 'ignoble' they might appear, the bladder, anus and intestines were essential for survival, and thus 'principal' members in a way that the hands and feet, or even the eyes and ears, were not.[51] This particular hierarchy was often headed by the stomach, in recognition of the cook's sterling work in feeding rich and poor alike, but there was little chance of it usurping power from its 'noble' and 'spiritual' superiors, among which the heart (either alone, according to Aristotle, or in partnership with the brain and liver, as the Galenists believed) reigned supreme. The heart owed its hegemony not just to the central, dominant position which it occupied within the body, but also to the inherent 'spirituality' which it shared with other parts of the upper thorax and the arteries. This was because it produced a life-giving substance known as *pneuma*, or 'spirit', which was manufactured out of air from the lungs, transported through the arteries along with blood to the base of the brain and then transformed into those 'animal spirits' (from *anima*, a comprehensive Latin word meaning either breath, life, mind or soul) which made possible movement, thought and sight.[52]

In his great work of legal theory, *De Laudibus Legem Anglie*, Sir John Fortescue (d.1479) compared the mixture of blood and *pneuma*, 'by which the body is maintained and quickened', to the will of the people, and the nerves, or motivating force, to the law.[53] Here, his insistence that the head could neither deny the bones and members sustenance, nor change the workings of the nervous system, struck a powerful blow against absolute monarchy; but most theorists relied upon medical metaphors for the conventional purpose of defending social inequality. Thus, for example, in 1483 Bishop Russell, the Chancellor of England, penned an ingenious defence of high taxation, in which he likened the royal Court not, as was commonly the case, to the head or the heart, but (as the sixth-century *Epistula Ypogratis* had done) to the chief of the 'principal' members, the stomach. On the face of things, a comparison between the monarch and the digestive system might not seem the happiest of literary conceits, but Russell was well schooled in medical theory:

> That bodye is hole and stronge whois stomake and bowels is ministered by the utward membres that that suffiseth to be wele digested; for if the fete and hondes, whyche seme to doo most paynefulle labour for mannys lyvyng, wolde complayne ageynste the wombe [abdomen] as ageynste an idelle and slowthfulle parte of the bodye, and denye the provysyon of syche necessarye foode as the stomake calleth for, hyt might sone happe, that faylynge the belye for lake, the guttes and intestines compressed and shut by drynesse, alle the other membres shold nedes peryshe togedyr. And therfor hyt ys undoubted in nature that thys middelle membres of the body . . . be not unoccupied, but hafe ryght a besy office; for when they be fed they fede agayne, yeldynge un to every parte of the bodye that withoute the whyche no man may leve. . . . What ys the bely or where ys the wombe of thys grete publick body of Englonde but that and there where the kyng ys hym self, hys court and hys counselle? For there must be digested alle maner metes, not onely servyng to commyn foode but alleso . . . some tyme to medicines, such as be appropred to remedye the excesses and surfettes committed at large.[54]

Sometimes, however, the body politic became infected with dissent, and more desperate measures were required. Undesirables might have to be purged from society, just as the physician set about eliminating evil humours from his sick patient. Not surprisingly, references to amputation, extraction and evacuation proliferated during periods of civil conflict. The *Somnium Vigilantis*, a Lancastrian propaganda document produced in defence of the proscriptions of 1459, compared the Yorkist lords to 'a roten tothe' which had to be pulled out before it caused 'confusioun and undoying' to all the rest.[55] Richard, Duke of York, countered by likening his opponents to a wasting fever or pernicious cancer, and appealing to the parliament of October 1460 as a physician enlisting the help of his apothecary:

> I, beyng the partye greved, and complaynaunt, can not minister to my self the medicine that should helpe me (as experte leches and chyrurgians may) except you be to me both faithful ayders, and also trew counsaylors. Nor yet this noble realme, and our naturall countrey shall never be unbukeled from her quotidian fever, except I (as the principall physician) and you (as trew and trusty appotecaries) consult together, in makyng of the pocion, and trye out the clene and pure stuffe, from the old, corrupt and putrified dregges. For undoutedly, the rote and botome of this long festered cankar is not yet extripat. . . .[56]

All too often in the fifteenth century the political equivalent of major surgery seemed the only answer to the nation's ills: just as the human body might require far more drastic treatment than was envisaged in the comforting pages of the *regimen sanitatis*. For no amount of care in the matter of diet, environment and all the other non-naturals so crucial for survival could be guaranteed to ensure a long and healthy life. Indeed, as medical authorities were themselves the first to point out, an obvious disadvantage of the individually produced *regimen* was that it took a long time to devise, even longer to put into practice and months, at the very least, before significant improvements became apparent. What, then, could be done in the short term to restore the precarious equilibrium of phlegm, bile and blood once it had been disturbed? The practitioner's first step was, of course, to establish the nature and cause of the malady, paying particular attention to the balance of the humours, not simply in order to establish the patient's overall 'complexion', but more specifically with regard to the afflicted part of his or her anatomy.

Far from being crudely ascribed to an excess or deficit of one particular humour, most serious disorders were believed to result from a complex interplay of physical and environmental factors. A disease might, in one individual, arise from a superfluity of choler, or yellow bile, while in another the very same problem could easily be caused by too much phlegm. Successful treatment, at least in contemporary terms, required an extremely sensitive reading of the patient's symptoms, which made considerable demands upon the diagnostic skill of the physician. Retention of the menses (seen as a particularly threatening condition, which obstructed the natural process of purgation, and could lead to dropsy, heart disease, haemorrhoids or even leprosy) might, for example, be caused by an excess of any one of the four humours in the uterus, although an examination of the woman's urine would soon reveal to the practised eye which one had to be eliminated. If the specimen seemed highly coloured and greasy the physician would prescribe a series of remedies designed to reduce the level of choler; 'feble colour' accompanied by a white discharge obviously denoted too much phlegm; an unhealthy surplus of black bile could be detected in thin, cloudy urine, full of tiny particles; and any evidence of bleeding pointed unmistakably to corrupt 'sykenesse of the blode'.[57] Here, as was usually the case, little or no distinction was made between the symptoms of a disease and the actual ailment itself, since the practitioner regarded both as the products of humoral imbalance, which he had to rectify.

Uroscopy (the examination of urine) was one of the principal diagnostic tools employed by the medieval *medicus*, who is generally depicted in contemporary iconography with his flask or 'jordan', earnestly scrutinizing a patient's sample (colour plate 6). 'I pray to God to save thy gentil cors', cries Chaucer's affable Host after hearing the Physician's tale on the way to Canterbury, 'and eek thyne urynals and thy jurdones.' Others were less complimentary, regarding the practice as an ingenious confidence trick on the part of the medical profession. It was, as satirists never tired of pointing out, easy enough for the 'false fisicien' to 'wagge his urine in a vessel of glaz',

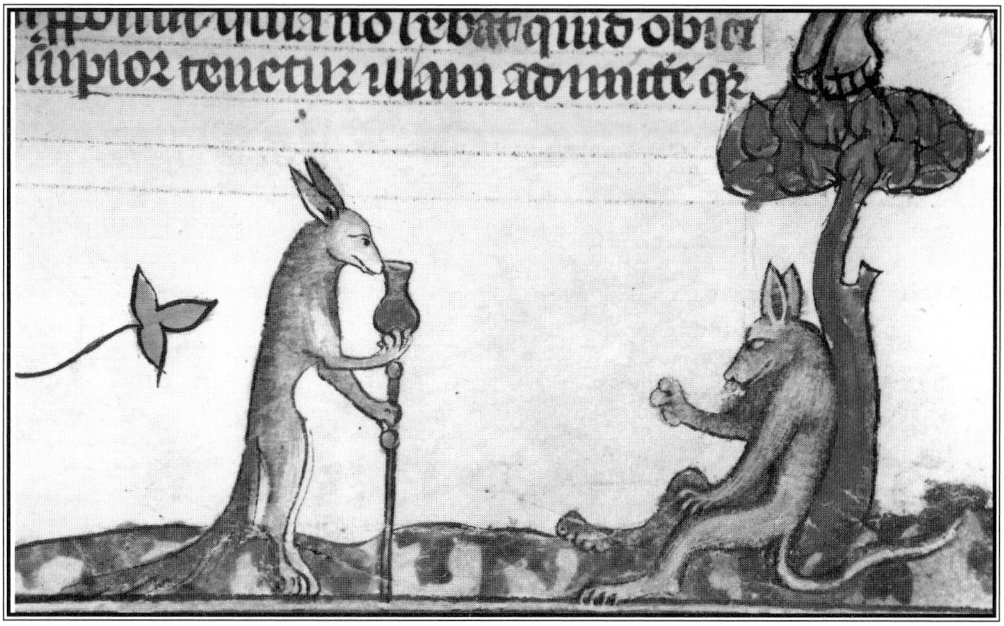

Medical procedures and practitioners easily lent themselves to satire. In this copy of the Decretals of Gregory IX, the artist enlivens a serious text with animal imagery from popular tales. Disguised as a physician, Reynard, the wily fox, tricks his enemy, Isegrym, the wolf, pretending to test his urine.

make gloomy pronouncements about the patient's chances of survival and extort large sums of money from worried relatives.[58]

Yet most people retained a trusting belief in uroscopy as the most accurate and effective means of diagnosis available. By the beginning of the fifteenth century simplified English versions of scholarly Latin texts on the subject were circulating widely among surgeons and other interested parties who could not understand the originals. One of the earliest known translations of a substantial medical work, made in about 1379 by the Dominican friar, Henry Daniel, offered readers an impressive compendium on uroscopy, culled over a long period from 'the books of many authors and the sayings of commentators on them'. And another, allegedly 'contryvyd and made by the wysest clerkys of phisik of Inglond, and translatyd owte of Latyn in to Englysch at the instaunce and prayere of oure lyege lorde, Kynge Herry the 4te', found its way, some fifty years later, into the same small volume as a thirty-four page *Liber de Iudiciis Urinarum*, also clearly set out in the common tongue.[59] This growing interest in the practical aspects of uroscopy has been ascribed to the fact that basic information about colour, quality and smell could easily be conveyed in manuscript form, often with the use of illuminated diagrams.[60]

Given that the artists who illustrated all but the finest medieval medical manuscripts had a limited palette and frequently compensated for their lack of expert knowledge with wild flights of imagination, it seems likely that such charts served as a very elementary guide to what was, in practice, a much more subtle procedure. Many, even so, identified twenty or more different types of urine, as well as drawing attention to possible gradations of colour, sedimentary deposits and degrees of 'substaunce' within each (colour plate 5). They also briefly listed what disorders might have given rise to such coloration, which part of the body was likely to be affected, and what remedies the physician might consider. Usually the accompanying text provided more detailed and specific help:

> Now in every man is body is foure qualitees: hete and colde, moyste and drye. Hete and colde they ben causers of colours. Drynes and moystenes they ben cause of substaunce. Hete is cause of rede colour; drynes is cause of thyn substaunce; moystenes is cause of thycke substaunce. As thus, if the uryn of the pacient be rede and thicke it signifieth that blode is hote and moyste. If it be rede and thynne hit sheweth that colere hath dominacioun, ffor why [because] colere is hote and drye. If the uryn appere white and thicke hit betokeneth fleume, ffor fleume is colde and moyste. If the uryn shewe white and thynne, it sygnifieth malencoly, ffor malencoly is colde and drye. When thu hast considerid wel as this, then beholde the diversite of colours of the uryns. . . .[61]

There would follow a verbal description of each colour: 'rubicunda', for example, seemed 'lyke to a flaume of fyre sentte oute' and usually accompanied 'a fever acute and sharpe'; while 'lactea', which derived its name from cow's milk, was produced during a protracted fever or dropsy, and sometimes gave an ominous warning of early death. Some authorities went so far as to suggest tests for determining a person's chastity (or lack of it) by this means. 'Stedfast virginite' naturally manifested itself in 'lyght water and ful bryght', but, if the contents of the urinal seemed troubled, corrupt or tinged with lead, sexual promiscuity might well be to blame. Few guilty secrets escaped the physician's observant eye.[62]

In theory, then, the medieval physician could diagnose, prescribe and even offer moral guidance on the strength of one or two urine samples produced by the patient; and although he obviously needed further information (such as 'the dyete of the seke body' and the duration of his or her illness) all this could be supplied by an intermediary. As early as the tenth century a set of medical aphorisms, compiled for a sophisticated Arab readership by Isaac Judaeus, had warned against the indiscriminate use of uroscopy for diagnosing disorders outside the urinary tract, and had particularly attacked 'fools who would base prophecies on it, without seeing the patient, and determine what disease is present, and whether the patient will die, and other foolishness'.[63] None the less, many late medieval practitioners prided themselves on their ability to treat the sick at long distance, giving advice about diet and assessing the success or failure of medication through uroscopy alone; and some medical authorities confidently assumed that such a service would be offered as a matter of routine.[64]

Affluent city dwellers and gentry families living on the outskirts of towns regularly dispatched samples of urine to be examined by their physicians. Some did so as a preventative measure, hopeful that steps could be taken to deal with any incipient humoral problems before they assumed life-threatening proportions. Others, such as Agnes Stonor, were already ill, and anxiously sought a favourable prognosis. In 1480 it was reported that she had 'sente here water unto Master Derworthe to undirstonde his conceite, ande howe he demyth by here water whedir she be in wey of mending'. Specimens from wealthy patients arrived almost daily while treatment was in progress so that the physician could see how far the wayward humours had responded to medication; and the nurses or servants who actually cared for the invalid were under orders to despatch a fresh one as soon as any changes occurred ('as this meydsans wyrkyth on hym so send word ayen with his watter').[65]

Members of religious communities were just as preoccupied with the need to have their urine

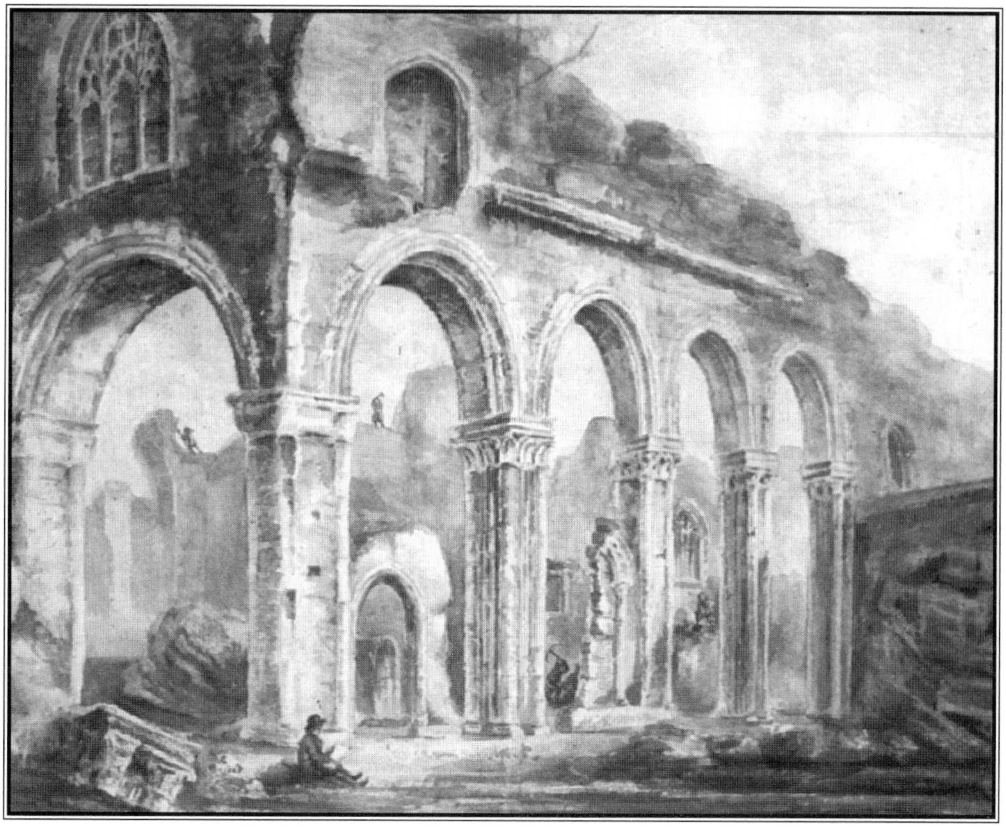

The ruins of the infirmary of Norwich Cathedral Priory, painted at the time of its demolition in 1805. This large building boasted its own chapel, and a separate chamber for monks who were being phlebotomized.

properly inspected. The thirty-eight surviving infirmarers' accounts from Norwich Cathedral Priory record routine payments for glass phials for this purpose at a cost of a few pence a year, although in 1400 the outlay on urinals, flasks and measures rose to four shillings. Local physicians had always been employed on an *ad hoc* basis to treat the monks, but two decades later it was decided to retain Master Mark, a university-trained practitioner, at 13s.4d. a year, specifically 'for the examination of urine'. He served the sick brothers until 1460 or thereabouts, when the annuity was first reduced and then cut altogether, perhaps because the infirmarer himself assumed this task.[66]

Uroscopy offered the medical profession a reassuring degree of certainty, which, in turn, made them appear knowledgeable and confident to their patients. The rudiments could easily be mastered with the help of a coloured chart and some practical guidance from a senior colleague. Moreover, as a diagnostic technique it boasted the added advantages of being both painless and discreet, especially for women, who were expected to remain modestly covered at all times during consultations, and could thus do little more than describe any embarrassing disorders. Great importance was still given to the proper assessment of external symptoms, but urine provided the best means of understanding and thus correcting the patient's humoral balance. For obvious reasons, this particular aspect of the physician's practice was seen as fundamental, if not to his success, then at least to his credibility:

Maximan the maistre of phisike
Seeth the urin of the peple;
He can saye to them
Wherof they be seke:
Of the heedache;
Of the payne of the eyen,
Of the eres;
Yf they have tothache,
Atte the breste, at the pappes;
He can hele and cure
Dropesye, blody flyxe,
Tesyke [phthisis], mormale [gangrene],
Feet, nayles,
Fever quartayn and tercian,
Of the Jaundyse
(Wherof God kepe us),
And of all that
That may greve us.[67]

The university curriculum for medical students also included short, classically based texts on diagnosis by pulse. Building upon Galen's list of nine 'simple' and almost thirty 'complex' pulse-rates, Arab and western commentators had developed a complicated theory and vocabulary influenced by the attractive idea that 'human music', or the rhythm of the pulse, corresponded to the harmony of the heavenly spheres. Most practitioners (including the otherwise formidably learned Bernard Gordon) had only a hazy grasp of this recondite and essentially impractical branch of study, but were well aware of the importance of taking the pulse carefully during a consultation, and using it as a guide to health. They sought to identify the extremely subtle variations of beat described by Galen (using comparisons with animals, such as the gazelle, the ant or the worm), and to evaluate them in terms of the patient's 'complexion', age, sex and way of life. Having little idea of the workings of the heart and insufficiently precise means of measuring time, they could put this information to only limited use, but were none the less sometimes able to make a surprisingly accurate assessment of the patient's general condition.[68]

Treatises on the examination of blood and faeces also circulated quite widely in the Middle Ages, adding in no small measure to the medical practitioner's unsavoury association in certain quarters with bodily impurities, 'disagreeable to the smell, foul to the sight and unsettling to the stomach'.[69] The English surgeon John of Arderne (b.1307), who specialized in treating disorders of the lower bowel, stressed the importance of inspecting fecal matter, especially after the administration of clysters. As well as looking for such obvious signs of superfluous humours as 'blode or putrid flemme', his colleagues were advised to check the sample for intestinal parasites, which were all too common, and note any unusual hardness, fluidity, odour or coloration. In some cases, where it was impossible to achieve a satisfactory diagnosis by this means alone (as, for example, when distinguishing between advanced cancer of the rectum and dysentery), Arderne recommended a rectal examination, but this would have been carried out only in special circumstances.[70]

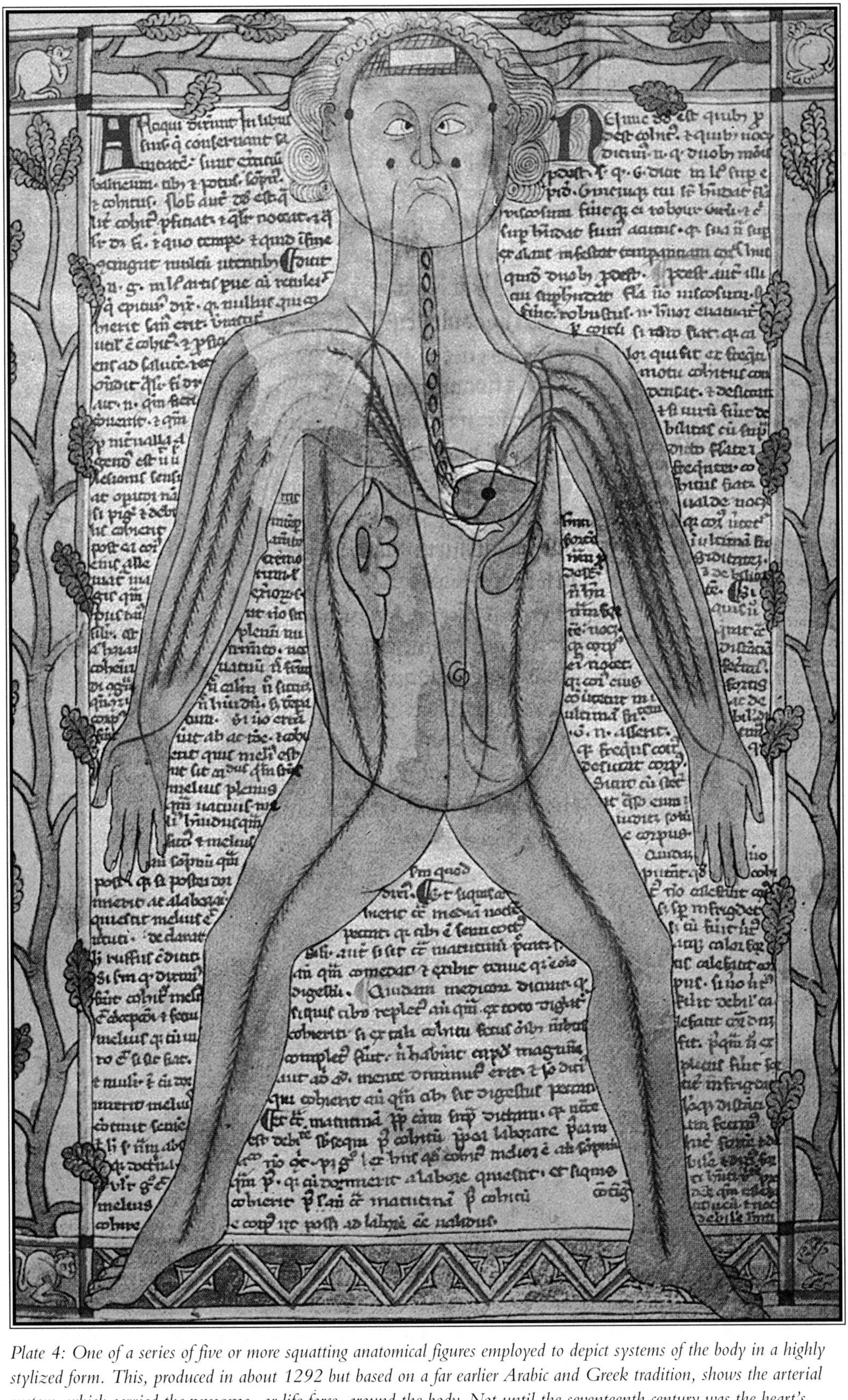

Plate 4: One of a series of five or more squatting anatomical figures employed to depict systems of the body in a highly stylized form. This, produced in about 1292 but based on a far earlier Arabic and Greek tradition, shows the arterial system, which carried the pnuema, *or life force, around the body. Not until the seventeenth century was the heart's function as a pump fully understood or the closed nature of the circulatory system discovered. The veins, from which blood was let, were traditionally coloured red in this period and the arteries blue.*

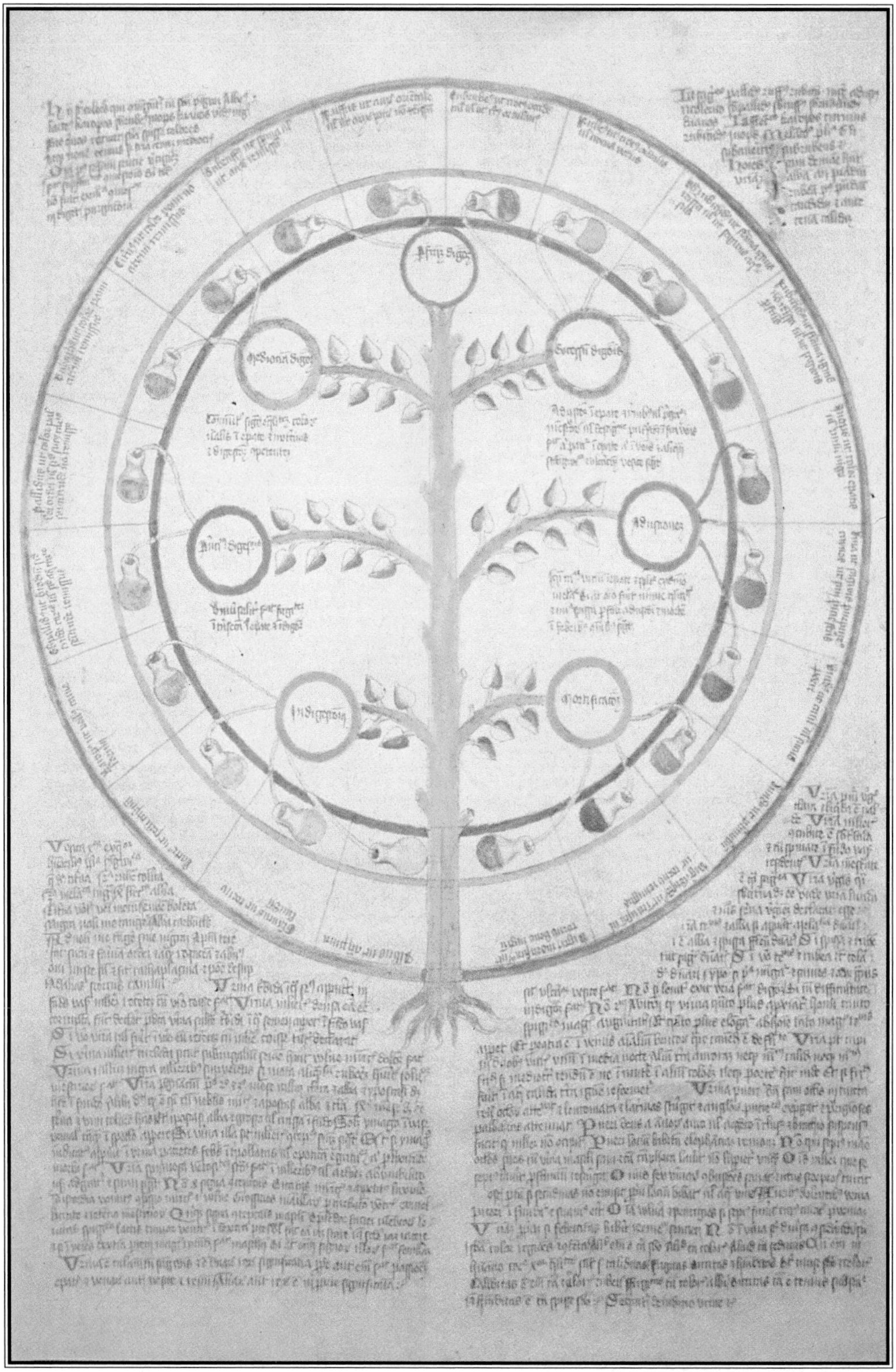

Plate 5: Information about the colour, smell, sedimentation and viscosity of urine, presented in diagrammatic form, helped the physician to determine the 'complexion' of his patients and to prescribe accordingly. The 'tree' of samples, contained within this wheel, further explains how urine is produced, the healthiest type being at the top.

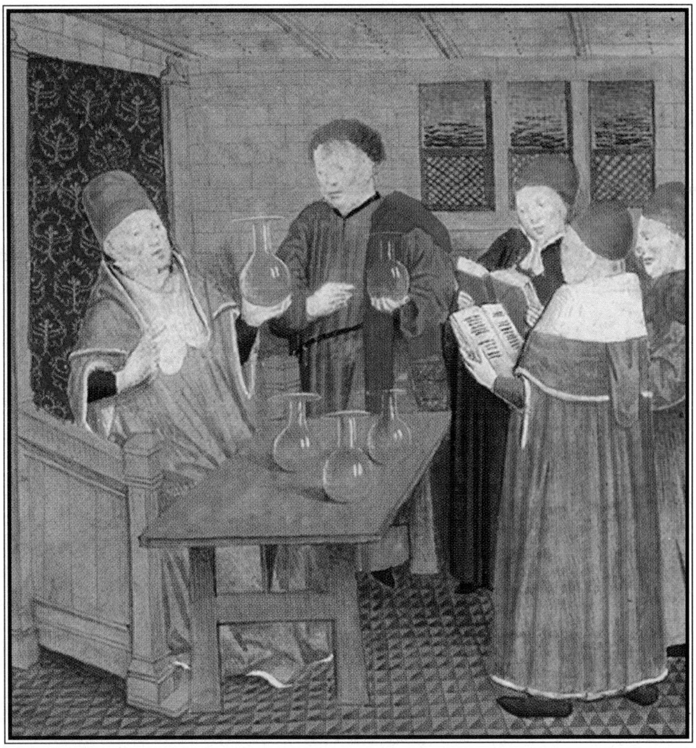

Plate 6: The examination of urine samples constituted one of the principal diagnostic and prognostic tools available to the medieval practitioner, who might even prescribe without seeing the patient.

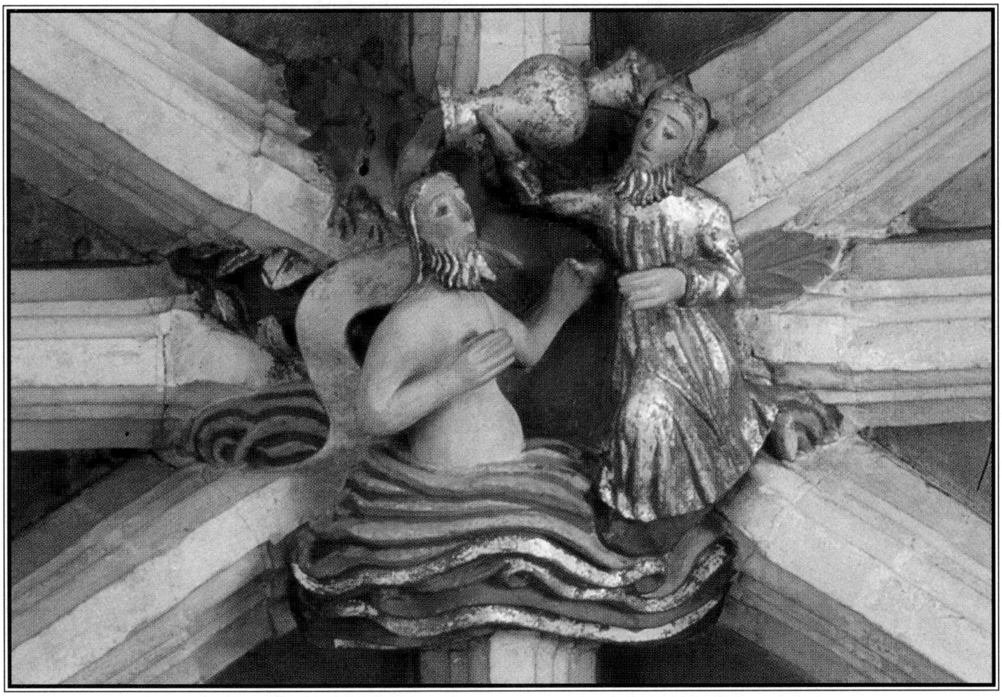

Plate 7: The 'jordan', or glass phial, used to examine urine took its name from the river where Christ was baptized. Barbers often enacted this scene in mystery plays, and the river was invoked in charms to stop bleeding.

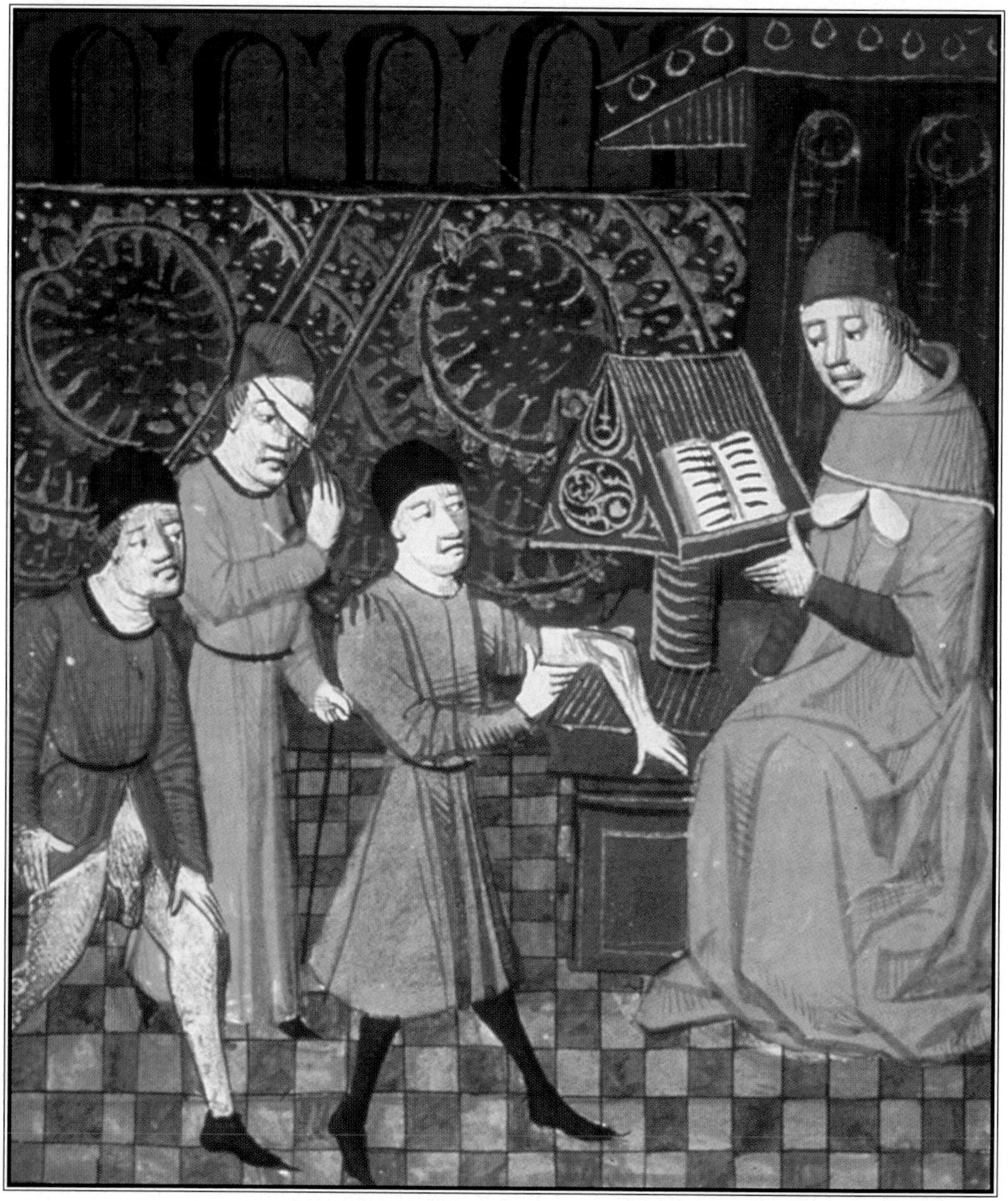

Plate 8: His status as a magister *clearly denoted by a canopy, lectern and academic robes, Guy de Chauliac holds a consultation. The battered patients, as depicted in this illustration from his* Grande Chirurgie*, display the kind of injuries and ailments regularly encountered by medieval surgeons whatever their academic credentials.*

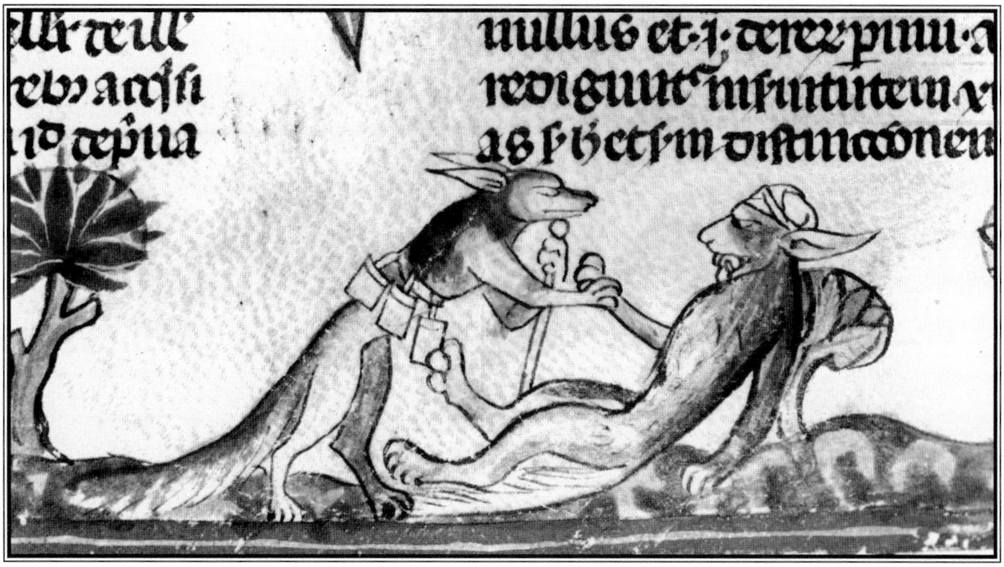

Reynard, the vulpine physician, checks the pulse of his patient, Isegrym, before leaving him for dead at the roadside. Like many human practitioners, he carries charts and materia medica *in pouches around his waist.*

As we shall see, the widespread practice of phlebotomy meant that samples of blood were readily available for scrutiny by the physician or surgeon, who once again sought to determine the balance of his patient's humours through the colour, heat, texture and smell of the sample. Sometimes he might even taste the blood, which in a healthy person was supposed to be slightly sweet, but could become bitter, sour or saccharine if the balance had been disturbed. Having described Christ on the cross as a patient being 'leten bloode' (to purge the sins of the world), the *Ancrene Riwle* notes, in passing, that 'no man ne may wel iugge bloode atte Barbours ar it be colde'. This guide for female recluses contains numerous references to the common practices of daily life, and we may assume that such tests were a routine affair. The technique involved was quite similar to that employed in uroscopy, although the process of coagulation was also carefully observed; and in certain cases the sample had to be 'washed' in order to discover the tell-tale sediment or grease which provided one of the principal indications of leprosy.[71] It must have been difficult to master the nuances of colour and 'substaunce' without magnification:

> Gode blode is that that is noght to grete in substaunce ne thenne, but it is able to breke and wel temperate, in colour rede and bright, and lovesome in smelle and in savour. Evel blood is that that goth oute of wayee fro this: as that that boweth to thenesse and to yelownesse and to bittrenesse and hath scharpe smelle, it is cleped colerik blood. That forsothe that boweth to gretnesse and to blakkenesse or to yelownesse and to sourenesse and to soure savoure is melancolik blood. That forsothe that boweth to gleymynesse and to whitenesse and hath swete smel and swete savour and is also watery is fleumatyk blood. That blode that hath moche of watrinesse and of uryne bytokeneth mykel drynke or feblenesse of the reynes [kidneys]. That forsothe that is fulle of greynes and of asshen bytokeneth the lepre. . . .[72]

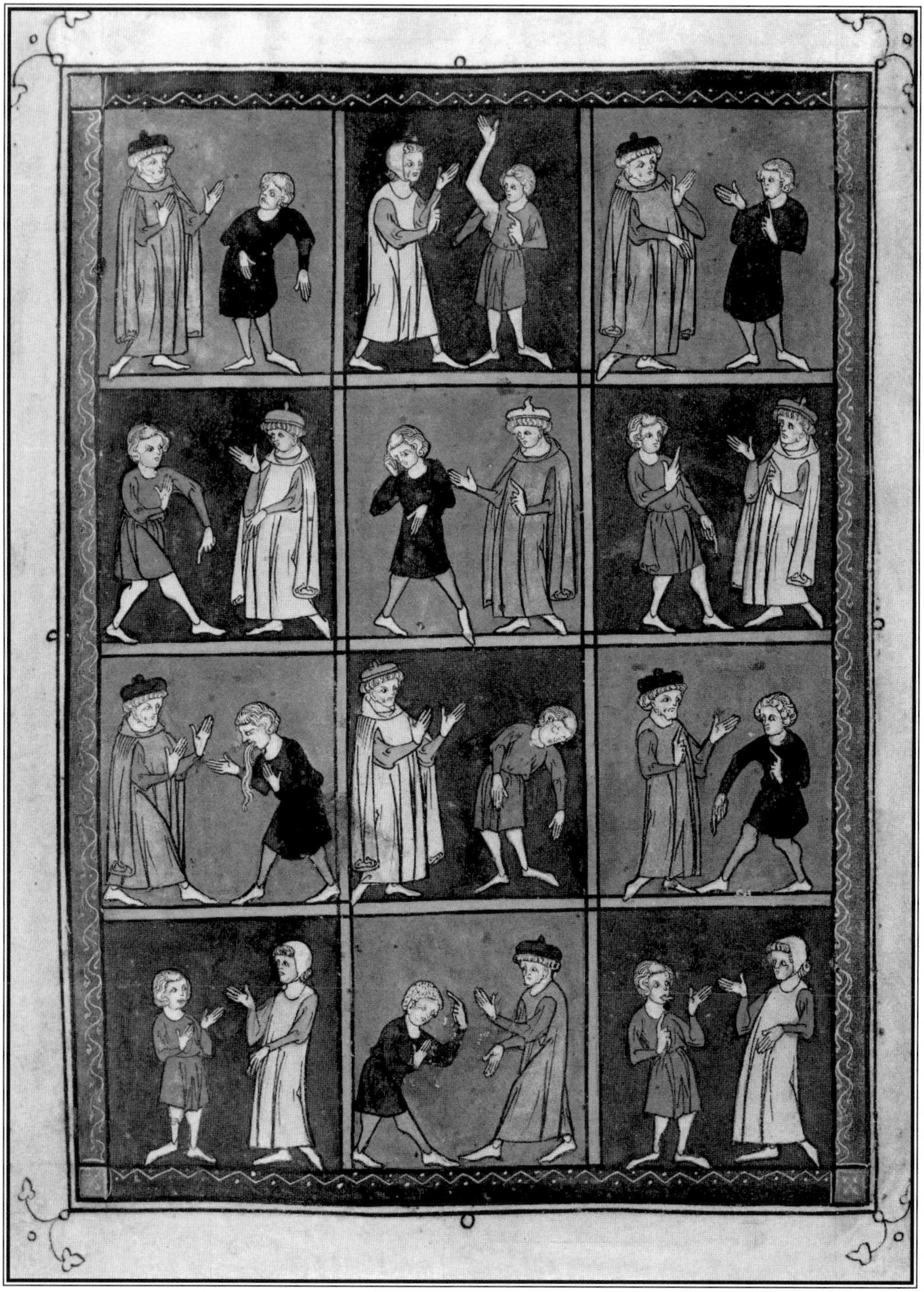

Although physicians could diagnose at long distance by urine sample alone, an examination of the patient and discussion of his or her symptoms was extremely important. Here, a variety of problems, including head lice, vomiting, toothache, dizziness, dislocations and headaches are presented.

Having talked to the patient, taken his or her pulse, conducted an external examination (so far as decency allowed) and inspected a quantity of urine, if not blood and fecal matter too, the physician was at last in a position to consider his diagnosis and embark upon a course of therapy. This would usually involve a combination of dietary measures and medication (often barely distinguishable from each other), accompanied by purgation in the form of laxatives, clysters, diuretics, phlebotomy, cautery, fumigation, hot baths or cupping, as seemed necessary to restore the humoral balance. As we shall see in Chapter IV, due regard had also to be paid to the influence of the heavens at each stage of treatment; but even without the added complication of horoscopes and difficult astrological calculations considerable skill and judgement were required to devise a suitable regime:

> To gyff a conveniabull and trew medicyn aganes seknes and perillus, a gode ffesicyan nedes to loke welle a bowte and be full well warra, and full wel avysed. For nothyng lettes more helthe of seke men than unconyng and neclygens of phisicians. Also, to hele and save effectuelly hym nedes to know complexions of men, composicions, myxtyous and medlynke, bouthe of members and of humours, and disposicyons of tymes and condiconse of male and female and age. For one medicyn helpes in wyntur and anodur in somour; and one in the begynnyng of the evyll, and anodur in the full, and an odur in passyng ther off; one in chyldehode and yn youthe, and an odur in full age, and an odur in th'elde; one in the male kynde and odur in female kynde. And hym nedys to know causes and occasyons of evylse . . . for medcyn may never be securly takyn gyf the cause of the evyll is unknowen. Also, hym nedes to know complexions, vertues and wyrkynges of medcynable thynges. For [unless] he know what medsyne is symple, what componed, what colde and what hote, what helys seknes, what herdyth and constraynes, what nesshes [softens] and laxis he may never securly passe furthe and wyrke in medycens.[73]

Surgical techniques will be discussed in the next chapter, but it is worth emphasizing here that surgeons placed just as much value on diet and medicine as did physicians. Exactly the same criteria obtained in judging how best to treat external sores and injuries as came into play when assessing suitable types of treatment for internal disorders. Indeed, ulcerated or otherwise damaged tissue was believed to respond with exceptional sensitivity not just to whatever hot, cold, dry or moist preparations might be applied locally, but also to foodstuffs and potions consumed by the patient.

In his *Science of Cirurgie*, compiled in 1296 and subsequently translated into English, Lanfrank of Milan stressed that two men suffering from identical wounds in the arm, inflicted at exactly the same time, should not necessarily be given similar treatment. On the contrary, the surgeon would have to adopt a radically different *modus operandi* if, say, one were sanguine in temperament and the other proved to be melancholic. Whereas the former's injury might give rise to 'an hot swellynge' and attendant fever, to be counteracted by a combination of phlebotomy, laxatives and 'streit dietynge' in order to reduce the body temperature and expel dangerously hot humours, the latter would be urged to replace much-needed blood by consuming meat, wine and other delicacies noted for their heat. Nor could both wounds be dressed in the same way. Since the great risk while nursing a sanguine patient was that the afflicted area would become suffused with corrupt blood, a 'medicyn defensif' or desiccative agent was recommended to dry out the surrounding skin. The melancholic, on the other hand, needed 'moister medicyn' to encourage the growth of healthy flesh on what was fundamentally a 'drie lyme'.[74]

Practitioners had thus to familiarize themselves with the relative levels of heat, cold, dryness and moisture inherent in all forms of medication, whether internal or external, as well as learning the particular 'virtues' or attributes of each. Every single animal, vegetable or mineral product customarily employed for therapeutic purposes was qualified, according to Galenic principles, in terms of three or four 'degrees' or grades of increasing intensity, ranging from one (relatively mild) to four (in some cases inimical to human life). Lettuce, for example, was held to be cold and moist in the third degree, and thus useful as a means of cooling and soothing overheated skin. On the other hand, celandine, being equally hot and dry, was able 'to dissolve and to consume and draw out of a man wikkyd humors, both colore and flemme and melencoly and eke roten blode'.[75] Other herbs, such as fenugreek (dry in the first degree and hot in the second) and camomile (hot and dry in the first degree), possessed more temperate qualities which made them invaluable for gentler types of medication. Moreover, when mixed together in compound remedies they served to modify or dilute the effects of more aggressive 'simples', unsuitable for use alone. Some of the stronger chemicals reserved for external application required very careful preparation with other ingredients beforehand: mercury and arsenic, which Guy de Chauliac suggested (not quite convincingly) as an alternative to surgery for those who 'ben dredefulle and wolde rather dye' than submit to the knife, had still to be mixed three or four times over with 'colde herbes' to reduce their 'wylde fire'.[76]

Herbals and medical recipe books, compiled for ordinary domestic use during the fourteenth and fifteenth centuries, listed and categorized the most common of these 'simples', while the reference works kept by physicians, surgeons and apothecaries (discussed in Chapter VII) were far more technical and academic. Awareness of the 'virtues' if not the precise numerical 'qualities' of plants was thus fairly widespread, as was a basic grasp of the humoral theory, which, on the written page at least, dictated how they should be administered. By using a wider and more esoteric range of commodities, selected with a mathematician's regard for 'degree', the trained professional could, however, confidently achieve exactly the right combination of dessicating, moistening, warming and cooling agents appropriate to each stage of treatment. The composition and purpose of these remedies, not to mention the type and amount of purgation or surgical intervention recommended at any given time, might vary from day to day, or even hour by hour, as the patient's humoral balance swung precariously up and down. But the practitioner was well armed for his task with a positive battery of cures, and we shall now see how he applied them.

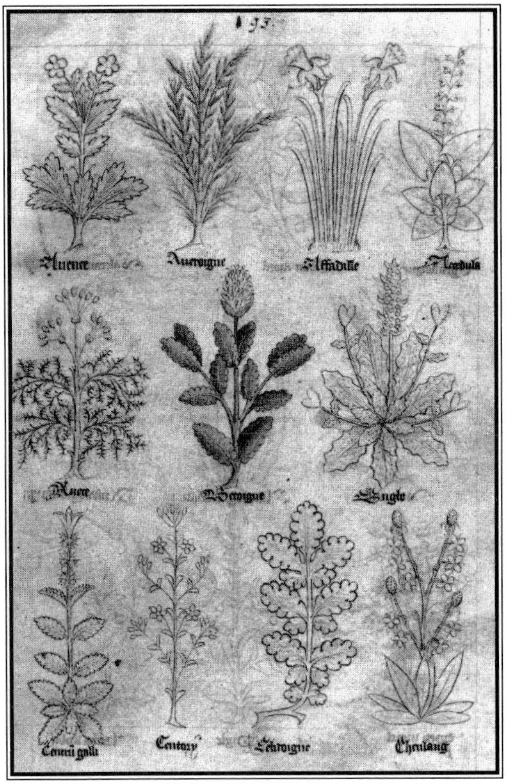

This page from a fifteenth-century English herbal depicts each simple or plant, from wood avens to hound's tongue (chenlang)*, in a clear line drawing before listing its respective degrees, qualities and uses.*

NOTES

1. *Secular Lyrics of the Fourteenth and Fifteenth Centuries*, ed. R.H. Robbins (Oxford, 1952), pp. 95–6. For a discussion of the 'Lettre d'Hippocrate', a pseudo-Hippocratic medical compilation which enjoyed great popularity in lay circles during the Middle Ages, see T. Hunt, *Popular Medicine in Thirteenth-Century England* (Woodbridge, 1990), pp. 101–41.

2. The literature on Greek medicine is vast, but an accessible introduction to the subject may be found in E.D. Phillips, *Greek Medicine* (London, 1973), *passim*; and *Hippocratic Writings*, ed. G.E.R. Lloyd (pbk, London, 1983), pp. 7–60.

3. R. Jackson, *Doctors and Diseases in the Roman Empire* (London, 1988), pp. 59–64, provides a lively sketch of Galen. For greater detail see R.E. Siegel, *Galen's System of Physiology and Medicine* (New York, 1968), *passim*.

4. *Hippocratic Writings*, op. cit., pp. 53–5.

5. L. Demaitre, *Doctor Bernard de Gordon: Professor and Practitioner* (Toronto, 1980), pp. 112–15.

6. C.H. Talbot, 'Medicine', in *Science in the Middle Ages*, ed. D.C. Lindberg (Chicago, 1978), pp. 329–96. For a reassessment of the view that medicine entered a 'dark age' between the fall of the Roman Empire and the eleventh century, see J.M. Riddle, 'Theory and Practice in Medieval Medicine', *Viator*, V (1974), pp. 157–84.

7. D.C. Lindberg, 'The Transmission of Greek and Arab Learning to the West', in *Science in the Middle Ages*, op. cit., pp. 52–90. Among the 'people of some eminence' observed by Dante in his passage through Limbo at the start of *The Divine Comedy* are Hippocrates, Galen, Avicenna and Averroes, 'the great commentator', as well as Dioscorides, the compiler of a celebrated work on herbal medicine. But although they occupy the 'noble castle' of human wisdom, they are, as unbaptized pagans, denied entry to heaven (Dante Alighieri, *Hell*, trans. S. Ellis (London, 1994), pp. 21, 25).

8. A general discussion of the university curriculum, which differed little from place to place during the later Middle Ages, may be found in N.G. Siraisi, *Medieval and Early Renaissance Medicine* (pbk, Chicago, 1990), Chapter III.

9. S. Flanagan, *Hildegard of Bingen, A Visionary Life* (pbk, London, 1990), p. 95.

10. *Hippocratic Writings*, op. cit., p. 54.

11. Geoffrey Chaucer, *Works*, ed. F.N. Robinson (Oxford, 1970), pp. 20, 22.

12. John of Arderne, *Treatises of Fistula in Ano*, ed. D. Power (Early English Text Soc., CXXXIX, 1910), p. 60. R. Porter, *Mind Forg'd Manacles: A History of Madness in England from the Restoration to the Regency* (pbk, London, 1990), pp. 39–41, gives a lucid account of the history of melancholia and its natural child, 'the spleen'.

13. *The Cyrurgie of Guy de Chauliac*, ed. M.S. Ogden (Early English Text Soc., CCLXV, 1971), p. 377.

14. L.R. Mooney, 'A Middle English Verse Compendium of Astrological Medicine', *Medical History*, XXVIII (1984), pp. 411–12. The English physician, John of Gaddesden, notes the widely held belief that apostumes, or swellings, caused by excessive humours had four stages: 'inception, increase, statis and decrease'. (*Rosa Anglica, sev Rosa Medicinae Johannis Anglici*, ed. W. Wulff (Irish Text Soc., XXV, 1929), p. 175. This edition, a translation from medieval Irish, is the only one currently available in modern English.)

15. *The Cyrurgie of Guy de Chauliac*, op. cit., p. 31.

16. John Gower, *The English Works*, ed. G.C. Macaulay (Early English Text Soc., LXXXI, LXXXII, 1900), vol. II, p. 245.

17. British Library, Dept of Mss, Sloane 983, ff. 81v, 82v, 89v–90.

18. *Healing and Society in Medieval England: A Middle English Translation of the Pharmaceutical Writings of Gilbertus Anglicus*, ed. F.M. Getz (Wisconsin Publications in the History of Science and Medicine, VIII, 1991), p. xxxiv; M.C. Pouchelle, *The Body and Surgery in the Middle Ages*, trans. R. Morris (Oxford, 1990), p. 169.

19. *Rosa Anglica*, op. cit., pp. 163–99, 227.

20. L. Thorndike, *Science and Thought in the Fifteenth Century* (New York, 1929), pp. 127–8.

21. S.R. Ell, 'The Two Medicines: Some Ecclesiastical Concepts of Disease and the Physician in the High Middle Ages', *Janus*, LXVIII (1981), pp. 15–25; L. Garcia-Ballester, 'Changes in the *Regimina Sanitatis*: The Role of the Jewish Physicians', in *Health, Disease and Healing in Medieval Culture*, ed. S. Campbell, B. Hall and D. Klausner (Toronto, 1992), pp. 119–20.

22. British Library, Dept of Mss, Sloane 4, ff. 127–209.

23. John Lydgate, *The Minor Poems: Secular Poems*, ed. H.N. MacCracken (Early English Text Soc., CXCII, 1939), pp. 703, 704–5.

24. Garcia-Ballester, op. cit., p. 121.

25. The ever-popular *Secreta Secretorum*, for example, warned readers: 'if a man ete and drynke out of tyme or ovyr moche, it makith him febille, and to falle into dyverse seeknes and many other inconvenientis; and if a man ete and drynke moderatly and temperatly he shalle fynde helthe to his lyf, strengthe to his body and helthe of alle his lymes' (*Three Prose Versions of the Secreta Secretorum*, ed. R. Steele (Early English Text Soc., extra series, LXXIV, 1898), p. 22).

26. *Healing and Society in Medieval England*, op. cit., pp. xxxii–xxxiii; Chaucer, op. cit., p. 21.

27. *The Lisle Letters*, ed. M. St Clare Byrne (5 vols, Chicago, 1981), vol. IV, no. 898.

28. T. Scully, 'The Sickdish in Early English Recipe Collections', in *Health, Disease and Healing in Medieval Culture*, op. cit., pp. 135–7.

29. W.P. Baildon, 'Notes on the Religious and Secular Houses of Yorkshire', *Yorkshire Archaeological Soc.* (Record Series, XVII, 1894), p. 78.

30. British Library, Dept of Mss, Add. Ms. 27582 (ff. 70 *et seq.* is a treatise on the sweating sickness dedicated to Henry VII by the Norman physician, Thomas Forestier), f. 76; Egerton 2572, f.67; *Lanfrank's 'Science of Cirurgie'*, ed. R. von Fleischhacker (Early English Text Soc., CII, 1894), p. 75.
31. *Rosa Anglica*, op. cit., pp. 91–3; British Library, Dept of Mss, Sloane 983, ff. 35, 86v. John of Arderne (op. cit., p. 59), lists overindulgence as one of the main potential causes of haemorrhoids. The others were: 'scharpnes of blode and over mych hete brennyng the blode, as in colorick men that ben of hote nature' (again possibly aggravated by diet); a naturally sanguine 'complexion'; and, conversely, blood that was 'subtile or watry, as in tham that useth rawe fruytez [which] gendreth watry blode'.
32. Fynes Moryson, *An Itinerary* (4 vols, Glasgow, 1907–8), vol. IV, p. 39.
33. Ibid., pp. 468–9.
34. U. Ranke-Heinemann, *Eunuchs for Heaven: The Catholic Church and Sexuality*, trans. J. Brownjohn (London, 1990), p. 165. For a fuller discussion of the theory of conception, see below, pp. 171–4.
35. Cited in J. Harvey, *Medieval Gardens* (pbk, London, 1990), p. 6.
36. Robert Burton, *The Anatomy of Melancholy*, ed. T.C. Faulkener and others (2 vols, Oxford, 1989–90), vol. I, p. 234.
37. *A Litil Boke the Whiche Trayted and Reherced Many Gode Thinges Necessaries for the . . . Pestilence* (John Rylands Facsimiles, III, 1910), pp. 3v–4. The relevant passage from the *Aphorisms* reads: 'South winds cause deafness, misty vision, headache, sluggishness and a relaxed condition of the body. When the wind is prevalent these symptoms occur in illness' (*Hippocratic Writings*, op. cit., p. 213).
38. J. Henderson, 'The Black Death in Florence: Medical and Communal Responses', in *Death in Towns: Urban Responses to the Dying and the Dead, 100–1600*, ed. S. Bassett (Leicester, 1992), pp. 136–50, provides a stimulating discussion of ideas about contagion.
39. British Library, Dept of Mss, Add. Ms. 27582, f. 72.
40. *Memorials of London and London Life in the Thirteenth, Fourteenth and Fifteenth Centuries*, ed. H.T. Riley (London, 1868), pp. 614–16. Questions of public health in medieval London are examined in three articles by E.L. Sabine: 'Butchering in Mediaeval London', *Speculum*, VIII (1933), pp. 335–53; 'The Latrines and Cesspools of Mediaeval London', *Speculum*, IX (1934), pp. 303–21; and 'City Cleaning in Mediaeval London', *Speculum*, XII (1937), pp. 19–43.
41. Pouchelle, op. cit., p. 152; R.I. Moore, *The Formation of a Persecuting Society* (Oxford, 1987), pp. 58–9.
42. British Library, Dept of Mss, Add. Ms. 27582, f. 75; *A Litel Boke*, op. cit., pp. 4v–5 (which advised 'lett your hous be made with fumigacion of herbes, that ys to saye with levys of baye tree').
43. D.W. Amundsen, 'Medical Deontology and Pestilential Disease in the Later Middle Ages', *Journal of the History of Medicine*, XXXII (1977), pp. 412–13.
44. *The Correspondence of Erasmus, Letters 1523–24*, trans. R.A.B. Mynors and A. Dalzell (*The Collected Works of Erasmus*, Toronto, X, 1992), p. 471. For background, see P. Krivatsky, 'Erasmus' Medical Milieu', *Bulletin of the History of Medicine*, XLVIII (1973), pp. 119–20.
45. G.R. Owst, *Literature and the Pulpit in Medieval England* (Oxford, 1961), p. 587.
46. Thomas Starkey, *A Dialogue between Cardinal Pole and Thomas Lupset*, in *England in the Reign of King Henry the Eighth*, ed. J.M. Cowper (Early English Text Soc., extra series, XII, 1871, and XXXII, 1878, reprinted 1973), p. 58. Most of this work is based on the idea of the state as a body, beset by various economic and social ills.
47. M. James, 'Ritual, Drama and Social Body in the Late Medieval English Town', *Past and Present*, XCVIII (1983), pp. 3–29.
48. *Twenty-Six Political and Other Poems*, ed. J. Kail (Early English Text Soc., CXXIV, 1904), pp. 64–9.
49. For a full exposition of this theory, see G. Duby, *The Three Orders: Feudal Society Imagined*, trans. A. Goldhammer (Chicago, 1980), pp. 264–6.
50. Pouchelle, op. cit., pp. 119–20.
51. Ibid., pp. 121–2.
52. Siraisi, op. cit., pp. 101, 107–9.
53. John Fortescue, *De Laudibus Legem Anglie*, ed. and trans. S.B. Chrimes (Cambridge, 1949), pp. 31–3. See A. Gransden, *Historical Writing in England II: c. 1307 to the Early Sixteenth Century* (London, 1982), p. 319, for a discussion of 'the analogy of the state with the human body' as a commonplace of late medieval thought.
54. S.B. Chrimes, *English Constitutional Ideas in the Fifteenth Century* (Cambridge, 1936), p. 175.
55. J.P. Gilson, 'A Defence of the Proscription of the Yorkists in 1459', *English Historical Review*, XXVI (1911), p. 517.
56. Edward Hall, *Hall's Chronicle Containing the History of England during the Reign of Henry the Fourth and the Succeeding Monarchs* (London, 1809), p. 245.
57. *Medieval Woman's Guide to Health*, ed. B. Rowland (Kent, Ohio, 1981), pp. 61–7.
58. Chaucer, op. cit., p. 148; *The Political Songs of England*, ed. T. Wright (Camden Soc., VI, 1839), p. 333.
59. F.M. Getz, 'Charity, Translation and the Language of Medical Learning in Medieval England', *Bulletin of the History of Medicine* LXIV (1990), pp. 12–16; Wellcome Library, Western Ms. 784. The translation of the *Liber de Iudiciis Urinarum* may have been made by John Lelamour, a master at Hereford School in 1373, who also rendered Macer's *Herbal* into

English (*Catalogue of Western Manuscripts on Medicine and Science in the Wellcome Historical Medical Library*, ed. S.A.J. Moorat, vol. I, *Mss. Written before 1650 A.D.* (London, 1962), pp. 578–9).
60. P.M. Jones, *Medieval Medical Miniatures* (London, 1984), pp. 58–9.
61. Wellcome Library, Western Ms. 537, ff. 16–16v.
62. Ibid., ff. 18v, 20–20v.
63. S. Jarcho, 'Guide for Physicians (Musar Harofim) by Isaac Judaeus', *Bulletin of the History of Medicine*, XV (1944), pp. 180–8, no. 35.
64. Siraisi, op. cit., p. 125.
65. *Stonor Letters and Papers*, ed. C.L. Kingsford (Camden Soc., third series, XXIX, XXX, 1919), vol. II, nos. 188, 275.
66. Norfolk County RO, DCN1/10/1–38.
67. William Caxton, *Dialogues in French and English*, ed. H. Bradley (Early English Text Soc., extra series, LXXIX, 1900), pp. 41–2.
68. Siraisi, op. cit., pp. 125–6; Demaitre, op. cit., p. 66; Jones, op. cit., pp. 57, 60. For some, however, the practitioner's efforts were misdirected. 'Lord!' remarked one Lollard preacher, 'sith a fysisyan lerneth diligently his signes in uryne, in pows [pulse] and othre thingus, whethur a mannys body be hool, how myche more schulde he knowe syche signes, that tellon helthe of mannys sowle, and how he hath hym to God' (*English Wycliffite Sermons*, ed. A. Hudson (3 vols, Oxford, 1983–90), vol. I, p. 459).
69. Thorndike, op. cit., pp. 123–32.
70. Arderne, op. cit., pp. 39, 77.
71. *The English Text of the Ancrene Riwle*, ed. A. Zettersten (Early English Text Soc., CCLXXIV, 1976), pp. 41–2. Pouchelle, op. cit., p. 73; *The Cyrurgie of Guy de Chauliac*, op. cit., pp. 381–2.
72. *The Cyrurgie of Guy de Chauliac*, op. cit., pp. 544–5. It is significant that Bernard Gordon's treatise, *De Flebotomia* (1308), was written because of his curiosity about the 'off-white, ashen colour' of the blood samples taken from natives of the Montpellier region. He attributed this symptom of endemic leukaemia to an idle and self-indulgent way of life, which prevented the proper transformation of digested food into blood; and he prescribed a change of diet and *regimen* (Demaitre, op. cit., pp. 6, 8).
73. British Library, Dept of Mss, Sloane 983, ff. 92v–93 (a passage taken almost verbatim from John Trevisa's translation into English of Bartholomaeus Anglicus' *De Proprietatibus Rerum*. This text has been edited by M.C. Seymour and others (3 vols Oxford, 1975–88), vol. I, pp. 435–6). It is interesting to compare the quotation with advice given in Book I of the treatise *Epidemics* in the Hippocratic corpus: 'First we must consider the nature of man in general and of each individual and the characteristics of each disease. Then we must consider the patient, what food is given to him and who gives it – for this may make it easier for him to take or more difficult – the conditions of the climate and locality both in general and in particular, the patient's customs, mode of life, pursuits and age. Then we must consider his speech, his mannerisms, his silences, his thoughts, his habits of sleep or wakefulness and his dreams, their nature and time. Next, we must note whether he plucks his hair, scratches or weeps. We must observe his paroxysms, his stools, urine, sputum and vomit. We look for any change in the state of the malady, how often such changes occur and their nature, and the particular changes which induce death or a crisis. Observe, too, sweating, shivering, chill, cough, sneezing, hiccough, the kind of breathing, belching, wind, whether silent or noisy, haemorrhages and haemorrhoids. We must determine the significance of all these signs.' (*Hippocratic Writings*, op. cit., p. 100).
74. *Lanfrank's 'Science of Cirurgie'*, op. cit., pp. 12–14.
75. *A Leechbook or Collection of Medical Recipes of the Fifteenth Century*, ed. W.R. Dawson (London, 1934), p. 89; British Library, Dept of Mss, Sloane 5, ff. 13–60v.
76. *The Cyrurgie of Guy de Chauliac*, op. cit., p. 608, and, for a list of simples and their use, pp. 616–31.

CHAPTER THREE

TREATMENT

Christ comes as a good physician to heal us. Christ acts like a physician in the following way. A doctor investigates the condition of the sick person and the nature of his sickness by such methods as taking his pulse and inspecting his urine. Thus when Christ visits a sinner, he first enlightens him with his grace to understand himself and his own sin, so that he may repent of his sins and shun them. . . . Second, after diagnosing the sickness he gives the sick person a diet as he requires and prescribes what he should eat and what he should avoid; this means that Christ teaches us to avoid the occasions of sin and to seek the occasions for practising the virtues. Third, after he has prescribed and worked out a diet, he gives the sick person some syrup, an electuary, or some other medicine against the sickness to expel it; that is, Christ gives him contrition of his sins, which is made from bitter herbs. . . . Fourth, when the sick person is healed, he warns him against relapsing, and teaches him how to live, so that he fosters in him a good intention to lead a good life. Christ further heals us in many additional ways as if from physical illness: First through the sweat of contrition, which one gets by hard exercise. . . . Second, through the bloodletting of confession. . . . Third, through the diet of fasting and penance, by which according to Jerome illnesses of the body are cured. Fourth, through the plaster or ointment of devout prayer. Fifth, through draining excessive body fluids, which means giving alms from all our goods. . . . Sixth, through the surgical removal of evil companionship, through the cautery of charity.

Fasciculus Morum: A Fourteenth-Century Preacher's Handbook

Late medieval preachers, anxious to instil into their congregations a rudimentary understanding of theology, had frequent recourse to the metaphor of Christ the Physician. Drawing upon a common experience of physical suffering and a shared, if sometimes limited, understanding of how the practitioner sought to combat disease, they expounded the basic tenets of Catholic dogma in terms of a long and intensive course of therapy. Since an invalid could only recover his strength after submitting to a carefully balanced regime of diet, exercise, medication and possibly surgery, it followed naturally enough that the Christian soul was unlikely to free itself from sin without first undergoing a parallel course of spiritual healing. This analogy seemed particularly appropriate, reflecting as it did not only the diversity of contemporary medical treatment, but also something of the effort and discomfort involved. Moreover, just as the humble penitent could never be entirely sure of the efficacy of his devotions, so the patient must often have turned desperately from one projected cure to the next, in a vain search for relief.

'When the ffesicyan commythe', explained a fifteenth-century sermon on the theme of spiritual well-being, 'he is in full purpose for to gyfe [the patient] medycyns, the whiche scholde be cawse of his helthe. Fyrste he yevithe hym a preparatyffe, secundary a purgatyfe, and aftyr that a proper sanatyff.'[1] And, indeed, the practitioner took as much care over the order in which both internal and external preparations were prescribed as did the priest with regard to the administration of the sacraments. His initial aim was to bolster the body's mechanisms for self-defence, only then proceeding to eliminate corrupt matter with more aggressive remedies. Finally, restorative foodstuffs and drugs would be recommended to speed convalescence and maintain the recently recovered humoral equilibrium.

Hardening of the spleen could not, for example, be treated immediately with 'hote medicyns that mowen dissolve the mater of the sekenes right as the hete of the sunne dissolueth th'is or snowe into watir', since the effect of too much heat upon such a coagulated mass would be to bake or consolidate it even further.[2] It had first to be gently softened or 'neisshed' through the agency of a 'mollificative', or potion of 'mene hete', designed to temper the effects of what was to come:

> Thou shalt gyve him no laxatif medicyn thoroughe his mouth, ne duretike medicyn, ne no medicin that is ful dissolutif, ne within, ne withoute, til thou have y-gove him mollificatives to make the spleen neisshe; for elles the mater that is sotel wolde vanisshe awei and the spleen waxe harder then it was. Ne suffre him to lete blode til the mater be y-made neisshe bi mollificatives, and that he be purgid, lest the spleen waxe harder than he was.[3]

As this quotation shows, medicines were commonly categorized 'by operation', that is, according to the effects which they produced upon the human body. Within the four basic classes of 'calefactives' (warming), 'infrigidatives' (cooling), 'humefactives' (moistening) and 'dessicatives' (drying) there were scores of preparations ranging from the gentlest 'lavatives' and 'lubrifactives', which cleansed and soothed the skin, to 'cauteriatives', noted, as the name implies, for their powers 'to bieste the flesch for to frette it and forto brenne the skynne so that it drye and hardene it'.[4]

Theoretically, at least, each individual symptom of a disease was customarily isolated and treated as a a humoral disorder in itself. This meant, for instance, that in a case of pneumonia the physician mindful of his academic training would give one prescription to control extreme fluctuations in temperature, another for lividness of the skin, a third for chest pains, a fourth for blood-stained urine, and so on, until all the patient's symptoms had been addressed. But such an approach demanded a combination of intellectual rigour and unlimited pharmaceutical resources: as Lanfrank of Milan confessed, 'ther is no man that can telle alle the noumbre of medicyns but oonli God'.[5]

Nor, indeed, could any physician, however learned, systematically apply the complex, often arcane, corpus of medical theory he had mastered at university to a living, breathing, suffering human body. And since he was, moreover, likely to be constrained by the availability and cost of *materia medica*, we may assume that a good deal of theoretical teaching was either abandoned or ignored by those who regularly dealt with the sick. Even the distinguished writer and teacher, Bernard Gordon, had to accept that simple folk remedies were sometimes more successful:

> It happened to me one time that a certain very old surgeon suffered an intolerable earache. The universal purgings and particular treatments according to the teachings of Galen, Avicenna and all the other authors proceeded, but they were utterly without effect. Then I applied camomile oil and in truth he was cured.[6]

Bernard's near contemporary, Henri de Mondeville, was far more of an iconoclast, perhaps because of his long experience as a military surgeon. Years spent in the field led him to re-evaluate the formal medical education he had received as a young man and to question the uncritical acceptance of classical authorities by scholars and laymen alike. He actually went so far as to compare the ancients to a decrepit, malodorous old dog, whose sentimental owner simply cannot face the prospect of replacing him with a fitter animal. But, as a recent study of de Mondeville points out, he had still to function within the intellectual confines of his age, and never cast doubt upon the fundamental importance of humoral theory.[7]

Whatever reservations may have been voiced by individual writers, the basic tenets of Galenic medicine continued to exert a profound and lasting effect upon day-to-day practice. Vernacular texts, compiled either for domestic use in gentry households or as reference works for leeches and surgeons who had not enjoyed the benefits of a university education, contain an interesting mixture of herbal and folk remedies alongside simplified accounts of the theoretical principles of uroscopy, phlebotomy and other standard procedures. Quite often the empirical and scholastic combined, as in one recipe for a 'mervelous drinke and a blessed' made of locally grown herbs. 'It doth a way scabbes in parte of the body, and hit consumeth venemous humores and clenseth crofulus and al manere of superfluytes of the body that comes of venymous humours,' explained the author, anxious to establish his academic credentials.[8] Classical ideas about health and disease thus filtered down through society, dictating when, why and how more traditional types of treatment would be used.

As a first step towards curing his patient, the physician or surgeon might well suggest a 'confortative' to temper the relative heat or cold of the afflicted part of the body, using a cool medication to retain the warm humours needed for physical regeneration, or perhaps one that was slightly warmer and drier than the diseased member to reduce the level of humidity. In accordance with the teaching of Averroes, 'aromatike thinges', such as musk, were often employed at this stage, as a means of reviving the vital organs and the flow of *pneuma* around the system. 'Gode savour forsoth dilateth the soule and reparaileth the spiritez and the vertuez,' urged the author of one English leechbook, adding that 'odoriferous medicynez bene moste sovereyn of al medicynez which conforteth the principale membrez'.[9]

The body could also be encouraged to defend itself against corrupt humours through the external application of 'maturatives', which generated natural heat and had, therefore, to contain a blend of ingredients whose inherent 'warmth' was just slightly greater than that of the limb or organ undergoing treatment. Customarily made of 'swynez gres and oile and emplastre of whete', they were moist and viscous in appearance, 'stoppyng the porez of the body and concludyng the spiritez and the hete inward, that the hete and the spiritez be noght evapored outward, bot holden with in and be comforted and augmented in thair werkes naturel'.[10] As the cure progressed, however, the practitioner had to go on the offensive by increasing the strength and variety of his prescriptions.

He might, for instance, consider it necessary to try a more intensive means of either retaining or diffusing heat through the use of 'repercussives'. Because of their relative coldness, medicaments of this kind were believed to prevent 'humours boilyng bi hete' from escaping through the epidermis, driving them back into the 'depnes of the centre' so they could break down any internal blockages. For this reason they seemed a particularly effective method of dispersing matter which had solidified in the principal organs, threatening the life of the patient. The mildest sort, known as 'mitigatives', were made of such anodyne substances as milk or various types of oil, and did little more than soothe aches and pains. But at their most powerful (as 'stupefactives') they induced total numbness and could cause death. Understandably, the latter were used only in cases of excruciating pain, and then with great caution.[11]

Plasters, ointments and salves were consequently employed not just as a means of curing skin diseases (although these figure prominently in most practical treatises and collections of remedies), but also for the treatment of serious internal disorders. According to their composition, they either encouraged or prevented the loss of heat and moisture, thus enabling the body to recover its humoral balance, and perhaps also providing a measure of comfort as well, at least in their less drastic forms. During the serious illness of Sir William Stonor's business partner, Thomas Betson, in the autumn of 1479, the physician, Master Brinkley, was called in by Stonor's mother-in-law. 'And or he departed', ran the report, 'he gave him plasters to his hede, to his stomake, and to his bely, that he alle that nyght was in quiete rest: and he came to hym ayene on ffriday and sye his water'.[12] Betson survived for another seven years, so even if it did no positive good, the treatment cannot have caused too much damage.

More long-term harm was probably inflicted by the contemporary preoccupation with purgation, which encouraged the healthy, as well as the sick, to rid their bodies of unwanted humours through vomiting and defecation. The ubiquity of laxatives in popular medical compilations testifies not so much to the prevalence of chronic constipation as a nervous anxiety about the disastrous effects that it *might* have. In this respect, Fynes Moryson's advice to early seventeenth-century travellers has a truly medieval ring:

> Touching the purgation of the body, as all repletion is ill, and Socrates well advised to take heed of those matters, which invited men to eate when they were not hungry, so when the humours are growne through intemperancy, it is good to purge them. . . . In the morning and noone let him offer thus to purge naturally, in whiche nature, for the most part yeelds to custome. Nothing is a more certaine signe of sicknesse growing, then the obstruction of the body, against which in Italy I tooke each morning, while I was so disposed, a spoonefull of the sirrop of Corinthian Currants. Damasco Prunes boyled, and other moist things, as Butter and Hony, are good for this purpose. . . .[13]

Other, more unpleasant and aggressive remedies (linseed fried in hot fat or a stew of mallow leaves in ale can hardly have been consumed with relish) clearly took their toll on the patient, so it is not surprising that in cases of serious illness or acute, prolonged constipation practitioners considered enemas (known as clysters) to be more suitable.[14]

The surgeon John of Arderne, who must have administered hundreds of enemas in his time, disapproved of the costly and elaborate concoctions favoured by his predecessors, preferring a simple, all-purpose one of water, mallows, green camomile, wheat bran, salt, honey (or oil), assorted herbs and soap; this could, if necessary, be reduced to just three basic ingredients. The mixture was to be gently squirted into the anus through a greased pipe attached to a clyster bag made of a pig's or neat's bladder while the patient lay 'grovelyng' on his bed, rubbing his abdomen with his hand.[15] Arderne was, no doubt, justifiably proud of his method, which he claimed had earned him 'grete honour with lucre in diverse places'. This may explain his belief in the curative powers of clysters: at all events, he advocated their use for nutritive purposes, too, in cases where the patient could not eat and might benefit from a 'norischyng' enema of potage or 'mylke of almandes':

> Therfor witte thou that clisteries noght only availeth to seke men and constipate, as of the colic or of sich other, bot it availeth to al men beyng in the febres . . . and to every inflacion

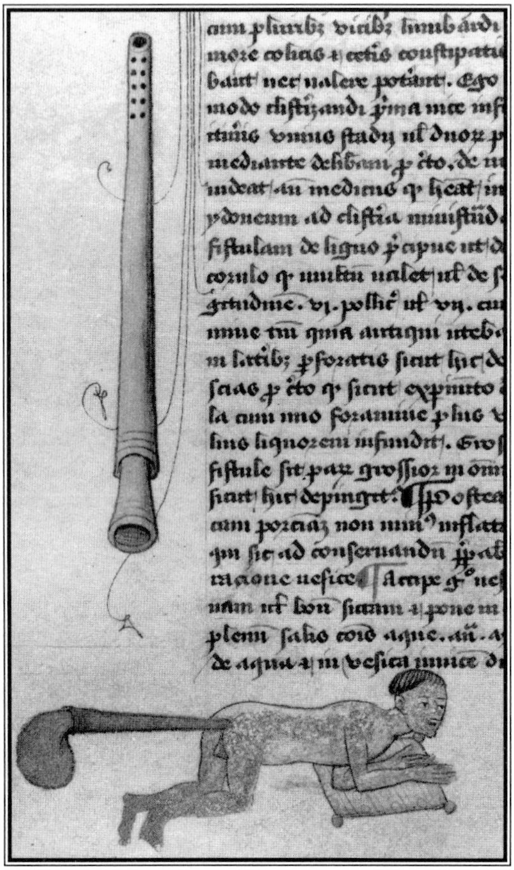

Clysters, or enemas, were recommended for purging the healthy as well as the sick. The mixture was customarily administered by means of a pig's bladder attached to a greased pipe, as this illustration and the accompanying text by John of Arderne explain.

> of the wombe [abdomen], and to every ventosite of it [flatulence]. . . . And som-tyme it availeth mych in som fluxes of the wombe. And for certayn it availeth mich to hole men, constipate and noght constipate, if thai be purged twyse at lest or 3 or four tymes in a yere with the forseid clisteries; that is tuyse in wynter, and in vere [spring] as it war after lentyn ones, in somer ones, or ofter tyme if nede be. For why [Because] the benefite of it may no man noumbre.[16]

In common with most of his contemporaries, Arderne recognized the therapeutic value of 'ane hote bath of swete watre', to be prescribed along with medication and purgatives as a means of steaming out impurities and easing pain. A long soak in pleasantly scented water must sometimes have provided the only available relief for patients suffering from fever, bruising, persistent gynaecological disorders (for which bathing was frequently recommended) or the torments of the bladder stone. Victims of this excruciating complaint were urged to sit up to the navel in a hot tub strewn with mallow, violets and other herbs: one piece of medical advice which they were presumably delighted to accept.[17] However much he may have disapproved of bathing as effete and degenerate, even Ailred, the saintly Abbot of Rievaulx (d.1167), was driven to abandon his principles:

> The agony was intense, for very often his urine contained fragments of stone as big as a bean, the passage of which was so unbearable that if in his suffering he had not tempered and softened the obstruction in the bath to ease its course he would have incurred sudden death. One day after no fewer than forty [another source has twelve] visits to the bath, he was so incredibly exhausted in the evening that he looked more dead than alive. And you dare to talk about the bathings of Ailred! Do you suppose that he took delight when there was so much frustration?[18]

The theoretical distinction whereby physicians assumed responsibility for the *inside* of the body, as regulators of its humoral balance, and surgeons for the *outside* inevitably broke down in practice (colour plate 12). The business of healing wounds, sores, broken limbs and other

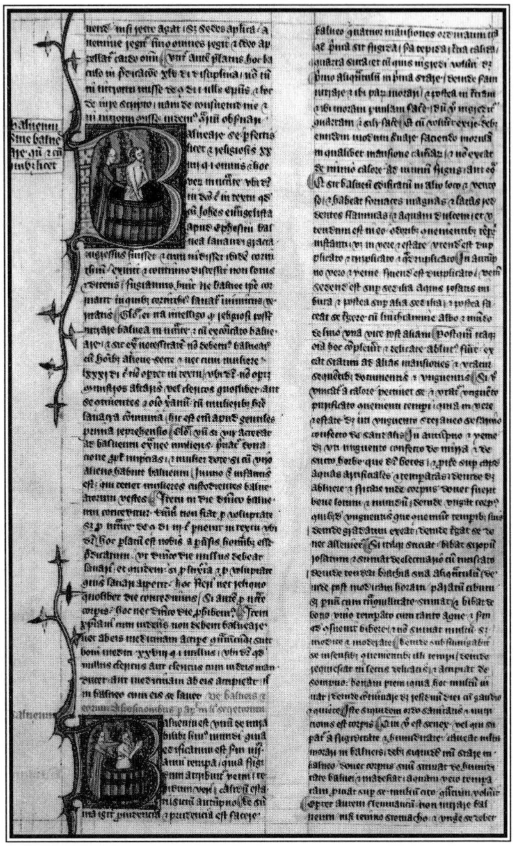

Bathing, an important part of the regimen of health, was still regulated on moral grounds. This text limits Sunday bathing to cases of pressing necessity, forbids Christians from bathing with Jews and gives details of the best syrups and electuaries to be taken with medicinal baths.

external injuries generally fell to the surgeon, but so too did the treatment of diseases such as leprosy, erysipelas and certain types of cancer.[19] He also performed manual operations whose sole purpose was to rid the body of superfluous humours, usually in conjunction with a course of medication recommended either by himself or by a physician. Cauterization, cupping and phlebotomy, which involved burning, scarifying or cutting the flesh, were perceived as requiring skill rather than academic training (not for nothing did surgeons, proud of their dexterity, liken themselves to carpenters, and physicians to theoretically minded geometricians), although a sound working knowledge of Galenic medicine was clearly required to undertake this kind of therapy effectively and at the right time when a physician could not be found to give instructions.

The three physicians and two surgeons who received formal permission, in April 1454, to attend Henry VI during his first bout of serious mental illness, were clearly expected to work together, each assuming responsibilty for specific medical or surgical procedures according to his own area of expertise. It would be interesting to know if these distinguished practitioners, noted for their 'faith, learning and wisdom', did, in fact, actually see eye to eye over the diagnosis and treatment of the royal patient. Their brief was certainly wide enough to allow for debate over the administration of:

> electuaries, potions, [distilled] waters, syrups, confections, laxative medicines in whatever form seems most effective, clysters, suppositories, medicines for clearing the head, gargles, baths, either complete or partial, poultices, fomentations, embrocations, shaving of the head, ointments, plasters, waxes, cupping, with or without cutting the skin [and] inducements to bleeding, in whatever way may best be arranged.[20]

The remit of these letters, which effectively gave the recipients a free hand so far as the king was concerned, suggests that he was subjected to the sort of regime proposed a century earlier by John of Gaddesden for the treatment of acute lethargy. To combat 'forgetfulness', 'confusion of reason' and 'much false sleep' he had suggested a number of procedures designed to restore lucidity and expel evil humours. Quite probably the royal consultants chose to replace the recommended poultices of pigeons' droppings and honey with something more appropriate for a reigning monarch, but they must have employed most of the following measures, all of which had sound classical antecedents:

> It is necessary for lethargics that people talk loudly in their presence. Tie their extremities lightly and rub their palms and soles hard; and let their feet be put in salt water up to the middle of their shins, and pull their hair and nose, and squeeze the toes and fingers tightly, and cause pigs to squeal in their ears; give [them] a sharp clyster at the beginning . . . and open the vein of the head, or nose, or forehead, and draw blood from the nose with the bristles of a boar. Put a feather, or a straw, in his nose to compel him to sneeze, and do not ever desist from hindering him from sleeping; and let human hair or other evil-smelling thing be burnt under his nose. Apply, moreover, the cupping horn between the shoulders, and let a feather be put down his throat, to cause vomiting, and shave the back of the head, and rub oil of roses and vinegar and smallage [wild celery] juice thereon. . . .[21]

Lesser mortals (especially those living outside the main medical centres of Oxford, Cambridge and London) are unlikely to have enjoyed the uncertain benefits of such intensive humoral therapy, although those who could afford professional or semi-professional services submitted themselves to a similar combination of cures involving both minor surgery and medication. By far the most widespread surgical procedure of this kind was phlebotomy, or blood-letting, which had, indeed, become so common that unqualified individuals often practised it as a profitable sideline. Lanfrank of Milan blamed his own colleagues for allowing 'barbouris and wymmen' to set up as phlebotomists because they were too proud to perform such a routine operation in person, although contemporary literary and medical sources suggest that the growing demand would, in any event, have encouraged freelance activity. Relatively humble laymen with few pretensions to medical knowledge felt it important to equip themselves with information on the subject. The commonplace-book of Robert Reynes, a parish constable at Acle in Norfolk during the late fifteenth century, contains instructions about blood-letting interspersed between a note of his duties as an officer of the watch and lists of taxes paid by the local community. Since he was also interested in the signs of the zodiac and their influence upon the human body, we may assume that he knew enough basic theory to determine the most auspicious times for phlebotomy, even if he did not attempt the operation himself.[22]

Because it was believed to perform an important prophylactic function in ridding the body of excessive humours, phlebotomy seemed just as necessary for healthy men and women, afraid of falling sick, as it did for those who were already ill. The promised rewards appeared incalculable:

> Blode lattynge in mesure it clerith thi thought, it closith thi bladder, it temperith thi breyn, it amendith thyn heerynge, it streyngth teres, it closith thy maw, it defieth [digests] thi mete, it clerith thy voyce, it sharpith the witt, it easith thi wombe, it gedrith thy slepe, it drawyth away angwysshe, it norisshith goode blode; wykkyd blode dystroyeth, and lenghtith thy lyve.[23]

As we have seen in the previous chapter, it was not until the eleventh and twelfth centuries that the work of leading Greek, Jewish and Arab medical authorities became widely available in the West. A few very basic texts on blood-letting had previously circulated among monastic communities and at Salerno, but a systematic exposition of theory and practice, set within the context of Galenic medicine, did not appear until then. Supported by unimpeachable classical authorities, and evidently offering a promise of health and vigour to those who practised it, phlebotomy came to be regarded as a fundamental aspect of medical treatment during the later Middle Ages.[24] But some of the masters who had preserved and transmitted Galen's teachings expressed reservations, at least with regard to the probity of certain practitioners. Isaac Judaeus, whose scepticism about the diagnostic merits of uroscopy has already been noted, was even more cynical on this score:

> It is a foolish and widespread custom that the sons of mankind band together and go to have their blood drawn, even if they need not. One tells the other that a certain day is good for blood-letting, and that all who are phlebotomized on that day are safe from a certain disease. And so they gather by the hundreds at the house of the blood-letter. After he draws their blood he tells them, in order to obtain an additional fee, that he sees by their blood that they will need another blood-letting. And the fools return to the phlebotomist as before, until their blood has poured out into his receptacles. . . .[25]

The dangers of losing too much blood at once or else of being phlebotomized too often were recognized by experts and well-informed laymen alike, albeit for what we today might consider the wrong reasons: as Robert Burton believed, phlebotomy 'unadvisedly, importunely, immoderately used' simply exacerbated the humoral inbalance, caused blindness and intensified melancholia.[26] Children, pregnant or menstruating women, pallid youths 'with fewe heeris in her browis' and very old men of uncertain health were generally considered too vulnerable, except in emergencies, as were those of a predominantly 'cold' temperament.[27] Surgeons also advised against bleeding at certain stages of treatment, during extremes of weather and at astrologically inauspicious times (discussed at length in the next chapter); yet phlebotomy still claimed its victims, either indirectly, as a contributory cause of death, or simply because of medical incompetence. Not for nothing did two late thirteenth-century Icelandic law codes exempt practitioners of phlebotomy and cauterization from the penalties normally imposed on persons found guilty of mayhem or murder.[28]

The English also seem to have accepted that blood-letting could prove fatal. Jurors at a London inquest of 1278, for example, reported that William le Paumer, a skinner, had collapsed and died in West Cheap, 'being greatly weakened' as a result of inexpert blood-letting performed on the previous day. Even so, the court held nobody to blame for his sudden demise, and did not think to name the person responsible, who had presumably severed an artery by mistake.[29] In his *Lilium Medicine* of 1303 Bernard Gordon describes how one of his colleagues fell into a coma and was phlebotomized on the instructions of the other masters. None, however, saw fit to supervise the operation, and the unfortunate man apparently bled to death at the hands of a careless surgeon. This event was probably still in Bernard's mind five years later when he cautioned students that 'it is safer to phlebotomize several times until the [harmful] matter is exhausted, rather than the patient: for I prefer the illness to be somewhat prolonged rather than a death be attributed to me'.[30] Given the risks involved, concern about the technical skills and physical aptitude of anyone attempting phlebotomy was more than justified:

> A man that schal be letere blood schal be yong, and he schal be no child, ne noon oold man, ne he schal not quake, and he schal have a good scharp sight; and loke that he kunne

> knowe veines, and that he kunne knowe hem from arterijs; and he schal have manie divers tool for to lete blood therwith, and thei schulen be clene and cleer, and not rusti; and summe of his tool schulen be longe, and summe schorte. . . .[31]

That many barbers and barber-surgeons, at least, took these injunctions seriously is evident from the spread, from the late fourteenth century onwards, of vernacular texts (sometimes with accompanying diagrams) on the subject of phlebotomy. At their most rudimentary, they listed and described the veins to be opened (which could number over thirty, depending on the sources used) and the ailments (such as eczema, headaches and sore eyes) likely to benefit in each instance. Often composed in rhyming couplets, they served as *aides-mémoire* for the master and as accessible guides for his apprentices, who would have had ample opportunity to observe the practical aspects of blood-letting, but might have found it hard to remember their theoretical application.[32]

A handsome drawing of a vein man, or blood-letting figure, preserved in a late medieval book belonging to the York barber-surgeons, marks nineteen potential targets for the phlebotomist's lancet, while an accompanying poem extends the total to a more specific thirty-three, eleven of which were in the head. Although it provides little more than a rough and ready indication of the points of incision, the diagram clearly and succinctly explains why, and sometimes when, each particular operation should be performed. Bleeding from the vein between the finger and the thumb, for instance, will alleviate migraine; diseases of the bladder and 'yvell humors' may generally be cured by blood-letting from 'the vayne under the ankle within the fute'; and, not without risk to the patient, the two veins 'in the nek hole' might be cut in cases of leprosy and 'straytnes of wynde'.[33]

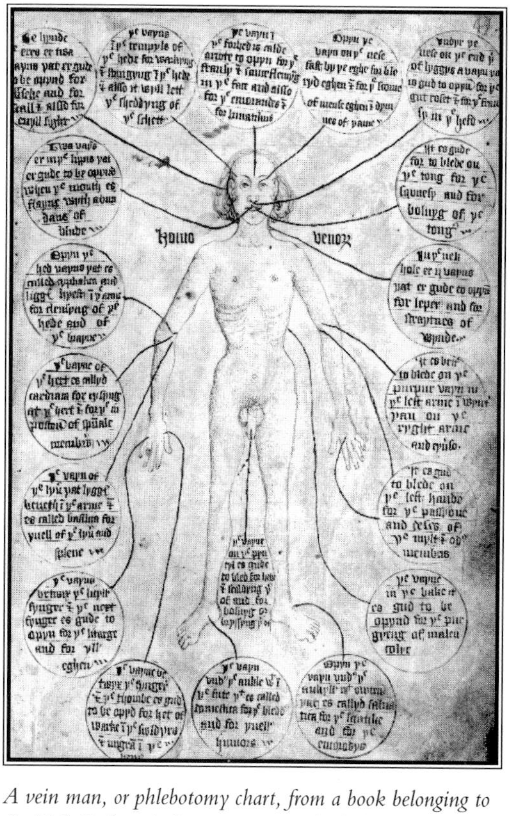

A vein man, or phlebotomy chart, from a book belonging to the York Barbers, indicates points on the body where bloodletting was recommended to ease specific ailments: 'the vayne in the bake' was, for instance, 'gud to be opynd for the purgyeng of malencolye'. In practice, however, some of these operations would have been difficult, if not impossible, to perform.

Translations of learned Latin texts, such as the collection produced by a clerk named Austyn for his 'dere gossip', the London barber-surgeon, Thomas Plouden (d.1413), made far greater demands upon the reader, even though they were often simplified and explained in the process. Austyn's offering includes an English version of a much earlier academic treatise on phlebotomy probably still in use at Oxford and Cambridge; and reveals a scholarly bent on the part of the recipient, who hoped to compensate for the lack of a classical education. His evident desire to obtain a 'betir entre into the worchynge of fisyk' was rewarded with readily accessible information about medical theory, including a discussion of the principles which dictated whether a patient should be bled on the same side of the body as his ailment or injury (metacentesis) or the opposite side (antipasis, a riskier undertaking which might infect healthy members with corrupt matter). Plouden and his more studious colleagues were clearly at one with Lanfrank of Milan in the belief that 'a man may be no good cyrurgian, but if he knowe phisik'.[34]

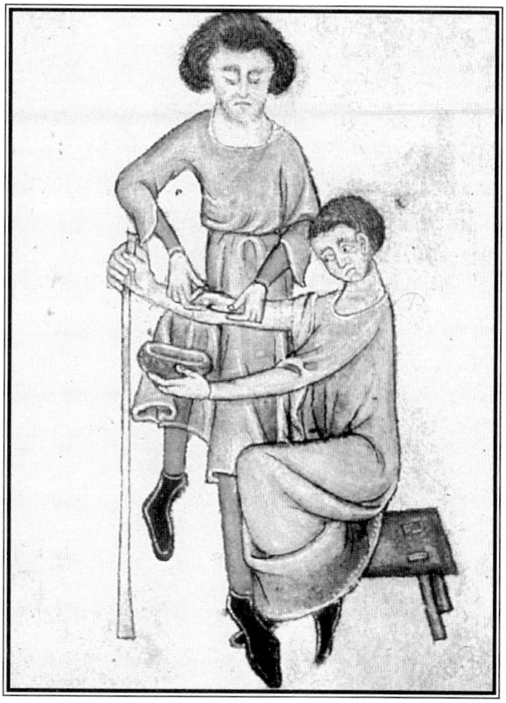

Generally, blood was let from the basilic vein, near the elbow, which was easily accessible to the phlebotomist. By lancing here, he or she could purge noxious humours from the liver and spleen, and thus perform the valuable prophylactic exercise of cleansing the blood.

Rhymes and diagrams notwithstanding, practical considerations of anatomy and expertise meant that blood was usually let from the arms and legs, most notably the basilic vein, just below the elbow. Bleeding from this point reputedly possessed the particular advantage of clearing the liver and spleen of impurities, so it could be used not only as part of the treatment customarily prescribed for patients with diseases of these organs, but also for routine phlebotomy carried out as a preventative measure for cleansing the blood.[35] The custumals and rules followed by religious houses provide a valuable insight into the prophylactic aspects of blood-letting, which, like all other facets of the monastic life, was precisely regulated. At the Augustinian priory of Barnwell, in Cambridgeshire, for instance, the brothers were bled on average seven times a year, being allowed to take three days' rest in the infirmary on each occasion. Since they were then exempted from the punishing round of liturgical practice, allowed a more generous and nourishing diet than usual and permitted to take as much gentle exercise as they wished, it is easy to see why they felt much better afterwards. The Benedictine monks of Ely may actively have looked forward to their sessions with the *minutor* (phlebotomist), which usually took place every six weeks. In theory, at least, they were forbidden to eat flesh, but while blood-letting was in progress beef, mutton, pork, veal, pullets, capons and fresh fish appeared on the infirmary table. Early in the fifteenth century a special building, or *minutorium*, was constructed in the precincts for the benefit of brethren undergoing phlebotomy, perhaps following the example of Bury St Edmunds, which already possessed one, as well as a vineyard, 'especially for the solace of sick monks and those who had been bled'.[36]

Just two days' recuperation, from Monday afternoon to Wednesday, were allowed to the Westminster Abbey monks, who presented themselves at the bathhouse in groups of ten for regular blood-letting. The 'seyney', as this operation was known, seems to have declined in frequency to about four or five individual sessions a year by the early sixteenth century, but since the monastic diet had by then grown so rich and carnivorous it is hard to tell exactly who ranked as a convalescent with extra privileges. Moreover, some members of the community paid for additional private 'seyneys', evidently preferring to undergo phlebotomy at a place and time of their own choosing, when the exercise might prove more beneficial.[37]

What, though, was to be done for individuals whose age or physical condition made phlebotomy too dangerous? Leeches could always be attached to the skin, although the practitioner had to distinguish carefully between the 'blak wormes like to a mouse taile', which were quite safe, and any discoloured or swollen specimens likely to poison the patient. Leeches had always to be taken from clear, running streams, not stagnant ponds or marshes, cleansed in fresh water and kept in a storage jar without nourishment for just a day before use. By and large, they were applied locally, as a means of drawing corrupt matter from open wounds, ulcers, haemorrhoids and the flesh around boils and swellings, and thus theoretically constituted an alternative to, rather than a substitute for, phlebotomy. They were considered the best means of cleansing blood 'bytwene the depenesse of the body and the skyn', and properly managed posed less risk of haemorrhage or infection. Since, however, leeches suck only blood, which they prefer to be fresh, their effectiveness as purifying agents must, at best, have been limited.[38]

Women, children and the very old were more commonly bled by cupping or 'ventosynge', which may, ironically, have proved far more of an ordeal than phlebotomy. As the name suggests, it involved placing heated glass, bone or brass vessels upon skin which had been scored or otherwise 'garsyed' with a knife (or even scratched by 'smytynge of the nayles'), thus stimulating a relatively gentle flow of blood through the creation of a vacuum. Because it required a reasonably large area of flesh, cupping was usually confined to the neck (in cases of eye trouble, halitosis and facial blemishes), the shoulders (chest infections and diseases of the 'spiritual members'), the lower back and buttocks (internal blockages, 'scabbe of the body' and problems with the liver or kidneys), the upper arms (arthritis or 'gowte') and the thighs (disorders of the bladder and reproductive organs).[39]

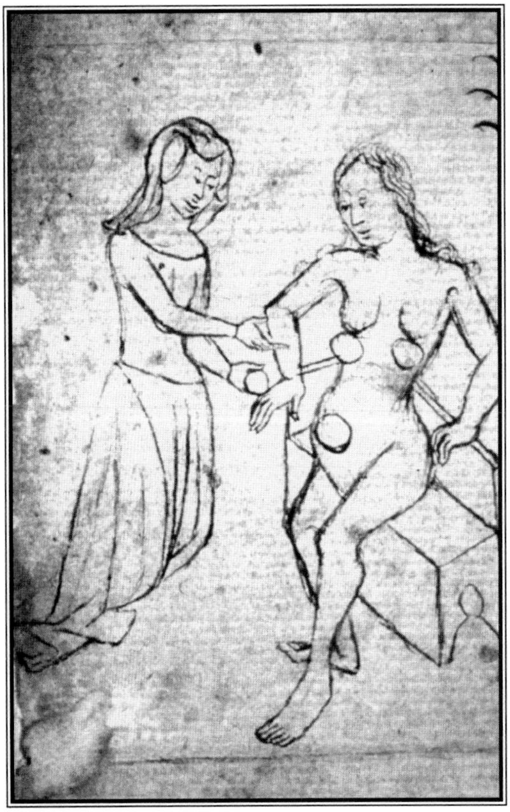

A female practitioner applies heated cups to bleed her patient, who may be pregnant and thus too vulnerable for phlebotomy.

'Drye ventoses withoute garsynge' were employed to extract dangerous fumes or venom from the body. The practitioner might, for example, seek to ease a painful attack of colic or flatulence by 'smekynge out the ventosite' into heated cups applied to the abdomen, or relieve a blocked nose through similar treatment of the head. Dry cupping was also believed to staunch nosebleeds and heavy menstruation by the simple process of 'drawing' blood in another direction. It should not be supposed,

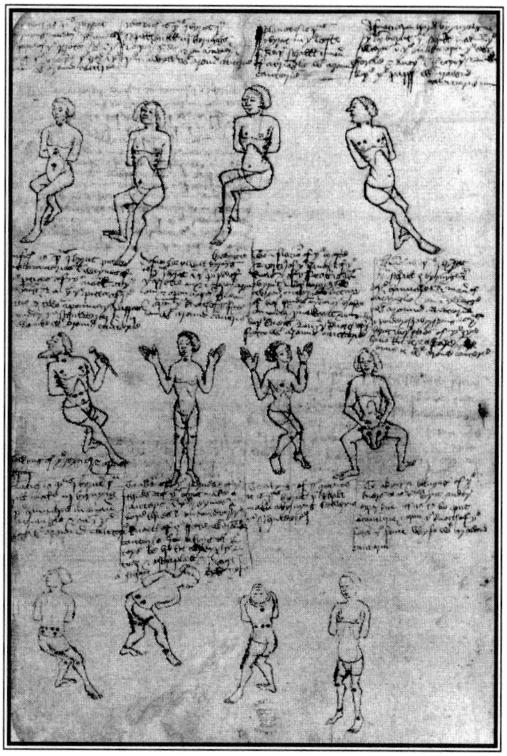

Twelve figures illustrating recommended points for the application of cauteries to ease or cure specific maladies. The bottom right-hand drawing, for example, shows how to treat aching or swollen knees.

however, that this process was any less uncomfortable than the other: Guy de Chauliac recommended putting 'a litel of drye towe withynn the ventose, and it is sette afire with a brennyng candel', then quickly placing the smoking cup on the exposed skin.[40]

Complaints about the ignorance and inexperience of empirics practising phlebotomy and cupping were understandably redoubled in the case of cauterization. As we have already seen, chemically based caustic medicines could be used to burn away flesh contaminated with evil matter, but whenever possible surgeons preferred to work with specially designed metal instruments, which could be heated to exactly the right temperature in a brazier, and were far easier to control, as well as being more predictable in their effects. Cauteries served not only to remove diseased tissue and seal wounds but also (when applied to designated points on the head or body) to eliminate the superfluous cold and moist humours responsible for stubborn headaches, dropsy, epilepsy, disorders of the eyes, throat, nose and ears, coughs, nosebleeds and 'flux of the wombe that cometh of the reume'. Used locally, on an ulcerated arm or leg, they were said, moreover, to prevent both the consolidation and spread of corrupt humours, restore 'good complexioun', staunch the flow of blood and eventually ease pain.[41]

Although there was some debate as to the value of cauterization in treating complaints caused by excessive bodily heat or dryness, Albucasis (d.1013), the great Arab authority on surgery, maintained that it had 'a universal application for every ill constitution', albeit only in the hands of experts, once other, less traumatic kinds of treatment had failed and (significantly) when the patient seemed fit enough to survive the shock.[42] A single multi-purpose operation, recommended by him for expelling 'excessive humidity and coldness' from the brain, and thus relieving many of the ailments described above, gives a good idea of the procedure involved, which began, as a matter of course, with the administration of laxatives:

> bid the patient open the bowels with an evacuant which will also clear his head, for three or four nights, according to the strength, age and habits of the patient. Then tell him to have his head shaved; then seat him cross-legged before you, with his hands on his breast. Then place the lower part of your palm upon the root of his nose between his eyes; and where your middle finger reaches mark that place with ink. Then heat an olivary cautery. Then bring it down upon the marked place with one downward stroke with gentle pressure,

> revolving the cautery; then quickly take your hand away while observing the place. If you see that some bone is exposed, the size of the head of a skewer or a grain of vetch, then take your hand away; otherwise repeat with the same iron or, if that has gone cold, with another, till the amount of bone I have mentioned is exposed. Then take a little salt in water; soak some cotton in it, apply to the place, then leave for three days.[43]

The number and depth of the punctures varied according to the ailment in question: a circle of about ten was, for instance, to be 'pricked' close around an aching ear; the entire length of the spine, as well as the chest and abdomen, received attention in cases of uncontrollable trembling; and a single crescent-shaped iron was used to burn the inguinal canal in order to arrest an incipient scrotal hernia or prevent the descent of an old one. Since, in the last case, the cautery had to be so hot that it actually gave off sparks (and would thus, paradoxically, inflict less pain in the long term), Albucasis' warnings about the possibility of causing death or permanent injury through carelessness were meant to be taken seriously. Followers of St Francis of Assisi (d.1226) recalled how he had astonished his surgeon by withstanding the agony of being cauterized from the ear to the eyebrow in a futile attempt to cure a chronic eye infection. The prospect of simply *watching* his ordeal had, in fact, caused them to flee while the instruments were still being heated. Possibly the shock may have served to stimulate the production of endorphins, the body's natural painkillers, which would explain why experts continued to recommend the procedure.[44]

Safety devices could be attached to prevent serious accidents, but sometimes things went badly wrong, as this Icelandic account of a bungled operation reveals. The practitioner had pressed a cautery to his patient's lower abdomen,

> but because there was no stop on the button iron, it ran so deep that to the patient who was being cauterized it seemed to plunge into his abdominal cavity. This impression of his was confirmed by a great bursting sound that occurred when the lesser membrane that was situated in the intestine burst apart. The man who was doing the cauterizing quickly drew away the cautery when he felt that nothing was stopping it. He then wished to squeeze the cauterized spot, but fat flowed out from it, which they believed was from the intestine. And when the patient stood up, he felt such great pain that to him it seemed to extend almost right back to his spine.[45]

Fortunately, miraculous intercession on the part of St Thorlakr Thorhallsson, to whose relics the victim had recourse, soon put things right: otherwise the mishap might have proved fatal. Albucasis had urged his readers that in certain cases it was best to leave well alone, lest the cautery did more harm than good; and most authorities redoubled his advice.

Without the benefits of blood transfusion, antisepsis or reliable anaesthetics, medieval surgeons had to consider hard and long before agreeing to perform all but the most routine operations on the strongest of patients. 'Ful ofte tyme men leie me to scorn that I lefte siche maner curis', confessed Lanfrank of Milan with regard to his nervousness about cutting for bladder stone (lithotomy). The candid admission that he 'coude not do it' and might thus lose both reputation and income by killing a wealthy patron serves to remind us that even the very best of surgeons were loath to take chances. Nor was he much more confident when obliged to remove fragments of bone by manual procedure from a fractured skull, preferring to use 'emplastris and medicyns' wherever possible. As one anonymous London surgeon advised, in 1392, it was best to shun dangerous and obviously terminal cases altogether 'in savynge of thi worschipe', but if 'pitee and charite' got the upper hand then every effort should be made to spare the knife. Conventional wisdom required that such patients ought rather to set their spiritual and temporal affairs in order and trust in the beneficent powers of Nature, who, after all, had some remarkable cures to her credit.[46]

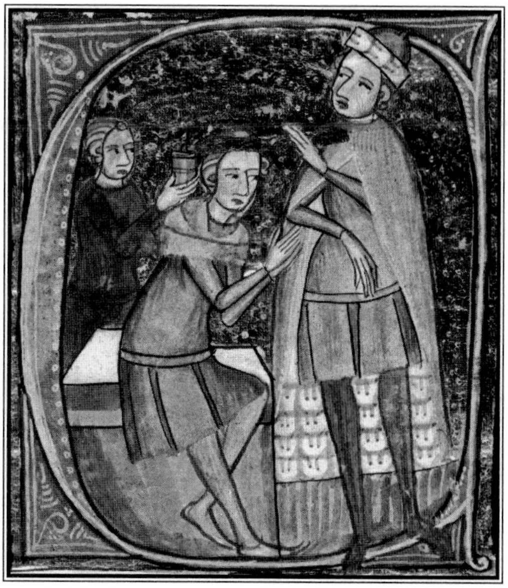

Surgeons were understandably reluctant to deal with fractures of the skull, although the widespread incidence of violence and accidents in medieval society made this unavoidable. The practitioner's fur robes show him to be a master of his craft, and thus presumably quite experienced in dangerous surgery.

To make matters worse, the practitioner might find himself in a difficult legal position in the event of death or mutilation. Such was the physical torment suffered by the York barber, John Cartmell, while 'languishing from a certain infirmity called *le stane*', in 1394, that one of his colleagues reluctantly agreed to perform the operation so dreaded by Lanfrank. Being understandably apprehensive about the outcome, he did however insist that Cartmell's wife and assigns should first appear before the civic authorities to discharge him from all responsibility, even if the patient expired.[47] In this instance, both men were well aware of the gamble involved; but layfolk with high expectations and deep pockets showed a natural reluctance to forgo their rights at law. It was largely to protect themselves from charges of malpractice that the surgeons of London insisted, in 1435, upon joint consultations when a patient seemed to be at risk. 'If ony persoone of the seid felowschip haue ony cure disperat of the which is lykli to falle into deth or mayme or to him unknown', ran the ordinance, 'he [must] schewe it to the maistris or to summe of hem withinne foure or fyve daies.' Failure to do so incurred a fairly steep fine, as did negligence on the part of the 'maistris' or wardens of the guild.[48]

Besides practical worries about loss of livelihood and professional status, the serious-minded practitioner must also have harboured deeper fears with regard to the welfare of his immortal soul. Might the Church regard him as an accessory to murder if his patient died under the knife or after taking medicine? In an influential treatise on penance, composed in about 1206, the theologian Robert Courson addressed the problem of medical culpability at some length, concluding that while physicians and surgeons were duty-bound to undertake cures with a reasonable chance of success, they ought never to try anything dangerous, especially in the hope of financial gain. Significantly, in the circumstances, he chose as his example a surgeon who had lost several lithotomy patients, but remained genuinely unsure of his own responsibility for their deaths. His moral dilemma, intensified by the fact that some of them were already dying in agony and had absolved him of all blame, was viewed with sympathy, at least to the extent that Courson recommended a light penance for medical men who showed due contrition for their mistakes. But such advice is unlikely to have reassured those who feared ecclesiastical censure, which inevitably fell most heavily on those who performed 'manual operacions'.[49]

Given that all surgery, especially when performed in such adverse conditions, carries some risk of permanent injury or death, what type of procedures were qualified practitioners of the craft generally prepared to undertake? The extraction of teeth, the manipulation of dislocated limbs, the lancing of boils and general treatment of scalds, burns and disfiguring skin diseases, the setting of bones and the suturing of wounds all fell to the surgeon's lot. In rural areas and among the urban poor most of these activities (as we shall see in Chapter VIII) were performed by empirics, some of whom were probably quite skilful. Certain operations, such as couching for cataract, became the preserve of itinerant specialists, whose manual dexterity and nerves of steel won them grudging praise, but with a few exceptions the medical élite remained hostile to such people.[50]

Nor were the authorities much kinder in their assessment of ordinary surgeons and barbers: claiming that most were little better than butchers, Bernard Gordon criticized them for spreading infections and causing many fatalities. It is, however, interesting to note that he often referred problematic, dangerous or uncertain cases to the handful of 'literate and experienced' surgeons whom he could trust. Conditions unlikely to respond to medication alone (such as fistulae, haemorrhoids, gangrene and scrofula) naturally figured high on his list, as did those where surgery appeared to be the last resort, a desperate gamble when all other alternatives had failed. His belief that, for example, sufferers from breast cancer, fractures of the skull or 'dropsy' (ascites, or the accumulation of free fluid in the peritoneal cavity because of colonic cancer or liver failure) might just possibly be saved by the knife was probably based on personal experience: as many of the surviving treatises by medieval surgeons reveal, compassion, curiosity, professional pride and the challenge of devising new experimental techniques sometimes overcame fear of the confessional, at least when the patient had otherwise been given up for lost.[51]

A sense of the powerlessness and frustration experienced by the medieval surgeon emerges from this account, set down in the late fourteenth century as evidence of the tenacity of 'cankerous humouris'. However they may be treated, the writer notes, they 'bringith wo and sorowe to the pacient by his lyve, and so wors and wors til he be ded':

> Ther was a worschipful riche wornman . . . in my tyme, the which hadde sich a cankre in her pappe [breast], to whom weren clepid the moste discrete worcheris of the cyte, bothe of fisik and of surgerie, among whom y was present, and worchinge in the same cause. Wherfore y seie that ther was no coste of expensis ne occupacion sparid. But y seie surely evermore the malice encreside fro day to day; and for al that we myghten do the syknesse was so fervent that it profitid ful litil to the pacient, so that agenstondynge al oure craft and kunnynge, at the laste it is woundid, and so the womman diede withinne schort tyme aftir. . . .[52]

If, on the whole, medieval surgeons were justifiably reluctant to attempt difficult operations on the sick or feeble, they had ample scope when faced with the battered victims of accidents, warfare and social violence (colour plate 8). It is a testimony to the skill of the medieval surgeon that so many badly wounded individuals actually lived to fight again. While escorting his step-father, Sir Thomas Brooke, to Westminster in 1404, Richard Cheddar fell victim to an '*orrible baterie et malfait*' which left him at death's door: his nose was almost completely severed, and the blows to the back of his head seemed so bad that he was not expected to survive for more than a few hours. A desire for revenge probably carried him through the worst of the ordeal, but the unknown surgeon who treated him must take most of the credit for a spectacular if unedifying

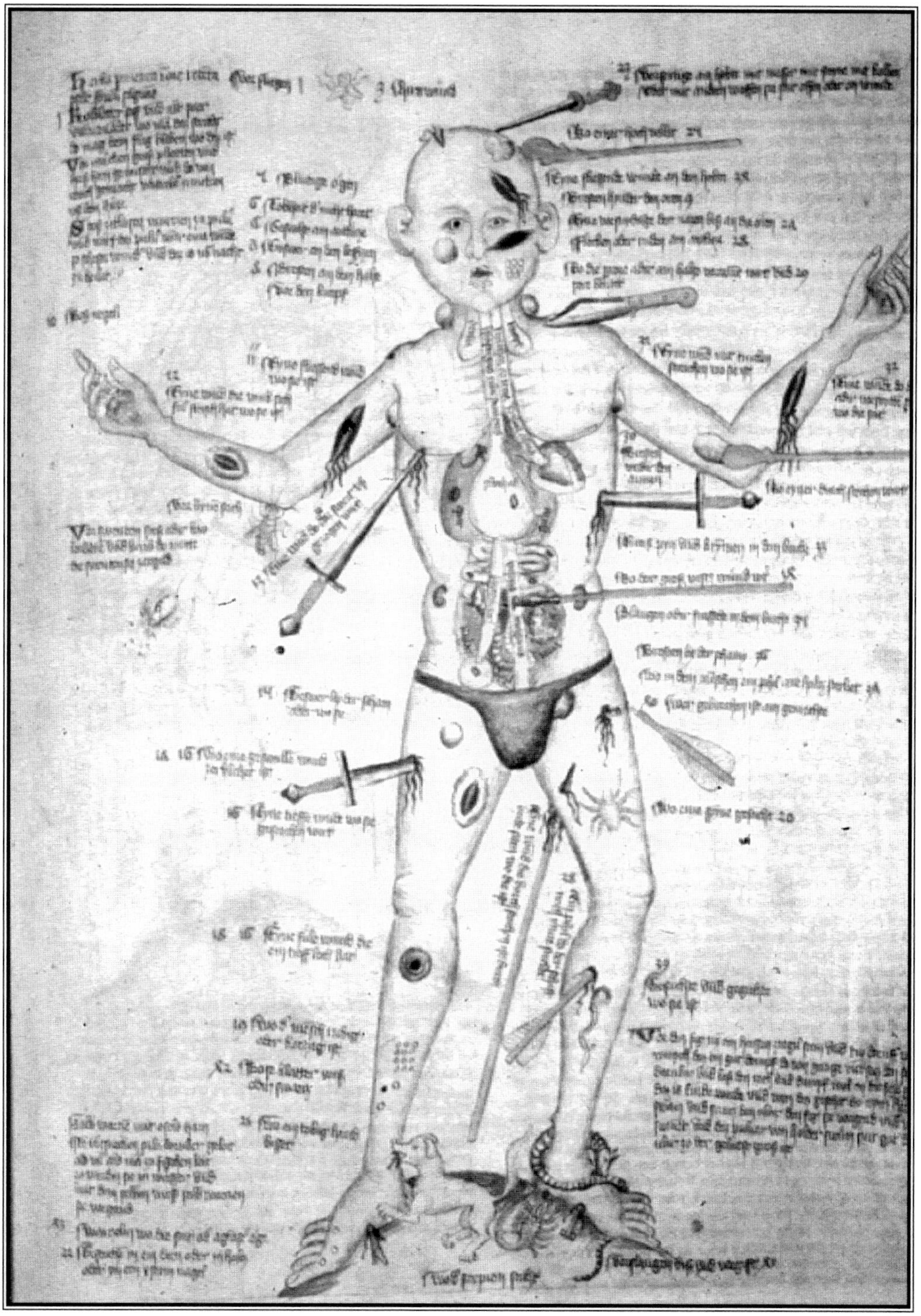

The wound man served as a mnemonic device to remind practitioners of the many different kinds of weapons and therefore of injuries which they might encounter (especially on the battlefield), and the need to select their instruments and medication with care.

recovery. By the end of the year Cheddar was well enough to lead one of many armed attacks on his assailant, his appetite for bloodshed heartier than ever.[53]

Advances in surgery have frequently been credited to practitioners working on the battlefield; and it may be that Cheddar's saviour had learned his craft while campaigning in France. The level of casual violence was, however, sufficiently high at home to provide even the most sedentary rural surgeon with a quota of serious head wounds and internal injuries upon which to develop and refine his skills. Such cases were treated, like all others, according to the principles of Galenic medicine, which practical, daily experience proved to be quite effective. Although the underlying theory was never questioned, the system did allow a certain amount of experimentation. As royal surgeons in the service of the Count of Valois, Henri de Mondeville and his teacher, Jean Pitard, had, for example, insisted upon applying dry, clean dressings instead of the cauteries, thick poultices and ointments customarily used to cultivate the 'laudable pus' through which evil humours were reputedly expelled. Lack of interest and even hostility on the part of their colleagues to this successful new technique has been taken as further evidence of the medical establishment's unquestioning attachment to an outdated academic tradition; but in this instance, at least, de Mondeville's critics were cautious pragmatists rather than blind reactionaries.[54]

The belief that premature cleansing, drying or closing of a wound would force corrupt matter inwards and poison the patient derived its justification from classical humoral theory, supported by the clinical experience of generations of surgeons. Modern, twentieth-century medicine recognizes that lacerations caused by blunt or dirty instruments must be kept open and allowed to suppurate in order to avert the dangers of an enclosed abcess and deadly infections, such as gas gangrene or tetanus, which breed in anaerobic conditions. Conventional medieval practices, designed for the same purpose, may thus actively have hastened recovery if foreign matter was present in a wound. De Mondeville (who cited Galen in his own defence) probably concentrated on relatively 'clean' sword and dagger wounds, which would have responded far better to his approach but may have been less common on the field. Surgeons were certainly well aware of the enormous diversity of cuts, blows and burns likely to come their way, and assumed that qualified members of their craft would 'knowen that wounde that is maad with a swerd, outhir with a knyf, muste othirwise ben heelid than that that is maad with a stoon, outhir with fallynge, or othere siche'.[55]

The writers of surgical treatises and manuals, who inevitably belonged to an élite group, had few inhibitions about recording their own achievements, presumably because the odds were so heavily stacked against them. John of Arderne's unique – and well-publicized – record in treating anal fistulae, which many authorities regarded as incurable, was due not so much to the novelty of the surgery involved (a combination of two separate and simpler procedures described by Albucasis) as in the remarkable extent of his anatomical knowledge and the restraint observed during post-operative care. After the fistula had been cut open, the incision was sponged, anointed with a mild styptic and wrapped in fresh bandages. Although he laid great stress on keeping the patient clean and dry after each movement of the bowels, Arderne did not advocate either the frequent removal of dressings or the use of any of the more aggressive preparations customarily applied to encourage suppuration. Like de Mondeville, he was ready to experiment with new ideas, while warning his readers against the dangers of disturbing the natural healing process.[56]

Pragmatism was certainly the hallmark of the military surgeon, who had constantly to alter his techniques and instruments to accommodate changes in tactics and weaponry. The London

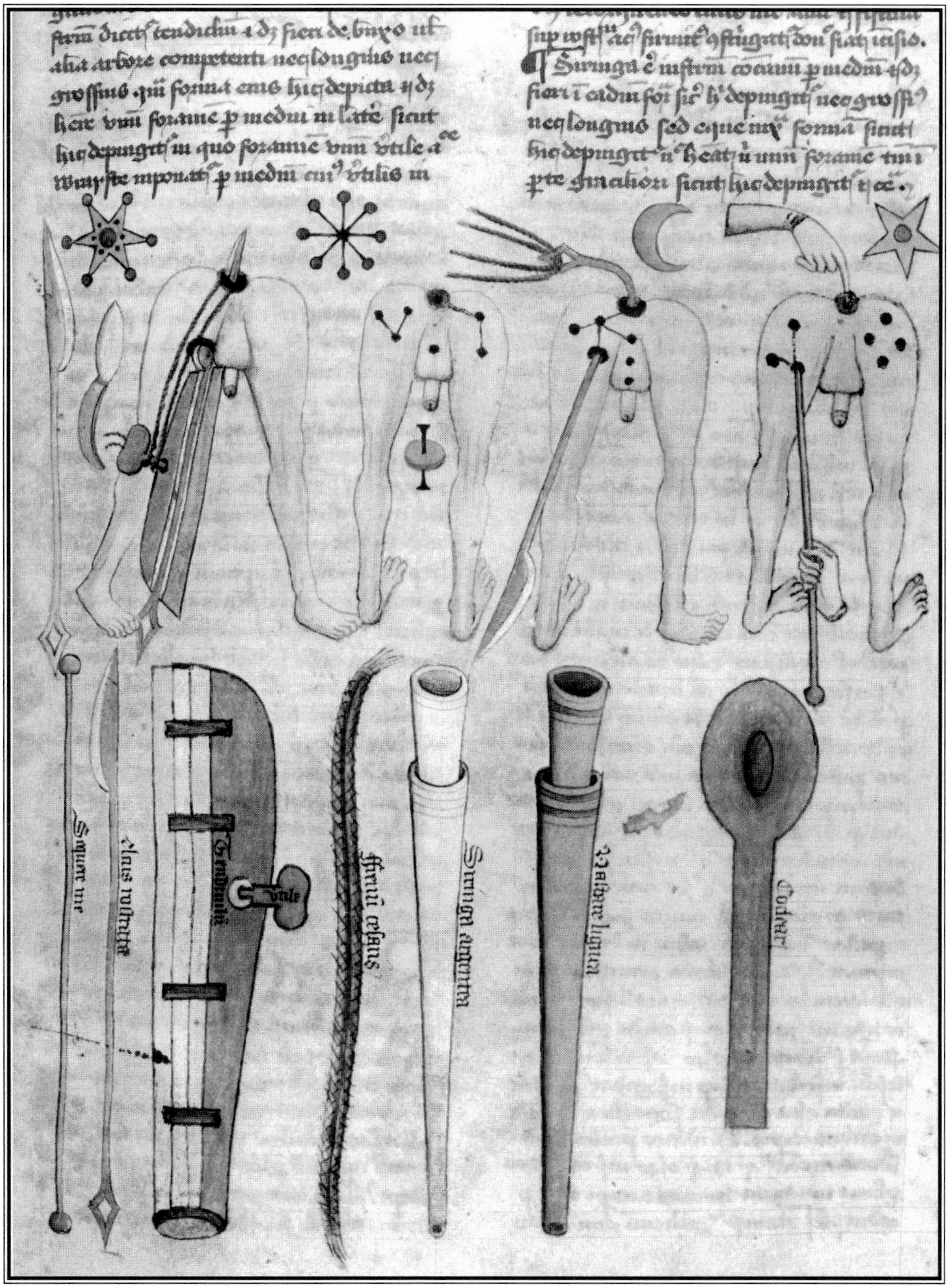

This fifteenth-century manuscript of John of Arderne's treatise on the cure of anal fistulae illustrates the technique for cutting the fistulae and the instruments used, both derived from the work of the Arab surgeon, Albucasis. The probe on the left was, however, devised by Arderne himself, for medieval surgeons often adapted or created their own instruments.

practitioner quoted above observed that 'everi dai ther ben maad arowe heedis and dartis of divers schap, and therfore it bihoveth that thou practise newe craft, and newe maner for to drawen out the same hedis'.[57] A fascinating example of the ingenuity and skill deployed in such cases comes to light after the Battle of Shrewsbury in 1403, when the Prince of Wales lay injured with a barbed arrow through his face. The head was embedded some six inches deep on the left side of his nose, and proved extremely hard to remove. After 'dyverse of wyse lechys' had attempted to draw it out 'with drynkys and odyr curis', the surgeon, John Bradmore, devised a special tong-shaped instrument with which he successfully performed the operation.[58]

Henri de Mondeville describes a less subtle, but mercifully quicker, procedure for expelling a crossbow bolt from a soldier's knee by employing a strong man to hit the point firmly with an iron hammer (the joint itself had to be carefully protected from the blow).[59] But however it was done, the extraction of foreign bodies was a dangerous undertaking for which the victim as well as the surgeon had to be fully prepared:

> And here you schalt undirstonden a general rule, that thou schalt nevere drawen out noon arowe ne darte ne noon that is lyk therto of no mannys body unto the tyme that he be clene schryven and have disposid alle hise erthely thingis or goodis aftir the desier of his herte; and also that it be outwardly the pacientis requeste in herynge of his freendis and of othere discrete personys, and he fully putte him silf to the grace of God and to the aventure that may bifallen. . . .[60]

Following the advice of Albucasis, most practitioners chose to postpone the surgical removal of arrowheads and the like until an abcess cavity had formed around the foreign body, which could then be lifted out with the minimum of cutting. John Bradmore may have owed some of his success to this natural process, since Prince Henry had already been wounded for several days when he began to treat him.

Medieval medical illuminations rarely even hint at the extreme discomfort, if not excruciating agony, experienced by patients undergoing surgery. The expression of serene detachment commonly worn by men and women depicted in contemporary illuminations as vital parts of their anatomy are lanced, probed, cauterized, stitched or sliced seems curiously at odds with the grim reality of the accompanying text, not least because of the repeated emphasis upon properly immobilizing the patient. The conventional lithotomy position required that he should be 'turnede up-so-down upon a disshe, or upon the knees of some stronge servant, be the thiges i-croked, and . . . bounden strongely with the nekke', which left him trussed like a turkey while the surgeon went about his work.[61] Greater problems arose in eye surgery, where the practitioner was himself partly responsible for securing the patient. Guy de Chauliac's instructions for couching for cataract reveal how difficult this must have been:

> Sette hym in a place that is ful clere, on the lighte side, in sittynge uppon a stedfast stole. And be there a good servaunt byhynde hym that schal holde his hede wel stille. And than the wircher [practitioner], after that he have chewede fenel sede or garlik or some sharpe thing, he schal sitte afore the pacient somewhat hyere than the pacient upon the same stole, in holdynge the pacientes hondes under the knees of the same paciente, and the wirchere schal byclippe the pacientes knees with his fete. And than open the eyghe of the pacient with that other honde. Wirche the right eyghe forsothe with the lefte hand and the lefte

eyghe with the right hand . . . commaunde the paciente that he turne his eyghe toward the nose and that he holde it stille.[62]

Although descriptions of them survive in large numbers, herbal remedies for inducing sleep or deadening pain were unreliable: some of the ingredients were potentially lethal, and since quantities and proportions were given in only the vaguest terms the dosage must often have been either inadequate or dangerously high. Whether they took the form of potions, powders, ointments, or inhalants, all such 'stupefactives' were designed to reduce the body's natural heat through the agency of ingredients noted for their inherent 'coldness', and were thus viewed with caution by members of the medical profession. John of Arderne recommended five different narcotic preparations to eliminate 'felyng or akyng', but some surgeons were unwilling to employ any because of the risks involved.[63]

This concern about the effect of drinks containing such soporifics as opium or hemlock, either of which could easily prove fatal, was not, however, shared by patients facing the terrifying ordeal of surgery without anaesthesia. For them the prospect of pain-free oblivion must have seemed positively enticing; and it is in medical recipe books for domestic use rather than surgical treatises that we can learn how such beverages were made. A popular one called 'dwale' included gall from a sow or a castrated boar (depending upon the sex of the patient), lettuce, briony, opium, henbane and juice of hemlock mixed in a large quantity of wine. The heady combination of alcohol, henbane and opium would have rendered the patient insensible, while the laxative properties of the henbane and briony would have ensured that the potion passed quickly through his body before it could do too much damage. Even a slight mistake over the dose of hemlock would, however, have paralysed the respiratory system, so enormous care was needed in getting it right.[64]

Even with the help of rudimentary anaesthesia, the surgeon had to operate quickly, avoiding loss of blood and damage to the vital organs wherever possible. Heavy bleeding was extremely difficult to control, and placed further limitations upon the range and duration of viable surgical procedures. The problem was, indeed, ubiquitous, since many badly injured patients depended for their survival upon techniques which, through no fault of the practitioner, must often have proved inadequate. Internal haemorrhages could rarely be staunched, and although surgeons were well versed in the use of torsion and cauterization when dealing with cleanly severed veins or arteries, alternative methods of treatment were far less reliable.

Where it was impossible to stitch or cauterize surgeons relied upon styptics (composed of such 'dry' commodities as egg white, gum, frankincense and aloes bound together with hair) to stop the flow of blood and encourage the tissue to knit. Lanfrank of Milan recounts at length his use of this preparation in saving the life of a small child who had accidentally severed his carotid artery, and was already falling unconscious when he arrived on the scene. After applying pressure to the boy's throat for well over an hour, Lanfrank dressed the wound with liberal quantities of the ointment, bandaged it carefully and left it alone for four days (a cause of great distress to the father). By then the preparation had formed a solid shell, and had gently to be loosened with oil, prior to its removal the following day.[65]

The battle fought daily by medical practitioners against death and disease was, more often than not, lost from the very start. In a depressing number of cases little could be done to prevent malignant humours from overwhelming the patient's 'animal spirits' and coagulating, fatally, within his heart. Chaucer's account of the wounded Arcite's last moments on earth, in *The*

Canterbury Tales, depicts just such a hopeless struggle, quite possibly based upon scenes which he would have witnessed himself at royal or baronial tournaments. In 1389, for example, the young earl of Pembroke had slowly and painfully succumbed to injuries sustained during a practice joust at Woodstock.[66] He had been thrown against his opponent's resting lance, which had speared his genitals and lower abdomen: like Chaucer's hero, he was beyond help.

> Swelleth the brest of Arcite, and the soore
> Encreesseth at his herte moore and moore.
> The clothered blood, for any lechecraft,
> Corrupteth, and is in his bouk ylaft,
> That neither veyne-blood, ne ventusynge,
> Ne drynke of herbes may be his helpynge.
> The vertu expulsif, or animal,
> Fro thilke vertu cleped natural
> Ne may the venym voyden ne expelle.
> The pipes of his longes gonne to swelle,
> And every lacerte [laceration] in his brest adoun
> Is shent with venym and corrupcioun.
> Hym gayneth neither, for to gete his lif,
> Vomyt upward, ne dounward laxatif.
> All is tobrosten [shattered] thilke regioun;
> Nature hath now no dominacioun.
> And certeinly, ther Nature wol nat wirche,
> Fare wel phisik! Go ber the man to chirche![67]

In this case, however, the attendant physicians could legitimately claim impotence in the face of a heavenly power quite beyond their control. For Arcite has been marked down in the lists by Saturn, the most cruel and vengeful of the planets, whose malign influence is to blame not only for his death but also for the extremities of his suffering.[68] As the medical profession knew only too well, Saturn was the planet of black bile and melancholy, disfigurement and plague: how could they be expected to defeat such an adversary?

NOTES

1. G.R. Owst, *Literature and the Pulpit in Medieval England* (Oxford, 1961), pp. 30, 36. For a development of this theme, see S.R. Ell, 'The Two Medicines: Some Ecclesiastical Concepts of Disease and the Physician in the High Middle Ages', *Janus*, LXVIII (1981), p. 16.
2. *Healing and Society in Medieval England: A Middle English Translation of the Pharmaceutical Writings of Gilbertus Anglicus*, ed. F.M. Getz (Wisconsin Publications in the History of Science and Medicine, VIII, 1991), pp. xl, 36.
3. Ibid., pp. xli, 237.
4. British Library, Dept of Mss, Sloane 6, ff. 22–32v.
5. J.M. Riddle, 'Theory and Practice in Medieval Medicine', *Viator*, V (1974), pp. 173–8; *Lanfrank's 'Science of Cirurgie'*, ed. R. von Fleischhacker (Early English Text Soc., CII, 1894), p. 328.
6. L. Demaitre, *Doctor Bernard Gordon: Professor and Practitioner* (Toronto, 1980), p. 123.
7. M.C. Pouchelle, *The Body and Surgery in the Middle Ages*, trans. R. Morris (Oxford, 1990), p. 56. De Mondeville also compared the Greeks to architects, whose work may have been admired when it was new, but which eventually has to be pulled down to make way for something 'in superior style' (ibid., p. 104).
8. York Minster Library, Ms. XVI. E. 32, f. 97.

9. British Library, Dept of Mss, Sloane 6, f. 28v.
10. Ibid., f. 27.
11. Ibid., ff. 22–32v; *Healing and Society in Medieval England*, op. cit., p. 38. For the use of 'stupefactives' to anaesthetize before surgery, see below, notes 63 and 64.
12. *Stonor Letters and Papers*, ed. C.L. Kingsford (Camden Soc., third series, XXIX and XXX, 1919), vol. XXX, no. 250.
13. Fynes Moryson, *An Itinerary* (4 vols, Glasgow, 1907–8), vol. IV, p. 393.
14. For some typical domestic remedies for constipation, see *A Leechbook or Collection of Medical Recipes of the Fifteenth Century*, ed. W.R. Dawson (London, 1934), pp. 70–5; and *The Liber de Diversis Medicinis*, ed. M.S. Ogden (Early English Text Soc., CCVII, reprinted 1969), pp. 27–9.
15. John of Arderne, *Treatises of Fistula in Ano*, ed. D. Power (Early English Text Soc., CXXIX, 1910), pp. 74–8. See *The Liber de Diversis Medicinis*, op. cit., p. 28, for a rather rough and ready explanation of how to use a clyster.
16. John of Arderne, op. cit., p. 78.
17. *Lanfrank's 'Science of Cirurgie'*, op. cit., p. 277. For baths to ease haemorrhoids, see John of Arderne, op. cit., p. 72; for wounds, Wellcome Library, Western Ms. 564, f. 80; for skin diseases, *The Cyrurgie of Guy de Chauliac*, ed. M.S. Ogden (Early English Text Soc., CCLXV, 1971), p. 398; and generally, *Early English Meals and Manners*, ed. F.J. Furnivall (Early English Text Soc., XXXII, 1868), pp. 67–9. John of Gaddesden often recommended baths, but not all can have been agreeable: in cases of paralysis a fox was to be boiled in the water first, while young cats were to be similarly stewed to cure the flux in hectic fevers. It was believed that the invalid would thus absorb the characteristics of the animals in question: hence the suggestion that paralytics should sleep in fox skins (*Rosa Anglica, sev Rosa Medicinae Johannis Anglici*, ed. W. Wulff (Irish Text Soc., XXV, 1929), pp. 110–11, 267).
18. Walter Daniel, *The Life of Ailred of Rievaulx*, ed. F.M. Powicke (London, 1950), p. 34.
19. Pouchelle, op. cit., p. 18.
20. *Foedera, Conventiones, Litterae et cuiuscunque Generis Acta Publica*, ed. T. Rymer (20 vols, The Hague, 1704–35), vol. V, part 2, p. 55. My own translation differs somewhat from that given by L.G. Matthews, *The Royal Apothecaries* (London, 1967), p. 48.
21. *Rosa Anglica*, op. cit., pp. 231–3.
22. *Lanfrank's 'Science of Cirurgie'*, op. cit., pp. 18–19; *The Common Place Book of Robert Reynes of Acle, an Edition of Tanner Ms. 407*, ed. C. Louis (Garland, New York, 1980), pp. 167–71. For women as phlebotomists, see below pp. 211–12.
23. *A Leechbook or Collection of Medical Recipes*, op. cit., pp. 62–3. The idea of phlebotomy as a cleansing, purifying operation occurs frequently in late medieval religious literature. Thus, for example, Thomas Hoccleve's 'Epistle of Grace Dieu' refers to a soul so poisoned with self-indulgence that 'the nature of thi maladye wil aske sothly a fleobotomye' (*Hoccleve's Works: The Regiment of Princes and Fourteen Minor Poems*, ed. F.J. Furnivall (Early English Text Soc., LXXII, 1897), p. xxiv).
24. L.E. Voigts and M.R. McVaugh, 'A Latin Technical Phlebotomy and Its Middle English Translation', *Transactions of the American Philosophical Soc.*, LXXIV (1984), pp. 5–6.
25. S. Jarcho, 'Guide for Physicians (Musar Harofim) by Isaac Judaeus', *Bulletin of the History of Medicine*, XV (1944), pp. 180–8, no. 47.
26. Robert Burton, *The Anatomy of Melancholy*, ed. T.C. Faulkener and others (2 vols, Oxford, 1989–90), vol. I, p. 232.
27. *Lanfrank's 'Science of Cirurgie'*, op. cit., p. 299; *A Leechbook or Collection of Medical Recipes*, op. cit., pp. 62–3; *Rosa Anglica*, op. cit., pp. 42–3.
28. I. McDougall, 'The Third Instrument of Medicine: Some Accounts of Surgery in Medieval Iceland', in *Health, Disease and Healing in Medieval Culture*, ed. S. Campbell, B. Hall and D. Klausner (Toronto, 1992), p. 64.
29. *Memorials of London and London Life in the Thirteenth, Fourteenth and Fifteenth Centuries*, ed. H.T. Riley (London, 1868), pp. 14–15. For a case of alleged negligence by a patient who failed to take the proper precautions after being phlebotomized and suffered terribly as a result see E.A. Webb, *The Records of St Bartholomew's Priory* (2 vols, Oxford, 1921), vol. I, pp. 403–4.
30. Demaitre, op. cit., pp. 35, 119. The use of excessive blood-letting as a punishment (for an unfaithful wife) is described by Pouchelle, op. cit., p. 77.
31. *Lanfrank's 'Science of Cirurgie'*, op. cit., p. 299. Some idea of the frequency with which a patient might be phlebotomized in cases where the blood was considered corrupt or over-abundant may be gained from *Rosa Anglica*, op. cit., pp. 34–5.
32. As, for example, C.F. Mayer, 'A Medieval English Leechbook and Its Fourteenth-Century Poem on Bloodletting', *Bulletin of the History of Medicine*, VII (1939), pp. 381–91.
33. British Library, Dept of Mss, Egerton 2572, ff. 50, 69–69v.
34. Voigts and McVaugh, op. cit., *passim*; *Lanfrank's 'Science of Cirurgie'*, op. cit., p. 298; and below, pp. 130–3. For similar productions in France, see D. Jacquart, *Le Milieu Médical en France du XIIe au XVe Siècle* (Hautes Études Médiévales et Modernes, series 5, XLVI, 1981), pp. 212–14.
35. P.M. Jones, *Medieval Medical Miniatures* (London, 1984), pp. 119–23.

36. *The Observances in Use at the Augustinian Priory of S. Giles and S. Andrew at Barnwell, Cambridgeshire*, ed. J. Willis Clark (Cambridge, 1897), pp. lxi–lxxiii; J. Harvey, *Medieval Gardens* (pbk, London, 1990), p. 12. The easy, relaxed atmosphere which obtained in monasteries at such times, leading monks to gossip more than they should, is described by Jocelin of Brakelond in his *Chronicle of the Abbey of Bury St Edmunds*, ed. D. Greenway and J. Sayers (pbk, Oxford, 1989), p. 14.
37. B. Harvey, *Living and Dying in England 1100–1540: The Monastic Experience* (Oxford, 1993), pp. 96–8.
38. *Lanfrank's 'Science of Cirurgie'*, op. cit., pp. 304–5; *The Cyrurgie of Guy de Chauliac*, op. cit., pp. 550–1.
39. *The Cyrurgie of Guy de Chauliac*, op. cit., pp. 545–50. Chauliac derived much of his information about cupping from the great Arab surgeon, Albucasis (*Albucasis on Surgery and Instruments*, ed. M.S. Spink and G.L. Lewis (London, 1973), pp. 656–70).
40. *The Cyrurgie of Guy de Chauliac*, op. cit., p. 549.
41. For the dangers of using chemicals for cauterization, see John of Arderne, op. cit., pp. 83–5, where he describes the near-fatal consequences of a mistake in dosage he made as a young man. The use of cauteries is discussed at length in *The Cyrurgie of Guy de Chauliac*, op. cit., pp. 566–75.
42. *Albucasis on Surgery and Instruments*, op. cit., pp. 8–9.
43. Ibid., pp. 17–18.
44. Ibid., pp. 28, 134–6, 158; *Scripta Leonis, Rufini et Angeli Sociorum S. Francisci*, ed. R.B. Brooke (Oxford, 1990), pp. 174–5.
45. McDougall, op. cit., pp. 67–8.
46. *Lanfrank's 'Science of Cirurgie'*, op. cit., pp. 127–9, 173, 281; Wellcome Library, Western Ms. 564, f. 176. Albucasis was critical of attempts by rash or ignorant surgeons to remove bladder stones, particularly from the elderly (*Albucasis on Surgery and Instruments*, op. cit., p. 4). Some surgeons could operate at great speed; but for a harrowing account of a bungled lithotomy in the early nineteenth century, which gives a good idea of what the patient might have endured at any time before successful anaesthesia, see R. Richardson, *Death, Dissection and the Destitute* (pbk, London, 1988), pp. 45–6.
47. *York Memorandum Book, 1388–1493*, ed. M. Sellars (Surtees Soc., CXXV, 1914), p. 17. D. Jacquart, *Dictionnaire Biographique des Medecins en France au Moyen Age* (Hautes Études Médiévales et Modernes, series 5, XXXV, 1979), p. 153, notes a similar case, in which the patient exonerated the surgeon from all blame in advance, '*ainsi qu'aupres de Dieu*'.
48. T. Beck, *The Cutting Edge: Early History of the Surgeons of London* (London, 1974), p. 132. These orders were, in fact, less strict than previous ones drafted in 1423 for a proposed joint college of physicians and surgeons. Had this institution ever materialized, 'desperate or dedly' cases would have to have been reported within two or three days by physicians and within three or four days by surgeons: in neither case was any cure to be essayed before consultations had taken place (ibid. pp. 64–5). Before this date, securities were pledged by London surgeons to the city chamberlain, binding them in very heavy sums (as much as £20) to report 'dangerous' cures to the wardens of their craft (*Memorials of London*, op. cit., p. 651).
49. V.I. Kennedy, 'Robert Courson on Penance', *Mediaeval Studies*, VII (1945), pp. 322–3.
50. N.G. Siraisi, *Medieval and Early Renaissance Medicine* (pbk, Chicago, 1990), p. 177.
51. Demaitre, op. cit., pp. 141–51. Tapping any part of the body for what medieval physicians loosely diagnosed as 'dropsy' was dangerous. As the ever-prudent Lanfrank advised: 'thou schalt take kepe [care] wher he be strong or no, and if he be not strong, thou schalt do no cure to him. Also thou schalt do no cure to olde men that be to-broke [feeble], for thou schalt not leeve the strenkthe of an oold man, for it is impossible for to fynde an oold man strong whanne the dropesie is confermed on him' (*Lanfrank's 'Science of Cirurgie'*, op. cit., p. 286).
52. Wellcome Library, Western Ms. 564, f. 175v.
53. *The History of Parliament: The House of Commons 1386–1421*, ed. J.S. Roskell, L. Clark and C. Rawcliffe (4 vols, Stroud, 1993), vol. II, p. 537.
54. Pouchelle, op. cit., pp. 5, 58–9. In championing de Mondeville, the author does not allow that his contemporaries may have been justified on clinical grounds in questioning his methods, at least with regard to the treatment of certain kinds of wounds. Siraisi (op. cit., pp. 169–70) takes these considerations into account when describing the controversy.
55. Wellcome Library, Western Ms. 564, f. 55v.
56. John of Arderne, op. cit., pp. 26–7, 87.
57. Wellcome Library, Western Ms. 564, f. 76v.
58. British Library, Dept of Mss, Harley 1736, ff. 48–48v. Part of this manuscript, including the account of Prince Henry's injury, appears in Beck, op. cit., chapter V, where its authorship is mistakenly ascribed to the famous London surgeon, Thomas Morstede (d.1450). For details of his and of Bradmore's careers, see below, pp. 140–1; and for a discussion of the authorship of Harley 1736, ff. 2–167, see S.J. Lang, 'John Bradmore and His Book Philomena', *Social History of Medicine*, V (1992), pp. 121–30.
59. Pouchelle, op. cit., p. 76.
60. Wellcome Library, Western Ms. 564, f. 75.
61. *The Cyrurgie of Guy de Chauliac*, op. cit., p. 525.

62. Ibid., p. 467.
63. John of Arderne, op. cit., pp. 100–1.
64. L.E. Voigts and R.P. Hudson, 'A Surgical Anesthetic from Late Medieval England', in *Health, Disease and Healing in Medieval Culture*, ed. S. Campbell, B. Hall and D. Klausner (Toronto, 1992), pp. 43–56.
65. *Lanfrank's 'Science of Cirurgie'*, op. cit., pp. 66–8. Some idea of the desperate measures taken to staunch blood may be gained from a court case of 1424, in which a patient sued his surgeons for mutilating his right hand through cautery. See p. 89 below.
66. Thomas Walsingham, *Historia Anglicana*, ed. H.T. Riley (2 vols, Rolls Series, 1863–4), vol. II, p. 195.
67. Geoffrey Chaucer, *Works*, ed. F.N. Robinson (Oxford, 1970), pp. 43–4.
68. P. Brown and A. Butcher, *The Age of Saturn* (Oxford, 1991), pp. 220–3.

CHAPTER FOUR

ASTROLOGY AND THE OCCULT

With us ther was a Doctour of phisik;
In al this world ne was ther noon hym lik,
To speke of phisik and of surgerye,
For he was grounded in astronomye.
He kept his pacient a ful greet deel
In houres by his magyk natureel,
Wel koude he fortunen the ascendent
Of his ymages for his pacient.

Geoffrey Chaucer, The Canterbury Tales

As Galian the full wies leche saith, and Isoder the gode clerk, hit witnessith that a man may not perfitely can the sciens and crafte of medessin but yef he be an astronomoure. And therefor thou shalt nothing don, and namly of that which appertenyth to the kepping of thy body, without consaill of astronomoure.

Secreta Secretorum

In October 1348 Philip VI of France requested the faculty of medicine at the University of Paris to provide him with a consultative document explaining the causes of the Black Death, then endemic throughout his kingdom. The ensuing report, which was drawn up by some of the leading medical authorities of the day, and represented the most scientific thinking in Europe, unequivocally – and perhaps conveniently – attributed the outbreak and severity of the disease to circumstances beyond the control of any human agency. Indeed, the fate of its victims had already been decided at one o'clock on the afternoon of 20 March 1345, when there took place

> an important conjunction of three higher planets in the sign of Aquarius, which, with other conjunctions and eclipses, is the cause of the pernicious corruption of the surrounding air, as well as a sign of mortality, famine and other catastrophes. . . . The conjunction of Saturn and Jupiter brings about the death of peoples and the depopulation of kingdoms, great accidents occurring on account of the change of the two stars themselves. . . . The conjunction of Mars and Jupiter causes great pestilence in the air, especially when it takes place in a warm and humid sign, as occurred in this instance. For . . . Jupiter, a warm and humid planet, drew up evil vapours from earth and water, and Mars, being excessively hot and dry, set fire to these vapours. Whence there were in the air flashes of lightning, lights, pestilential vapours and fires, especially since Mars, a malevolent planet generating choler and wars, was from the sixth of October 1347 to the end of May of the present year in the

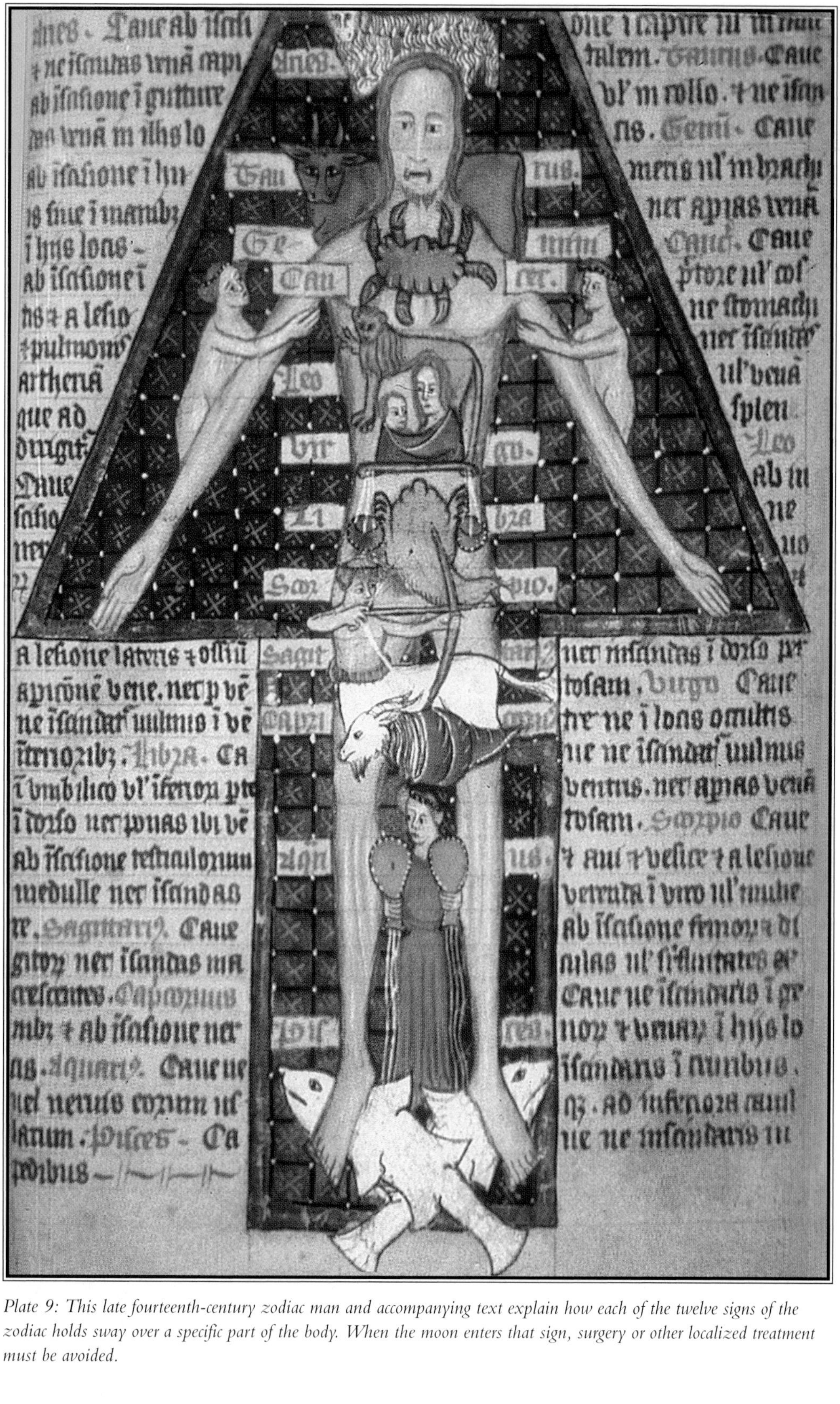

Plate 9: This late fourteenth-century zodiac man and accompanying text explain how each of the twelve signs of the zodiac holds sway over a specific part of the body. When the moon enters that sign, surgery or other localized treatment must be avoided.

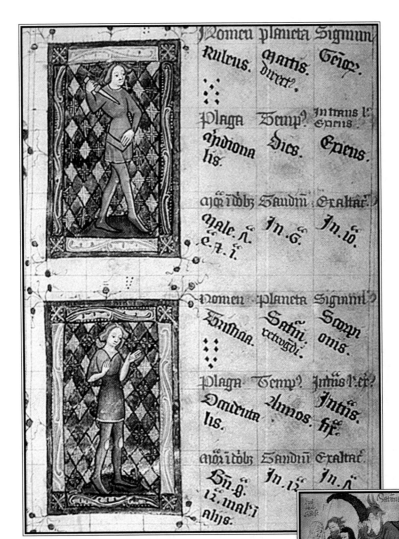

Plate 10: An illuminated book of prognostications and geomantic figures compiled as a presentation copy for Richard II in 1391. The geomancer makes his forecast from configurations of dots, derived from complex astrological calculations.

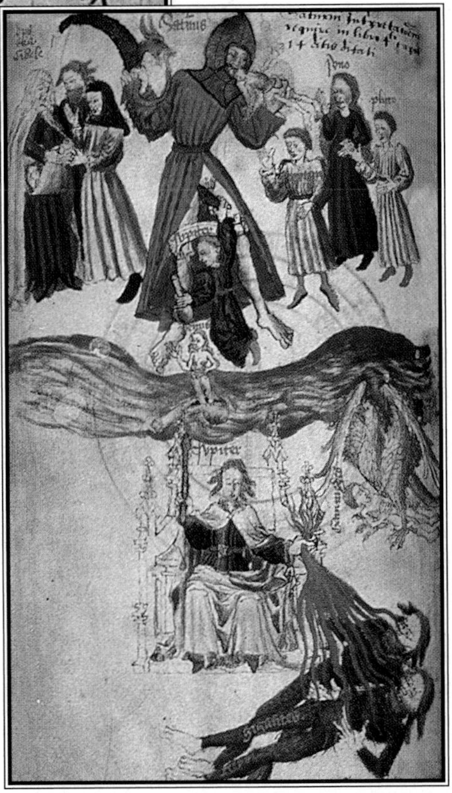

Plate 11: The outbreak of plague in 1348 was blamed upon a malign conjunction of Saturn and Jupiter three years before. Saturn, at the top of the page, eating his children, and Jupiter, at the bottom, casting thunderbolts, display the characteristics which made their planetary influence seem so terrible.

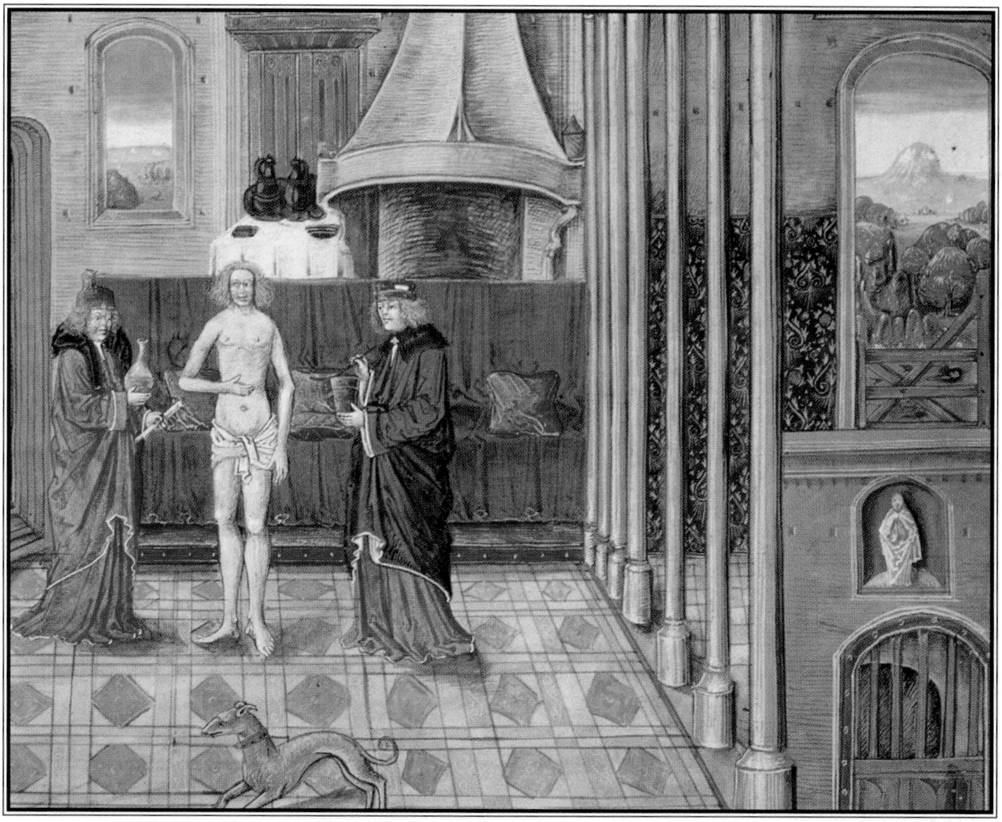

Plate 12: The twin brothers, St Cosmas, whose urinal shows him to be the patron saint of medicine, and St Damian, the patron of surgery, personify the division of practice and of the human body between the physician and the surgeon.

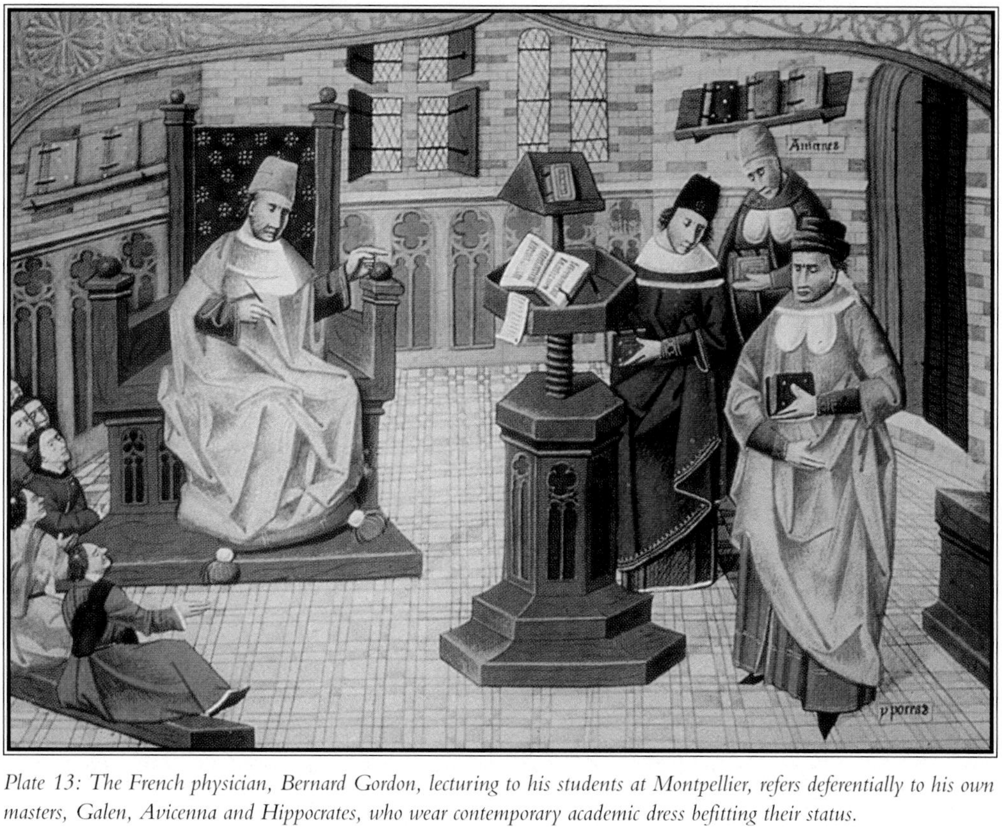

Plate 13: The French physician, Bernard Gordon, lecturing to his students at Montpellier, refers deferentially to his own masters, Galen, Avicenna and Hippocrates, who wear contemporary academic dress befitting their status.

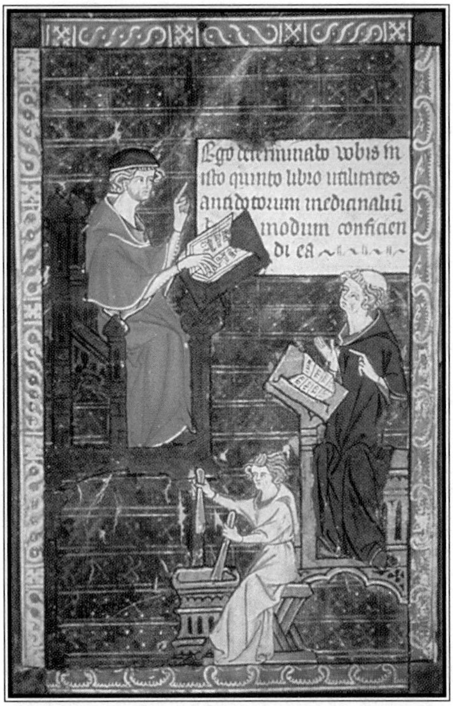

Plate 14: A master, probably at the University of Paris, lectures from Gerard of Cremona's translation of Avicenna's Canon. *At his feet an assistant prepares medicines with a pestle and mortar, while a student, already tonsured, follows from his own copy of this important text.*

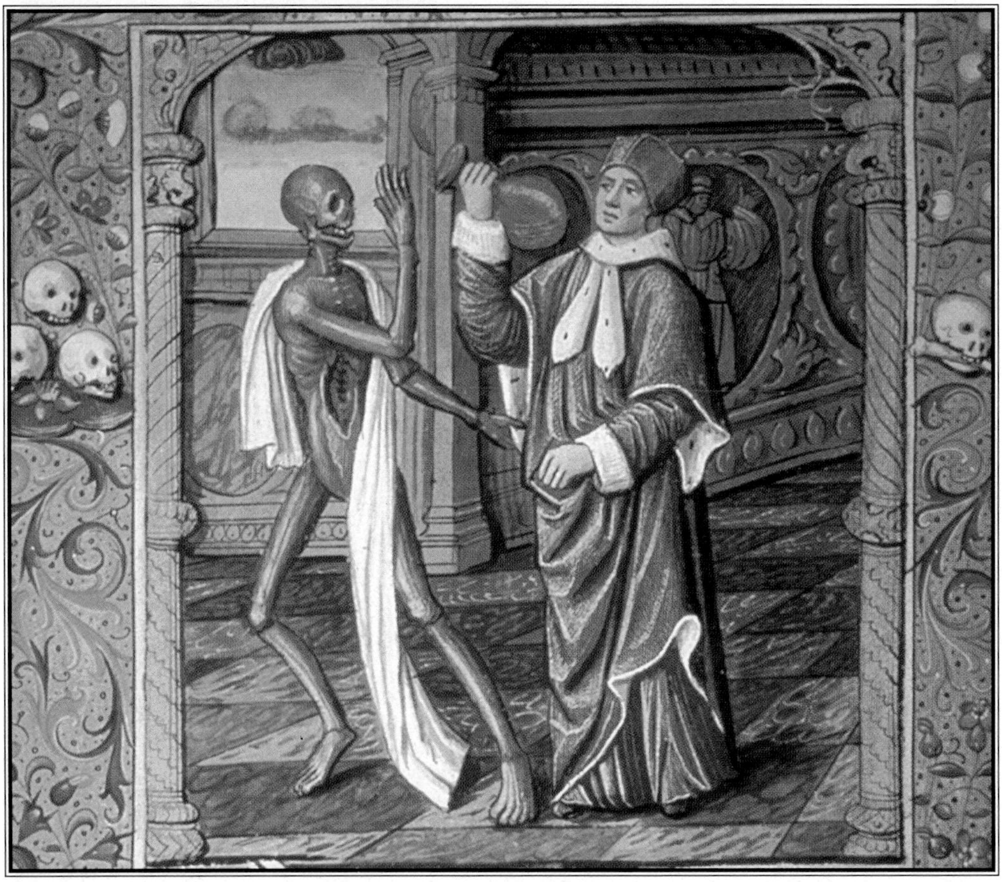

Plate 15: Stylish taffeta robes trimmed with fur and a large glass phial for the examination of urine samples together denote a rich and successful physician. But not even he can withstand the assault of Death.

> Lion together with the head of the dragon. Not only did all of them, as they are warm, attract many vapours, but Mars, being on the wane, was very active in this respect, and also, turning towards Jupiter its evil aspect, engendered a disposition or quality hostile to human life.[1]

This theme was elaborated further by a physician from the celebrated medical school at Montpellier, whose *Tractatus de Epidemia*, produced a few months later for the benefit of his colleagues at Paris, explained the uneven path taken by the plague through France in terms of extraterrestrial rays. Some places had been worse hit than others because they were more exposed to the evil influence of the planets: 'as when Saturn looks upon Mars with malignant aspect, or Mars with malignant aspect upon humane Jupiter, then the rays of these planets kill where they strike'.[2]

These two examples illustrate most effectively the importance which the disposition of the heavens had come to occupy not only in late medieval medical theory but also in shaping the ways in which contemporary men and women viewed their bodies and their lives. Yet the close connexion between astrology and medicine which fourteenth- and fifteenth-century practitioners took for granted was, in fact, a comparatively recent phenomenon made possible by the new spirit of intellectual inquiry abroad in Europe from the twelfth century onwards. As we have already seen, it was then that the great bulk of Greek scientific, philosophical and medical writing gradually began to exert an influence in the Latin West, thanks to the efforts of translators such as Constantine the African, and, significantly, that Christendom was also first exposed to major astrological texts by Greek, Hebrew and Arab scholars. These exciting and innovative works made possible the incorporation of what had hitherto been regarded as a morally questionable subject into the established *quadrivium*, or basic university curriculum, where it was soon studied along with its less controversial sister, astronomy.[3] This change in the climate of opinion had tremendous repercussions upon the development of medical theory, because the Church had previously been reluctant to condone any aspects of astrology, however potentially beneficial or 'natural' they might appear to be, or however rooted in tradition.

The intimate connexion between humoral theory and the latent or occult influence of the planets certainly boasted a long history, stretching back to the very earliest days of Greek thought. The tract *Airs, Waters, Places*, which formed part of the Hippocratic corpus and was known in Italy throughout the Middle Ages, had, for example, urged the physician to become 'familiar with the progress of the seasons and the dates of rising and setting of the stars' so that he could forecast climatic changes, and thus diagnose and treat his patients more effectively.[4] Assuming that man was, indeed, a microcosm of the universe in which he lived, it followed logically to the ancients that each season of the year would correspond to a particular bodily humour: people born in summer would incline to choler because of the dry heat, while an autumn birth date would induce melancholia, and a winter one a tendency towards the phlegmatic. Spring, the best time of year, when the sap began to rise, naturally invited a comparison with the sanguine, extrovert temperament. The very life cycle itself was divided into four similar phases, childhood being seen as hot and moist, youth hot and dry, middle age cold and dry and old age (which began at sixty) as a bleak period akin to winter.[5]

More specifically, each of the seven planets and twelve houses of the zodiac were held to play a crucial part in determining the health or illness of the individual: those unfortunate enough to be born when Saturn, that 'myrke and malesius planette', was in the ascendant (particularly in the

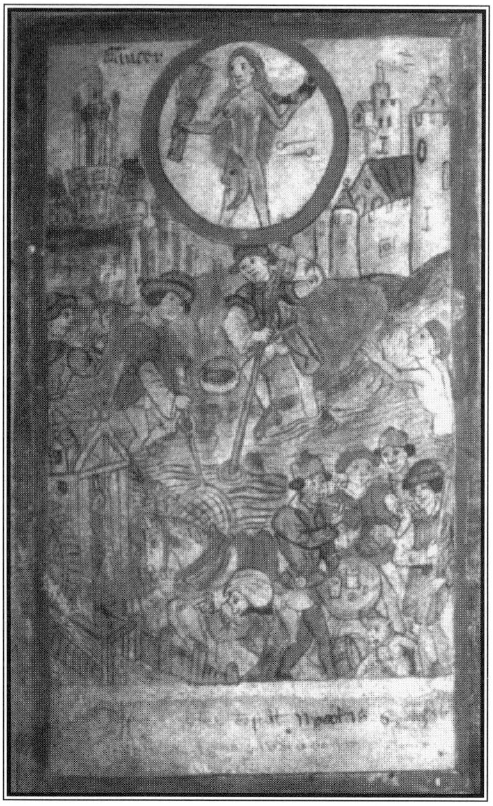

The children of the moon, a phlegmatic, feminine sign, are by nature as fluid and unstable as water. This astrological treatise was composed for non-specialist readers, and came into the possession of a sixteenth-century Norwich alderman.

sixth house, which ruled over a person's physical welfare) would be melancholic, swarthy of complexion, predisposed to disfiguring skin diseases and unclean in their personal habits (colour plate 11). The moon, on the other hand, being wet, cold and therefore intensely feminine, would predispose anyone born under its sway towards worry, irritability, indecisiveness, vulnerability to colds and other infections, and, in extreme cases, insanity. This was in marked contrast to the sun, the most masculine and glorious of the heavenly bodies, which bestowed a ruddy complexion and an impressive physique upon its children.[6]

None of the early Christian Fathers doubted for one moment the truth of these ideas, but because of their pagan and sometimes even demonic overtones they hastened to condemn any practices which questioned either the free will of the individual or the ultimate power of God to determine human affairs. Not for nothing were magicians and astrologers classed along with prostitutes, pimps and gladiators as being ineligible for reception into the ranks of the third-century faithful. While allowing that supernatural agencies could, indeed, play a notable part in the healing process, and, of course, accepting that miracles were still regularly performed through the agency of Christ and his saints, the patriarchs were reluctant to give any encouragement whatsoever to popular superstition. The unshakeable conviction that disease was inflicted by God upon the human race as either a test of faith or a punishment for sin, and could therefore be alleviated by divine grace alone ('for I am the Lord that healeth thee': Exodus 15: 26), already constituted a potential source of friction between the Church and practitioners of secular medicine, which fears about star-gazing and the occult only made worse.[7]

Ecclesiastical attitudes were further complicated by a system of belief which, on the one hand, saw Christ himself as the Great Physician, and the healing arts as a gift from heaven, yet, on the other, relegated these arts to an inferior position, reproaching men and women who put all their trust in physic rather than God's infinite mercy. No doubt with the fate of the Old Testament king, Asa, in mind ('in his disease he sought not to the Lord but to the physicians': 2 Chronicles 16: 12), writers like St Ambrose (d.397) and St Jerome (d.420) welcomed physical suffering as a means of casting aside the snares of the flesh and cleansing the soul of sin. Admittedly, only 'superior Christians' were considered strong enough to dispense entirely with medical treatment, but their weaker brethren were none the less encouraged to aim at such a goal. As late as the twelfth century Bernard of Clairvaux (d.1153), a staunch defender of traditional asceticism, criticized monks who bought special potions and sought out lay doctors to cure them of malaria on the ground that 'bodily medicine' was inimical to spiritual health. How much worse seemed the heretics and unbelievers who looked to the planets when their only hope lay in penitence and prayer.[8]

Yet, even as he wrote, the arrival in the West of such challenging and novel works as Ptolemy's *Almagest* and *Tetrabiblos* was opening up an irresistible range of intellectual possibilities, and the authorities soon began to modify their views. Some theologians may, in fact, have already accommodated themselves to the more scientific aspects of astrology, accepting the value of a discipline which could demonstrably extend the legitimate boundaries of human knowledge: whereas St Augustine of Hippo (d.430) had comprehensively denounced as blasphemous *any* attempt to pry into the workings of the Almighty, Isidore of Seville (d.*c.* 636) seems to have been far less alarmed by the idea of investigating man's relationship with the stars. Certainly, by the thirteenth century scholars of the stamp of Albertus Magnus (d.1280) and Robert Grosseteste (d.1253) were making a clear distinction between 'natural' astrology, as used by sailors in forecasting the weather or doctors in curing diseases, and the 'judicial' variety, which involved divination or soothsaying and was still regarded with deep suspicion.[9]

The lines of demarcation were established with great force and cogency in the following century by the French scholar, Nicholas of Oresme, whose *Livre des Divinacions* was translated into the vernacular specifically for the guidance of a lay readership, and whose remarkable output, in keeping with the mood of the times, also included a textbook on astronomy. But it was Oresme's friend, Philippe de Mezières, who laid down exactly how far medical astrologers could legitimately go, in a letter of advice written for the guidance of a fictional military commander:

> Now, as far as the rule concerning the acceptability of astrology which is authorized and necessary for human life, the General will have with him one or more doctors in medicine for the cure of the sick and the conservation of the health of the army, the which physicians, by the forecasts and elections of astronomy *as permitted by the Church*, will make cures and prescribe medicines for the well-being of the noble lord. But they will not ensnare themselves in any perilous predictions, which, contrary to the gospels, deal with what lies in the future, nor with [predicting] victories in battles, the which come alone from divine providence.[10]

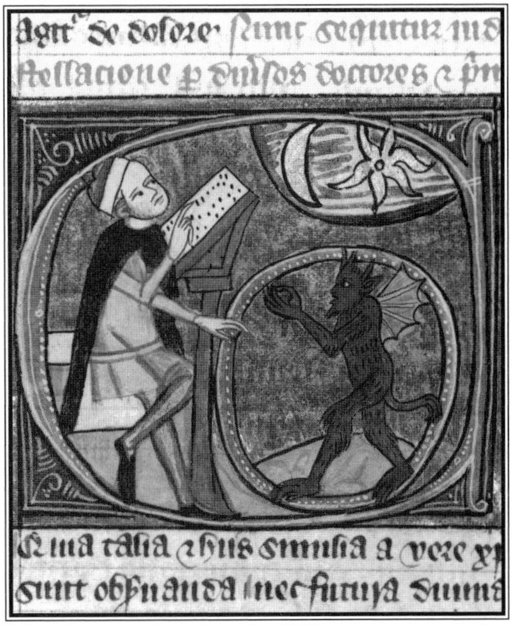

The devil lies in wait for those who use astrology to forecast the future. The text of this fourteenth-century encyclopaedia warns against the evils of divination from the stars, while the illustration depicts the practice of geomancy, which aroused especial concern.

Thus the late medieval physician was not only permitted but actually encouraged to put into practice much of the newly available teaching about the relationship between the cosmos and the human body – just so long as he did not stray into the forbidden world of divination or fortune-telling. Taking up the message conveyed in another 'Hippocratic' work on astrology, translated from both Greek and Arabic in the thirteenth century, scholars now began openly to argue that

> the physician cannot perform his duties well without a knowledge of the stars. He is like a blind man who must be led yet very often loses his way without such knowledge. . . . The physician that is not perspicacious in the science of the stars will discover that no one will entrust himself to him, because, as a blind man, he is unable to serve his patients with skill.[11]

The outbreak of the Black Death may well have given a further impetus to this development, since, as we have already seen, the epidemic was generally thought to have been caused by a malign conjunction of the planets. Quite a few physicians and surgeons were prompted to explain their theories in a simpler, more accessible way, presumably with a view to exculpating themselves and their colleagues from allegations that they had failed dismally to halt the spread of the disease. The eminent French surgeon, Guy de Chauliac, who survived the plague at Avignon, for example, composed a *Litel Book of Astrologie*, while the physician, Simon of Covino, ventured into verse, with a poem 'Concerning the Judgement of the Sun at the Banquet of Saturn'.[12] The foundation by Charles V of France, in 1371, of a joint college of astrology and medicine at the University of Paris, endowed with a fine collection of books and instruments, points clearly enough to the institutionalization of astrology as part of the medical syllabus. So too does the fact that his '*premier phisicien*', Gervaise Chretien, a clerk in holy orders, was celebrated throughout the kingdom as a '*grand et profond astrologien*', whose services were eagerly sought by the greatest in the land. Indeed, the subject now enjoyed something of a cult status, enhanced by its new-found intellectual respectability.[13]

Seminal in this respect was the *Introductorium in Astronomiam* of Abu Ma'shar (d.887), which helped to legitimize the hitherto distinctly questionable 'doctrine of the twelve signs' by establishing a precise and scientific correlation between parts of the body and the signs or houses of the zodiac. The work was available in the West from the twelfth century onwards, and had a profound influence upon the practice of medicine in the later Middle Ages. Aries, for instance, was believed to rule the head, Taurus, the neck and throat, Gemini, the shoulders, arms and hands, and so on down to the feet, which came under the control of Pisces. The identification of each sign with specific limbs or organs was based upon the idea of shared 'virtues' or characteristics. Thus, because the 'entire strength' of the lion lay in his heart, Leo was believed to preside over the chest, while the scorpion, whose sting lay in his tail, was associated with the genitals.

Whole nations, too, allegedly fell under the sway of specific signs, although the attribution of shared characteristics seems to have been more partisan than scientific. One English astrologer maintained that the Scots, a 'cruel, proud, excitable, luxurious, bestial, false and underhand' race, must, inevitably, be ruled by Scorpio. We do not know what manner of national horoscope his Scottish counterparts cast for their enemies in the south, but it is unlikely to have been any more flattering. Such a clear-cut and visually compelling physiological scheme naturally lent itself to pictorial representation, and the ensuing diagrams, known as zodiac men, constitute some of the most fanciful and attractive of all medieval medical illuminations. But, however pleasing to the eye, their purpose was essentially didactic: only through a proper understanding of the heavens could the physician establish exactly when such activities as herb-gathering, blood-letting, the administration of purges, surgical operations and even the cutting of the hair and nails might safely be performed[14] (colour plate 9).

The presence of the moon in a particular house made it extremely dangerous, if not potentially fatal, to treat the part of the body over which that house held sway. As one fifteenth-century compilation, specifically produced for a lay readership, warned: 'when thow takest a cure, be it of phisik or of surgery, take kepe [notice] of the mone, and of the tyme whan the sikenes toke and in what signe it bigan first'. Thus, when the moon was in Aries the physician had to be very careful not 'to do oght tyll a manny's hede, as wesche or to keme [comb] yt, or to shave or to do ony medicyne thir to or arise ony blode that be any maner of wyse. Or to blede at the nesse [nose] . . . or to receve ony purgacione'. He was also urged to watch out for those 'evil days', such as the *caniculares* or 'dog days' of summer, when the 'dobill heyt' in the heavens spelt doom for anyone who was unlucky enough to fall ill or sustain an injury. This period of 'perilus hette' seemed so ominous that even healthy individuals were warned to eschew 'lynge by women' and any other activities likely to upset the delicate humoral balance. Each lunar cycle, too, had its good and bad dates: whereas those who became sick on the second day after a new moon were promised a quick recovery, little if any hope could be offered to men or women succumbing on the third, while infants born on the fifth were expected to grow up as 'lunatyk or ellys folysch'.[15]

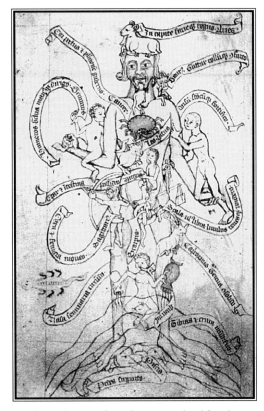

An elegant drawing of a zodiac man produced for a late fourteenth-century English astrological treatise. Because they could so easily be embellished, some of these guides to the influence of the heavens on the human body may, in practice, have been harder to use than the more mundane run of medical diagrams.

In order to reach a proper diagnosis, the physician ideally needed to consult horoscopes indicating the disposition of the heavens when the patient was born, as well as at the time he fell ill; and he had also to ascertain the precise conjunction of the planets at every stage of treatment. Given such information, medical astrologers such as Conrad Heingarter, who laboriously drew up charts for a variety of French notables, including Louis XI, believed that they could overcome the most pernicious diseases. Nor was there any shortage of self-help manuals, designed to assist and encourage the less experienced as they came to grips with the problem of interpreting a mass of difficult, sometimes esoteric data. Jean Ganivet's popular *Amicus Medicum* of 1431, for example, set out to direct physicians 'in the practice of medicine with reference to the influence of the sky as well in time of epidemic as at other times of the year so [they] may themselves know . . . when they ought to give medicines'.[16]

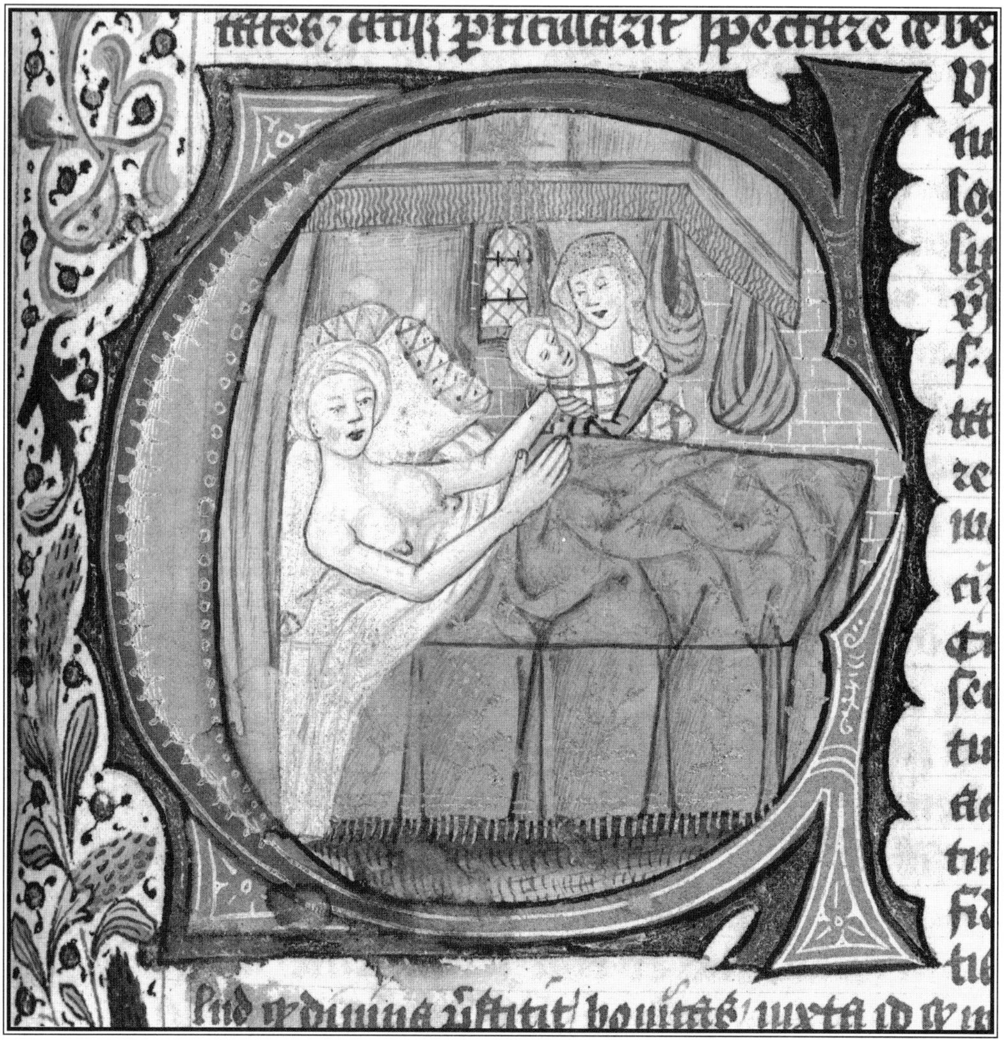

A child's natal star shines directly above the delivery room, determining, among other things, his or her vulnerability to disease. Note the swaddling bands employed by the midwife to retain the infant's moist humours and sprawling limbs.

Then, as now, however, the experts did not always see eye to eye. Although everyone agreed that phlebotomy and the administration of purges could be positively beneficial, even for the hale and hearty, there was some difference of opinion over the most effective dates for ridding the body of unwanted humours. According to one English vernacular source, dropsy could be prevented by letting blood on 17 September, migraine by a similar exercise on 3 April and blindness by a repeat performance eight days later. But in 1437 a lively controversy erupted at the University of Paris over the best time for taking laxatives in January. Two distinguished arbitrators (both of whom were theologians) were brought in to settle the quarrel: neither expressed a clear preference, yet they did stress that all physicians should equip themselves with proper sets of tables for calculating the position of the moon each day, as well as an astrolabe, 'in order to select for every day, every hour and fraction of the hour an ascendant sign corresponding to [that] in which the moon is found'. Some thirty years later Louis XI incorporated these recommendations into an ordinance 'for the good of the public weal and to maintain the health of the human body', which insisted that anyone practising medicine in France should possess an up-to-date almanac so they would know when best to offer treatment.[17]

Particularly at risk, and therefore of consuming interest to astrologers, were patients whose disease had reached a turning-point, and whose survival thus hung on a knife-edge. Medieval physicians, influenced by the teachings of Galen, were convinced that most illnesses followed a predictable pattern, culminating in a 'crisis', after which the invalid either died or began to recover. If the crisis happened to fall on an astrologically inauspicious day the prognosis must have seemed bleak, to say the least, perhaps even causing some people to give up the ghost in despair. But it is important to remember that, just as the average medical practitioner possessed a comparatively basic training in theory compared with senior members of the profession, so too a specialist knowledge of astrology was confined to an élite group. And, if the Italian scholar, Pietro d'Abano (who taught astrology, philosophy and medicine at Paris and Padua in the early fourteenth century), may be believed, even the experts betrayed a 'sloppy and superficial' approach to the subject, largely because they had no more than an elementary understanding of the ancient authors.

Quite probably the rest derived their rudimentary grasp of how the heavens worked from the vernacular textbooks which enjoyed wide circulation in the fifteenth century, and did no more than explain the bare essentials necessary for day-to-day use. It is, for example, unlikely that John Crophill, a leech who practised in the Essex countryside at the end of our period and assiduously recorded the birth dates of his patients in a notebook, was able to achieve anything very sophisticated in the way of astrological forecasts, although he clearly knew enough to establish what major planetary influences held sway at any given time. Regulations of 1505, listing the areas of expertise in which an Edinburgh barber or surgeon had to prove himself before gaining his licence to practise, included a demonstrable familiarity with the 'domination' of signs over bodily members, at least to the extent that phlebotomy and other common surgical techniques could be performed without risk to the patient.[18] A good deal of empirical knowledge must have been picked up by watching others cast horoscopes and interpret astronomical tables, since these too were readily available in a small, portable format.

The idea that the fate of his patient was, to a greater or lesser degree, predetermined by the stars and thus beyond his control can only have reassured the medieval practitioner, not least because it provided him with a fully comprehensive insurance policy in the event of death or mutilation. A suit for malpractice brought in 1424 by a Londoner against the three surgeons who had unsuccessfully attempted to cure his wounded thumb was thrown out of court on the advice of a distinguished panel of specialists on the ground that the complainant had been injured on 31 January, when the moon 'was consumed with a bloody sign, to wit Aquarius, under a very malevolent constellation', and that, even worse, some nine days later, by which time the moon had passed into Gemini (the sign governing the hands), no less than seven 'great effusions of blood' had taken place. In other words, the plaintiff could consider himself fortunate to have survived at all against such tremendous odds.[19]

Despite the warnings given by Oresme and other theologians, and the chilling example of such astrologer-physicians as Ceco d'Ascoli, who went to the stake in 1327 because of his supposed diabolism, or Jean de Marigny, executed '*pour ses demerites*' some thirty years later, many members of the late medieval medical profession were inexorably drawn into the business of astrological divination. After all, the techniques required for determining what planetary influences might affect a patient's health were no different from those needed to cast horoscopes for judicial purposes; and before too long practitioners were busy providing their patrons with advice of a more dubious nature, ostensibly so that they were fully apprised of the most favourable times for important undertakings such as marriage, the negotiation of diplomatic alliances or the launching of military campaigns. According to the French soothsayer, Simon de Phares, a third of the 114 most famous astrologers active in Europe between 1412 and 1495 were, like him, also medical practitioners. His purpose in compiling his *Receuil des Plus Celebres Astrologues* for his royal master, Charles VIII, shortly before the latter's death in 1498, was, however, to clear his name after charges of witchcraft had been brought against him by the Bishop of Lyon, forcing him to renounce 'all sorcery and divinatory acts, magical or mathematical, upon pain of life imprisonment'.[20]

Although the English hardly figure at all on de Phares's list, skilled astrologer-physicians flourished at Oxford, Cambridge and the king's Court at Westminster during his lifetime. The survival of a notebook belonging to the London practitioner and moneylender, Richard Trewythian (who did not hold a degree of any kind), suggests that by the mid-1440s, if not far earlier, medical and divinatory services could, in fact, be purchased together at one consultation by any reasonably affluent individual. We know most, however, about the royal and baronial patrons who employed academic specialists, sometimes with disastrous consequences. Whereas Continental universities, such as Paris and Bologna (which in 1405 stipulated that all medical students should study astrology for four years), placed increasing emphasis on the subject, neither Oxford nor Cambridge actively promoted astrology as a discipline in its own right. Even so, once the Court grew more receptive to the idea of judicial astrology, in the late fourteenth century, it became much easier for physicians and other learned men to venture down new, enticing intellectual byways, often with the direct encouragement of powerful lay amateurs.[21]

As befitted men with cosmopolitan tastes, the two royal bibliophiles, John, Duke of Bedford, and his brother, Humphrey, Duke of Gloucester, were both personally interested in astrology and medicine, commissioning special translations and compilations of important texts for their libraries. Bedford's collection included a *Livre du Jugement des Estoilles*, translated for him in 1430 from the Latin, and a *Physiognomy*, compiled by his physician and astrologer, Roland l'Ecrivain, with a fine frontispiece illustrating the influence of the heavens on the human body. The magnificent donation of 280 books made by Gloucester to Oxford University (thanks, largely, to the efforts of his physician, Gilbert Kymer) contained a number on astrology as well as medical theory, some of which had previously been in his possession for many years.[22]

Though Gloucester's fascination with the occult may have been innocent enough, that of his wife, Eleanor Cobham, was far more sinister. At her trial for witchcraft in 1441 it was revealed that her secretary, a talented Oxford scholar named Roger Bolingbroke, and the eminent physician Thomas Southwell (who had been one of the arbitrators in the above-mentioned lawsuit) had conspired through the practice of the black arts to discover when Henry VI would die. Southwell himself had allegedly helped to invoke 'demons and evil spirits' with the aid of magical figures, vestments, instruments and 'a book of necromancers' oaths and experiments'; and he certainly had a hand in casting a horoscope of the young king, which foretold his early demise. With some urgency, Henry's own physician, John Somerset, was despatched to commission an alternative and more optimistic reading, a feat achieved through the employment of another expert (quite possibly Roger Marshall, a fellow of Peterhouse, Cambridge, who later joined Edward IV's medical staff), equipped with a different set of astronomical tables.[23]

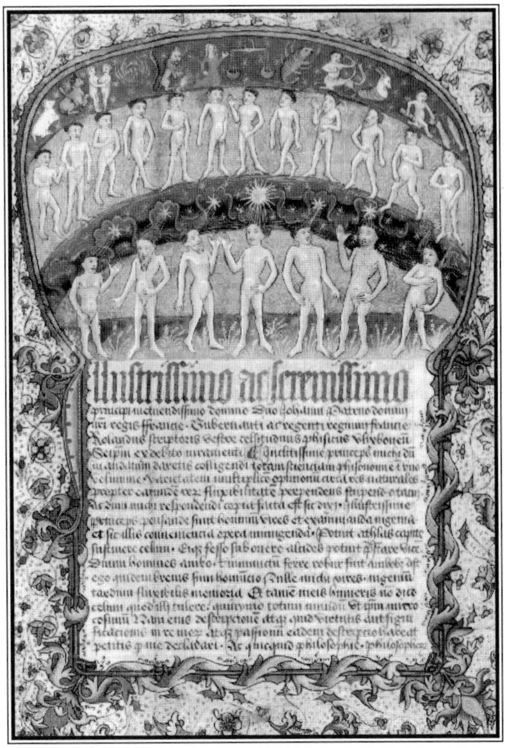

The frontispiece to Roland l'Ecrivain's Book of Physiognomy, *produced for John, Duke of Bedford, shows the twelve signs of the zodiac and the seven planets influencing the lives, characters and health of those born under their sway.*

A conviction that sickness or even death could be inflicted through sorcery was common at all levels of society, and, although allegations of witchcraft were sometimes levelled for purely political motives (a tactic profitably deployed by Henry V against his step-mother, whose property he coveted), a very real fear of necromancy made men and women ready to believe the worst. Contemporaries were only too eager to suspend their critical faculties in the case of Alice Perrers, Edward III's unpopular mistress, who was commonly held to have ensnared the elderly and increasingly feeble-minded monarch through enchantment. She owed her success, it was thought, to the skills of a Dominican friar, well known for his lucrative medical practice, but even more notorious as a magician ('*magus iniquissimus*'). He had reputedly provided Alice with wax effigies of herself and the king (as well as powerful herbs and ancient incantations attributed to the Egyptian necromancer, Nectanebus, and a magic ring just like the one owned by Moses), through which she had effected the seduction. Alice and the Court party came under attack during the Good Parliament of 1376, when two shire knights decided to take matters into their own hands by arresting the necromancer and thus depriving Alice of her influence. Through a clever ruse, they managed to capture the friar, who narrowly escaped being burnt at the stake, while Alice was apparently forced to swear an oath that she would stay away from the king. The account of the affair, narrated with undisguised glee in the *Chronicon Angliae*, provided the author (a member of the regular clergy) with an opportunity to play upon the stereotypes of both the wicked friar and the avaricious doctor, topics beloved of medieval satirists. Having disguised themselves as patients anxious for a consultation, the two knights had arrived at Alice's manor of Pallenswick in Fulham, where their quarry was lying low. They had produced two phials of urine for his inspection, although it was the lure of the fee rather than the challenge to his professional expertise which had actually proved his undoing. Greed overcame caution, and he was caught as a result.[24]

Given her remarkable hold over the king, Alice naturally tended to invite speculation of the wildest and most lubricious kind, and it is surprising that formal accusations of witchcraft were never brought against her. Others were less fortunate. In 1426, for example, a royal commission, comprising some of the most influential figures in the south-west, was set up to examine charges made by William, Lord Botreaux, that his uncle had employed sinister supernatural means to 'weaken and annihilate, subtly consume and altogether destroy' him. Botreaux must have had a strong case, because his uncle (who had represented Cornwall in several parliaments) was actually committed to the Tower of London, whence he was released only after surrendering pledges of £1,000 that he would cease his vicious practices. A few years later the court of Chancery heard a similar appeal against one of the Prior of Bodmin's priests, who stood accused of 'ymagenyng by sotill craftys of enchauntement wycche craft and sorcerye' the downfall of an opponent at law. The priest was said to have caused his victim to break a leg and to have threatened him with a broken neck, as well as inducing ill-health, lassitude and suffering, which, it was felt, would cease upon the delivery of a royal writ of *sub poena* ordering him to stop.[25]

Medieval litigants had few scruples with regard to the truth or accuracy of their evidence, and it is now impossible to tell how many allegations of this kind began as fabrications intended to defame an opponent. Men such as Botreaux, who suspected with good reason that his uncle sought to deprive him of part of his inheritance, were, moreover, predisposed to feel threatened, and came quite genuinely to see themselves as victims of diabolism. Concern about the work of '*sortilegii, magici, incantatores, nigromantici, divinatores, arioli et phitones*' in the diocese of Lincoln had, for example, reached such a pass by 1406 that Henry IV himself ordered a thorough inquiry by the episcopal authorities into the activities of evil persons who were causing harm to others. Such fears may, indeed, have been encouraged by calculating, unsuccessful or bewildered physicians, who found it expedient to blame their patients' decline upon evil forces.[26] In the absence of clear external causes, impotence, for example, was commonly diagnosed as being caused by curses or spells, and practitioners who otherwise distanced themselves from the supernatural were prepared to follow the advice set out by Arnold of Villanova (d.1311) in his treatise *On Bewitchments*. A variety of counter-measures, ranging from natural magic to full-scale exorcism were recommended by him as a means of effecting a cure, although some, such as fumigating the matrimonial chamber with the bile of a fish, may well have caused more problems than they solved.[27]

The unsavoury association in the mind of fifteenth-century governments between the occult and crimes against the state, dating from the days of Eleanor Cobham and that other royal witch, Joan of Navarre, can only have been reinforced by the activities of such physicians as the two Cambridge graduates, Lewis Caerleon and the 'nigromansier', Thomas Nandike, who were employed respectively by Margaret Beaufort and Henry, Duke of Buckingham, in 1483, on the eve of their abortive rebellion against Richard III. Yet both had shown a signal lack of clairvoyant skills by attaching themselves to the losing side, and they suffered accordingly, Caerleon with imprisonment and Nandike with attainder on a charge of high treason. John Argentine, the royal physician who cast horoscopes for Edward IV and his unfortunate son, Edward V, was probably too shrewd to play the dangerous game of forecasting the death of kings: certainly, the fall of the House of York seems to have taken him by complete surprise. A sycophantic desire to tell their patrons exactly what they wanted to hear may, perhaps, explain why so many late medieval astrologer-physicians made such a poor showing, and why the English Court maintained a healthy degree of scepticism, at least so far as divination was concerned. Witness the case of William Parron, a self-styled physician and professor of astrology from Piacenza, who left the service of Henry VII under a cloud in 1503 after the funeral of the queen, to whom he had recently promised another forty years of active life. His prediction that the future Henry VIII would enjoy a happy and fertile marriage fell equally wide of the mark, although the latter did at least oblige him by surviving into middle age.[28]

A more successful example of the dual practice of medicine and astrology may be found north of the border in the household of James III of Scotland, a keen patron of natural science. The physician Andrew Alaman (alias Andrews) had initially forged a reputation as a soothsayer in the Low Countries, where he was recruited by the king with the promise of fees, robes and other marks of royal favour. He evidently possessed uncanny powers of prognostication, being said not only to have foretold the death in battle, in 1477, of Charles the Bold, Duke of Burgundy, but also James's own violent end at the hands of a baronial faction led by his son, a fate which his mercurial temperament and reliance upon unsuitable favourites made, in retrospect, all too predictable.[29] Notwithstanding the risks involved, a preference for the society of dabblers in the occult seems to have been a Stuart family trait, since James IV, too, sought out the company of men whose activities did not always win the blessing of the Church. One such was the French physician and alchemist, John Damian, a figure strongly reminiscent of his contemporary, Leonardo da Vinci. Against considerable opposition, King James made Damian Abbot of Tungland in 1504 and installed him in a laboratory in Stirling Castle in the hope of discovering the philosophers' stone. Not surprisingly, the alchemist incurred a good deal of ridicule because of his attempts, 'lyk another Simon Magus', to demonstrate his magical powers:

> he causet the King believe that he, be multiplyinge and utheris his inventions, wold make fine golde of uther mettall, quhilk science he callit the quintassence; quhairupon the King maid greit cost, bot all in vaine. This Abbott tuk in hand to flie with wingis, and to . . . that effect he causet mak ane pair of wingis of fedderis, quhilkis beand fessinit apoun him, he flew of the castell wall of Striveling, bot shortlie he fell to the ground and brak his thee bane; bot the wyt thairof he asscryvit to that thair was sum hen fedderis in the wingis, quhilk yarnit and covet the mydding [dung heap] and not the skyis.[30]

As an amateur surgeon and dentist James would himself have been able to patch up the wounded aeronaut, who survived to continue with his experiments. He was not the first monarch earnestly to consult 'secret books, containing the sounder philosophy of alchemy', nor was he alone in employing university-trained physicians in searching out a permanent cure for his country's economic ills.

In point of fact, physicians were in many respects far better qualified to essay the transmutation of metals than other scholars or wealthy dilettantes, since the practice of alchemy required a sound working knowledge of astrology, as well as the kind of practical skills, such as distillation, which a *medicus* would have acquired in the course of his work. The idea that all matter could be reduced to four elements, and that these four, in turn, were somehow reducible to a single element or 'quintessence' was entirely in keeping with current medical theory, although the alchemist Thomas Norton, for one, felt that his art was infinitely more sophisticated and complex than that of a mere leech.[31] His defensive attitude is understandable in view of the number of charlatans and tricksters who continued to defraud the public, even after the kind of experiments so amusingly satirized by Chaucer in *The Canon's Yeoman's Tale* were made illegal early in Henry IV's reign. The prospect of paying off the government's not inconsiderable debts with freshly transmuted gold was, none the less, most attractive to Henry VI's leading advisors, who actually set up a couple of royal commissions in 1457 to investigate the possibility of achieving financial equilibrium in this way. To the same end, the royal Council agreed to exempt approved individuals, such as physicians, from prosecution should they elect to 'pursue the art of the transmutation of metals'.[32]

There was, however, another, more laudable reason besides its notorious 'special love of gold' for the medical profession's involvement in this rather grey area of occult practice. The belief that health and longevity could somehow be assured 'bi power of astronomye, alkamye and prospectief and of sciences ex-perimental' had been current in academic circles since the days of Roger Bacon (d.1294), and understandably continued to fire the imagination of those who followed in his footsteps.[33] Draft letters patent awarded in 1456 to the three prominent physicians, Gilbert Kymer, John Faceby and William Hattecliffe, along with a few other scholars 'most learned in natural science', outlined the many direct physical benefits expected to accrue from their researches. Hattecliffe had quite recently been empowered to treat Henry VI during his long period of mental collapse, and was later to sit on one of the alchemy commissions, so it may well be that the Court party was desperately hoping to stave off a further constitutional crisis occasioned by fears for the king's sanity. At all events, his licence referred in general terms to the quest for

> a most precious medicine, which some have called the mother of philosophers and Empress of medicines; others have named it the inestimable glory; others, indeed, have named it the quintessence, the philosophers' stone, and the elixir of life; a medicine whose virtue would be so efficacious and admirable that all curable infirmities would be easily cured by it; human life would be prolonged to its natural term, and man would be marvellously sustained unto the same term in health and natural virility of body and mind, in strength of limb, clearness of memory, and keenness of intellect; moreover, whosoever had curable wounds would be healed without difficulty; and it would also be the best and most perfect medicine against all kinds of poisons.[34]

The moral and theological ambivalence which surrounded so many areas of astrology and alchemy extended into other fields of medicine, too, notably with regard to the use of charms, spells, amulets and similar quasi-magical devices, the popularity of which posed another problem to the ecclesiastical authorities. Although it was commonly agreed that the three Magi, in prostrating themselves before the infant Jesus, had acknowledged the triumph of Christianity over all aspects of paganism and the occult, some physicians and surgeons and the great majority of practitioners without formal training continued knowingly to recite a whole litany of incantations over their patients. The trio of royal necromancers was, in fact, considered especially potent in driving out the demons associated with epilepsy, often as part of a ritual based upon the number three, which thus, implicitly, invoked the protection of the Trinity as well:

> Take blode of the lytyll ffyngre of hym that is syke of the ryzt hende and wryte with the blodde this iij names in parchment: Jasper, Meltizar, Baltezar. And close yt and heng yt a bout his nek; and er the close yt put therin golde, myr and encens, of ilkon [each one] a litel, and bid hym that halse the seknes blesse hym [when] he ryses of his bed iche day with thais iij names and sey for ther fader saules iij *Pater Nosters* and iij *Aves* and ylke a day a monyth.[35]

Charms to ease painful childbirth, prevent conception, cure impotence, frigidity or infertility, staunch the flow of blood, remove boils, banish the ringworm, heal broken limbs and soothe aching teeth appear repeatedly in the books of remedies used by laymen and professional healers alike.[36] Yet sceptics were to be found in the ranks of the former as well as the latter, and especially among the hard-nosed businessmen of medieval London. During the trial in 1382 of an illiterate quack who had tricked an equally ignorant victim into buying some old parchment reputedly bearing the words of a charm against fevers, the court of aldermen showed as much contempt for the *idea* that illnesses could be cured in this way as they did for the fraud itself. Having asked the accused to recite exactly what ought to have been written down, and having heard the words of a prayer invoking the body and blood of Christ, the judges told him that 'a straw beneath his foot' would have been about as much use under the circumstances, and had him paraded through the City as a warning to others.[37]

Nor were all medical men entirely convinced of the therapeutic value of prayers and incantations, however seemingly orthodox. Quite often the original meaning had been lost with the passage of years, so that only a few monosyllables or names remained. It is, indeed, hard to see how the refrain 'tarla + farla + tarla + arlaus + farlaus + tarlaus + on + on + on + Johannes + Lucas + Marchus + Matheus' chanted over and over again can have helped even the most suggestible of patients, unless intended to induce some sort of trance. This was probably the kind of charm which the medical writer and priest, John Mirfield (d.1407), had in mind when voicing his reservations on the subject. He certainly scorned the idea that a woman in labour could be helped by having a suitable prayer written out and strapped to her thigh, while carefully safeguarding himself from charges of impiety by transcribing the words for the benefit of his readers.[38]

This scepticism was evidently shared by Guy de Chauliac, who contemptuously dismissed '*emperiques* or charmers' as being unworthy of mention in any serious study of the surgeon's craft. A hint of chauvinism as well as professional pride may, perhaps, be detected in his criticism of 'all knyztes [knights] of Saxoun and . . . men folowynge batailles, the which procuren or helen all woundes with coniurisouns [conjurgations] and drynkes and with oyle and wolle and a cole [cabbage] leef', but his most scathing abuse was reserved for 'wommen and . . . many ydeotis or foles, the whiche remitten seke men for all manere of sekenesse onliche to seyntes, foundynge ham therfore up that: God gaf to me as it plesede hym; God schal take fro me when it schall like hym'.[39]

But most professional experts and an overwhelming proportion of the sick did retain their faith in the efficacy of charms. An anonymous treatise, composed in 1392 by a London practitioner, suggests that the religious ritual which customarily preceded surgery (for obvious reasons, the patient wished to confess his sins and prepare for the next world) might include the surgeon as well. Sometimes, as in difficult cases involving the removal of deeply embedded weapons, he actually abandoned his instruments, throwing himself upon the mercy of heaven:

> First, it is necessarie that thou and also the pacient to be clene schryven, and thanne seie thre *Pater Noster* and thre *Ave*, in worschipe of the Trinite, and sithen seie: '*In Nomine Patris*, etc. *adiuro te per Deum verum et per Agios et per Askiros ut exeas inde*.' And thanne putte therto thi two medicynable fyngres un to thei touche that yren, and it schal lightly come out, ffor this medicyne hath often tymes be proved of a knyght y-clepid Sir Richard Baskervile. . . .[40]

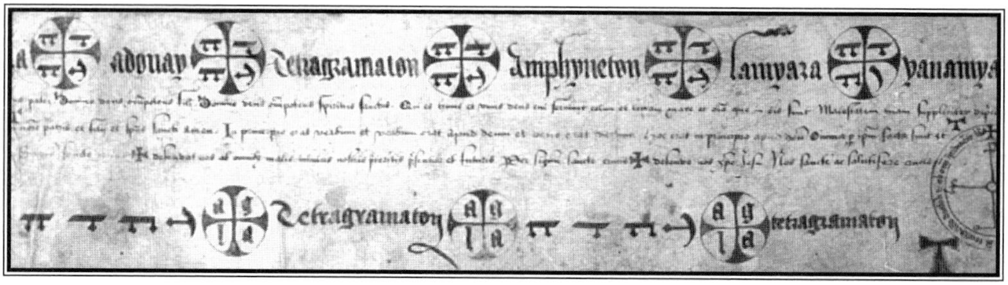

A section of an early sixteenth-century roll of Latin prayers and incantations used for medical purposes. The words along the top and bottom (Tetragram[m]aton, Adonay, etc.) are Hebrew names for God, which were believed to possess special occult properties and would be intoned while the reader made the sign of the cross.

Almost all the charms known to have been employed in late medieval England called upon divine intervention, often on the part of an appropriate saint or martyr. One such was St Apollonia, an elderly deaconess whose teeth and jawbone had been broken by the Romans before she was burnt, and who was thus commonly invoked by sufferers from toothache. Devout Christians who had given up hope of being cured by conventional means may thus have derived both comfort and strength from the constant murmur of friends and relatives gathered at their bedsides, and have been heartened to continue with painful treatment.[41] As we have already seen in the previous chapter, surgery in particular posed such a risk and offered such an uncertain outcome that it was simply not enough to rely on the skill of the practitioner. The ubiquity of charms to prevent heavy bleeding, for example, reveals how little could be done to staunch haemorrhages or serious wounds. Predictably, these are replete with images of holy blood and water: the miracle at Christ's baptism when the River Jordan stood still (a scene often enacted by barbers or barber-surgeons in mystery plays), or the piercing of Christ's side by the centurion's spear as he hung on the cross were by far the most common. The sanctity and power of these invocations had to be respected:

> First, the body hoveth to asske the name of hym that bledeth, and when you wilt seie the charme than go to the chirke and seie the charme, but loke thow seie it noghte but for seke man and woman. And by gynne: '*In Nomine Patris*, when Oure Lorde was doun on rode than come Longinus theder and smote Oure Lorde to the hert side; water and blood cam ought thereof; he wipen his eighen therwith, and saw onon aftir thrught the vertu of the goode heede [godhead]. I coniure the bloode that ne come oute of this cristen man or woman, *In Nomine Patris*.' Seie this charme iij tymys.[42]

A prayer written on a long scroll of parchment, whose length was based on calculations involving the height of Christ, likewise enjoyed great popularity across Europe, and was used as a medical charm, notably in childbirth, when it could be wrapped as a 'birth girdle' around the expectant mother. One, transcribed by a canon from Coverham Abbey in Yorkshire in about 1500 specifically claimed that:

> this crose XV tymes metyn is the trew lenth of our Lorde Ihesu Criste. And that day that thou lokes on it er beris it a-pone the, that day sall no wekid sprete haue pouer to hurte the.

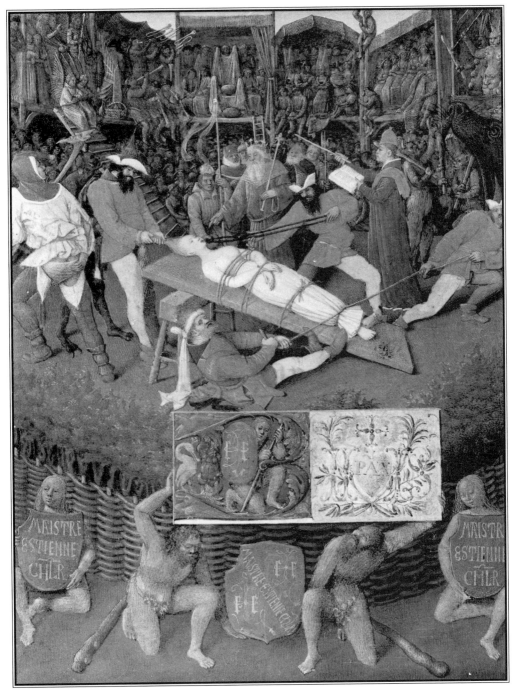

An illumination from the Heures d'Etienne Chevalier *depicting the martyrdom of St Apollonia, whose fate made her the patron saint of sufferers from toothache.*

> . . . And if a woman trawell of childe, take this crose and lay it one hyr wome and she shalbe hastely be delyuerde with joy with-outen perell, the childe to haue Cristendom and the moder purificacion of Haly Kirk.[43]

Passages from the Gospels, especially the '*In principio*' at the start of St John's Gospel, and St Mark's account of the exorcism of a daemoniac, were frequently carried by men and women as a means of fending off or curing disease. In vain *The Doctrinal of Sapyence*, a late medieval manual for parish priests, warned against the sin committed by these 'symple people' in refusing to forgo the 'brevettis and wrytynges' which, when strapped to their persons, brought a promise of health: not even the threat of 'admonycyon', 'perdycacyon' or 'excommynycacyon' could persuade them to risk losing such valuable insurance. Indeed, since many members of the clergy were themselves happy to provide their congregations with holy talismans, the authorities generally chose to turn a blind eye towards this controversial aspect of lay devotion. But at some point acceptable rituals, which might, for example, involve the blessing and distribution of wax, bread, water or salt as a defence against illness and epidemics, or the recitation of the Office of the Holy Name, 'which bestows sight on the blind, hearing on the deaf, makes the crippled walk, gives speech to the dumb and life to the dead', slid imperceptibly into something less orthodox.[44]

There was, too, a grey area where conjurations and rituals dating from pagan times had been superficially Christianized, or at least made relatively harmless. This tactic offered the Church a means of coming to terms with entrenched occult practices, at a time when direct confrontation had proved ineffective. In the early Middle Ages a good deal of constructive or 'white' magic had readily been absorbed in what one historian has described as a 'spirit of creative compromise', designed to eliminate far more sinister activities. If the distinction now seemed rather blurred, and the need for 'local negotiations' long past, the legacy of collaboration between priest and magus, particularly where medicine was concerned, still remained sufficiently strong to allow a limited degree of tolerance where the sick were concerned.[45]

Despite attacks launched by theologians in the sixth and seventh centuries against the magic rites performed by herbalists, for instance, the latter had continued with their observances, merely substituting one set of (Christian) names and directives for another. Throughout the Middle Ages the time, place and manner in which herbs were picked remained a matter of extreme importance, as also did the identity of the gatherer. One of many fifteenth-century verses on the medicinal properties of plants specified that betony should be plucked in August by a small child 'or the sonn ryse'; and another advised waiting until the moon had entered the house of Virgo, towards the end of the month, before cutting fresh marigold flowers. Even then, the herbalist, or the herbalist's assistant, had to be purged of 'dedly synne' after a suitable period of penitence and fasting, and make sure that he or she recited the appropriate prayers while at work. These helped to preserve the 'virtue' or curative powers of the plant, unless, of course, Jupiter happened to be in the ascendant, in which case nothing could be done to protect it.[46] A letter sent in 1396 to the wealthy Italian merchant, Francesco di Marco Datini, whose wife was suffering from malaria, illustrates a set of beliefs cherished at all levels of European society:

> If she would be healed speedily, let three sage-leaves be picked at morn before sunrise, and let the man who picks them do so on his bended knees, saying three Our Fathers and three Hail Marys in honour of God and the Holy Trinity, then send the leaves here in a letter, and I will write some words on each. And as the fever approaches let her say an Our Father

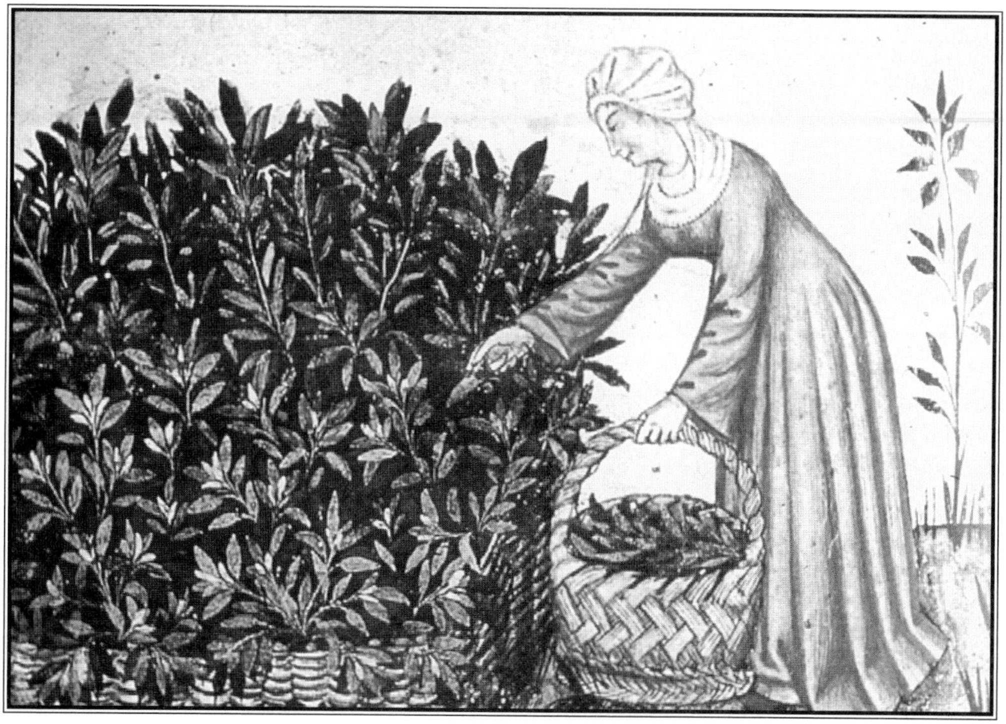

The gathering of medicinal herbs was highly ritualized. Some procedures had practical value, in guaranteeing optimum freshness and effectiveness, while others served a religious purpose. The woman who is here picking sage leaves can enhance their curative powers by reciting certain prayers.

> and a Hail Mary, and then eat a leaf, and so for each one of the three. . . . But she must have faith, for if she has not, they will be of no avail.[47]

Yet however piously intended, resort to latent spiritual forces of any kind made many churchmen nervous. They expressed particular reservations over the use of amulets, talismans and conjurations, but try as they might, the ecclesiastical courts had little success in weaning ordinary men and women away from their belief in the efficacy of appeals to the supernatural. In July 1481 one Richard Parkyn, 'unlerned of the parishe of Rotherham', was brought before the Archbishop of York to confess to having said prayers over garments taken from the sick, while also repeating their names, thereby conjuring up a spirit which explained to him exactly what was wrong with them. Richard's protestation that he regarded his visitor as a 'good angell' who enabled him to help others rings true enough, but he was still forced under oath to abjure all further dealings with such a 'gostly enmye', due penance being imposed upon him for his 'errour . . . agans . . . holy church'. The battle against lay ignorance was, indeed, nationwide, and continued to be fought for centuries to come. A number of 'sorcerers' indicted before the court of the commissary of the Bishop of London at the very end of our period included individuals who cured horses with incantations and signs of the cross, who recited charms over persons suffering from fever and, in one case, chanted prayers, such as the *Ave Maria*, while administering herbs. All were undoubtedly sincere Christians, whose simple faith may, ironically, have proved more effective than any quantity of physicians' potions in reassuring their patients.[48]

In such an atmosphere of fear and uncertainty, when even quite minor complaints could prove painful and hard to cure, and the prospect of death was never far away, patient and physician alike grasped anxiously at whatever straws came to hand. Predictions, based upon quasi-magical devices like the sphere of Pythagoras, aimed to forecast whether or not the sick would survive. They may quite possibly have bestowed some psychological benefit, at least if the outlook seemed optimistic; but most important of all they gave a warning of *mors improvisa*, sudden death, which struck before the victim had confessed his sins and been absolved by a priest. The concept of the sphere, as understood in layman's terms, involved placing three columns of numbers from one to thirty inside a circle, assigning each number to one of the letters of the alphabet ranged around the circumference and obtaining a total based upon the letters which made up the patient's name and the day of the lunar cycle on which he or she first became ill. Having then deducted the number thirty, the soothsayer was left with a figure which portended either life or death on the basis of its position above or below a line drawn right across the circle (eleven, for example, denoted *vita et felicitas*, but thirty was all too clearly *mors*).[49]

The practice of onomancy, or prognostication by names, developed along a variety of lines. One very simple method was described more out of curiosity than conviction by John Mirfield, who, having explained clearly and accurately the physiological signs of approaching death for the enlightenment of his readers, outlined a popular superstition as well:

> Take the name of the patient, the name of the messenger sent to summon the physician, and the name of the day upon which the messenger came to you; join all their letters together, and if an even number result the patient will not escape; if the number be odd then he will recover.[50]

The more sophisticated techniques demanded a working knowledge of judicial astrology, at least to the extent of being able to determine accurately the phases of the moon, and some assumed familiarity with geomancy, the ancient science of prognostication through a combination of astrology and numbers, as well. From a series of dots made at random on paper or sand the practitioner would, after a complex process of elimination, select and transcribe four figures, adding a further twelve derived from calculations of his own. These sixteen figures would then be applied to a chart of the heavens, thus providing an answer to whatever question had originally been posed. Pietro d'Abano, who died in prison in Paris in 1317 while awaiting

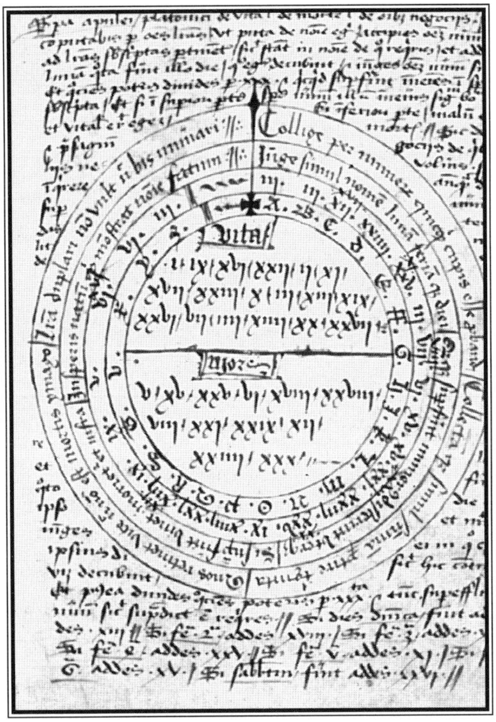

The sphere of Pythagoras and its use as explained in a fifteenth-century book of prognostications. To tell if a patient would live or die it was necessary to make a series of calculations based on names, dates and times. If the final total fell in the top half of the circle (1, 9, 16, etc.) the outcome looked hopeful. Otherwise (5, 15, 25, etc.) it was best to prepare for death.

trial on various charges of sorcery, considered geomancy to be a particularly difficult and demanding subject, although Nicholas Oresme characteristically dismissed it, along with other methods of fortune-telling, as 'nothing but the distinction between odd and even'.[51]

Like astrology, geomancy had become popular in the West once translations from Arabic works began circulating in the twelfth century, but it was never assimilated to the same degree by the academic establishment, partly because of its continuing association with necromancy. Even so, a number of highly respected physicians, including Roland l'Ecrivain, who spent years in the Duke of Bedford's service, attempted to justify it on moral and theological grounds. Among the other members of the English royal family to show an interest in geomancy were Richard II (probably under the influence of his brother-in-law, Wenceslas of Bohemia), and Bedford's brother, Duke Humphrey, who commissioned a set of *Tabulae in Judiciis Artis Geomansie*. Allegations made after Richard's deposition that he had been demented 'by sortilege or false and fallible calculations' were clearly the work of Lancastrian propagandists, however, for although a sumptuous book of divinations was produced for him in 1391, the compiler felt it necessary not only to justify the practices he described on theological grounds, but also, significantly, to explain everything as clearly and simply as possible because of the king's ignorance[52] (colour plate 10).

Of course, the great majority of practitioners and certainly of laymen had only the haziest grasp of these esoteric matters. They favoured easier methods of divination, which relied more upon folklore or tradition than complicated astrological tables or difficult calculations. A typical way of establishing if someone would live or die, for instance, required nothing more than a hen's egg, laid on the day that the patient first fell ill. On this the leech was instructed to write the letters 'i. so. s. p. q. x. s. y. s. 9. o.' (or a slightly different combination) before placing it outside in the fresh air overnight. If, on being opened the following morning, the egg contained blood, then there was no hope of recovery, and it would be advisable to send for the physician of souls.[53] Similar practices were employed to forecast the sex of an unborn child or determine whether or not a particular individual was sterile, being frequently explained in the vernacular for the use of unlearned men and women.[54]

In his description of the physician in the *Prologue* to *The Canterbury Tales*, which stands at the head of this chapter, Chaucer is at great pains not only to establish the academic credentials of his pilgrim by listing all the medical authorities with whom he was familiar, but also to stress the fact that he employed only 'magyk natureel' in making 'ymages' or charms for his patients.[55] Yet in an age when conventional medicine so easily and often overstepped the boundaries into the shady world of the soothsayer and even sometimes entered an unholy alliance with the black arts, it could be hard to tell exactly where one merged into the other. Despite the manifold 'official' pronouncements on the subject, contemporaries could be as uncertain about defining magic as they were in distinguishing between astrology and astronomy; and we should be careful not to fall into the trap of making too many anachronistic or artificial distinctions ourselves. Medieval practitioners were faced with a hostile and uncertain world upon which they sought to impose patterns of order and reason. To this end, they eagerly and promiscuously assimilated a wide range of astrological and alchemical ideas formulated by Greek and Arab thinkers who had found themselves in the same predicament centuries before. They attempted to harness the occult qualities of all manner of devices from charms and talismans to geomancy and other types of divination. In so doing they were able to satisfy the perennial human desire to understand and treat the human body, which is still the goal of medicine today.

NOTES

1. A.M. Campbell, *The Black Death and Men of Learning* (New York, 1931), pp. 39–42.
2. Ibid.
3. D.C. Lindberg, 'The Transmission of Greek and Arab Learning in the West', in *Science in the Middle Ages*, ed. D.C. Lindberg (Chicago, 1978), pp. 52–90. It is worth noting that some scholars, such as Adelard of Bath (d.1142) translated both medical and astrological texts.
4. *Hippocratic Writings*, ed. G.E.R. Lloyd (pbk, London, 1983), p. 149; P. Kibre, *Studies in Medieval Science, Alchemy, Astrology, Mathematics and Medicine* (London, 1984), article no. XIV, p. 134. Similar ideas were repeated, despite the teachings of the Church, throughout the Middle Ages, although lack of knowledge clearly hampered the physician in his astrological endeavours (L.C. Mackinney, 'Medical Ethics and Etiquette in the Early Middle Ages', *Bulletin of the History of Medicine*, XXXVI (1952), p. 26).
5. S.L. Thrupp, *The Merchant Class of Medieval London* (pbk, Ann Arbor, 1962), p. 195.
6. British Library, Dept of Mss, Egerton 2572, ff. 62–62v, 64–64v; P. Brown and A. Butcher, *The Age of Saturn* (Oxford, 1991), pp. 220–3.
7. J.A. Brundage, *Law, Sex and Christian Society in Medieval Europe* (Chicago, 1987), p. 73; S.J. Noorda, 'Illness and Sin, Forgiving and Healing', in *Studies in Hellenistic Religions*, ed. M.J. Vermaseren (Leiden, 1979), pp. 215–54.
8. D.W. Amundsen, 'Medicine and Faith in Early Christianity', *Bulletin of the History of Medicine*, LVI (1982), pp. 326–50; N.G. Siraisi, *Medieval and Early Renaissance Medicine* (pbk, Chicago, 1990), pp. 7–11, 14. The theological background to this debate is discussed at greater length in Chapter I.
9. J. Tester, *A History of Western Astrology* (Woodbridge, 1987), Chapter V; R. Kieckhefer, *Magic in the Middle Ages* (pbk, Cambridge, 1990), pp. 9–16, 34–41; V.J. Flint, 'The Transmission of Astrology in the Early Middle Ages', *Viator*, XXI (1990), pp. 2–12.
10. G.W. Coopland, *Nicole Oresme and the Astrologers* (Harvard, 1952), pp. 6–7, 29–31.
11. Kibre, op. cit., article no. XIV, p. 138.
12. *The Cyrurgie of Guy de Chauliac*, ed. M.S. Ogden (Early English Text Soc., CCLXV, 1971), p. 156; Campbell, op. cit., pp. 30–1.
13. H.M. Carey, 'Astrology at the English Court in the Later Middle Ages', in *Astrology, Science and Society*, ed. P. Curry (Woodbridge, 1987), p. 48; *Inventaires Mobiliers et Extraits des Comptes des Ducs de Bourgogne, 1363–1471*, ed. B. and H. Prost (2 vols, Paris, 1902–13), vol. I, no. 672.
14. C. Clark, 'The Zodiac Man in Medieval Astrology', *Journal of the Rocky Mountain Assoc.*, III (1982), pp. 13–38; H. Carey, *Courting Disaster: Astrology at the English Court and University in the Later Middle Ages* (London, 1992), p. 88; H. Bober, 'The Zodiacal Miniature of the *Tres Riches Heures* of the Duke of Berry', *Journal of the Warburg and Courtauld Institutes*, XI (1948), pp. 1–34.
15. Trinity College Library, Cambridge, Ms. R. 14. 52, f. 143; British Library, Dept of Mss, Egerton 2572, ff. 56v, 58v, 60; Sloane 775, f. 53; R.H. Robbins, 'Medical Manuscripts in Middle English', *Speculum*, XLV (1970), pp. 397–8; *The Works of John Metham*, ed. H. Craig (Early English Text Soc., CXXXII, 1916), pp. 148–56. For the classical background to the idea of unlucky days, which can be traced back to the second millennium BC, see A.J. Grafton and N.M. Swerdlow, 'Calendar Days in Ancient Historiography', *Journal of the Warburg and Courtauld Institutes*, LI (1988), pp. 14–42, and, for the subsequent popularity of the idea, V.J. Flint, *The Rise of Magic in Early Medieval Europe* (Princeton, 1991), pp. 322–3.
16. L. Thorndike, *A History of Magic and Experimental Science* (8 vols, London and Columbia, 1923–58), vol. IV, pp. 135–9, 375. The method used in casting a horoscope is described in Carey, *Courting Disaster*, pp. 117–19 and Appendix III.
17. *A Leechbook or Collection of Medical Recipes of the Fifteenth Century*, ed. W.R. Dawson (London, 1934), pp. 58–63; Thorndike, op. cit., pp. 139–42; Bober, op. cit., p. 12. For the types of instruments devised by astrologer-physicians, see L. White, 'Medical Astrologers and Late Medieval Technology', *Viator*, VI (1975), pp. 295–309.
18. Siraisi, op. cit., pp. 135–6; J.K. Mustain, 'A Rural Medical Practitioner in Fifteenth-Century England', *Bulletin of the History of Medicine*, XLVI (1972), pp. 469–76; *Extracts from the Records of the Burgh of Edinburgh, 1403–1528* (Scottish Burgh Records Soc., 1869), pp. 102–3; Robbins, op. cit., pp. 393–415. A good example of this kind of 'popular' treatise may be found in British Library, Dept of Mss, Egerton 2572, ff. 54v–66v.
19. *Calendar of Plea and Memoranda Rolls of London, 1413–1437*, pp. 174–5.
20. Symon de Phares, *Receuil des Plus Célèbres Astrologues et Quelques Hommes Doctes*, ed. E. Wickersheimer (Paris, 1929), pp. viii–xi and *passim*; Siraisi, op. cit., p. 36; *Extraits des Comptes des Ducs de Bourgogne*, op. cit., vol. II, no. 1863.
21. E. Poulle, 'Horoscopes Princiers des XIVe et XVe Siecles', *Bulletin de la Société Nationale de Antiquaires de France*, Feb. 1969, p. 69; Carey, *Courting Disaster*, Chapters V, VI and VII, *passim*.
22. For Bedford's books see J. Stratford, 'The Manuscripts of John, Duke of Bedford: Library and Chapel', in *England in the Fifteenth Century*, ed. D. Williams (Woodbridge, 1987), pp. 346–9, and plates 15 and 16; and for Gloucester's see *Duke*

Humphrey's Library and the Divinity School 1488–1988 (Bodleian Library, Oxford, 1988), Chapter III, and F.M. Getz, 'The Faculty of Medicine before 1500', in *The History of the University of Oxford, Volume II, Late Medieval Oxford*, ed. J.I. Catto and R. Evans (Oxford, 1992), p. 403. Sir John Fastolf (d.1459) also showed an active interest in astronomy: his secretary, William Worcester, compiled a table of 1,022 fixed stars on his instructions in 1440, as well as making extensive notes on medical subjects and collecting major texts (K.B. McFarlane, *England in the Fifteenth Century* (pbk, London, 1981), p. 222).

23. R.A. Griffiths, 'The Trial of Eleanor Cobham: An Episode in the Fall of Duke Humphrey of Gloucester', *Bulletin of the John Rylands Library*, LI (1968–9), pp. 381–99; Carey, *Courting Disaster*, Chapter VIII, *passim*; J.D. North, *Horoscopes and History* (Warburg Institute Surveys and Texts, XIII, 1986), p. 142; H.A. Kelly, 'English Kings and the Fear of Sorcery', *Medieval Studies*, XXXIX (1977), pp. 219–29.

24. *Chronicon Angliae 1328–1388*, ed. E.M. Thompson (Rolls Series, 1874), pp. 98–9; J.R. Maddicott, 'Parliament and the Constituencies', in *The English Parliament in the Middle Ages*, ed. R.G. Davies and J.H. Denton (Manchester, 1981), p. 80; G.A. Holmes, *The Good Parliament* (Oxford, 1975), pp. 136–7.

25. *Calendar of Close Rolls, 1422–29*, p. 363; *Calendars of the Proceedings in Chancery in the Reign of Queen Elizabeth*, vol. I, p. xxiv. For a graphic case of decline and death reputedly caused by the use of a lead image and a pin, see *A Contemporary Narrative of the Proceedings Against Dame Alice Kyteler*, ed. T. Wright (Camden Soc., XXIV, 1843), pp. xxiii–xxix.

26. Kelly, op. cit., p. 217. As late as 1716, for example, a physician is to be found blaming the death of an infant upon a 'curs', although the mother rejected this explanation in favour of a more rational one: namely, that the nurse had been negligent with her charge (Clywyd RO, Ruthin, DD/WY/6642).

27. D. Jacquart and C. Thomasset, *Sexuality and Medicine in the Middle Ages* (Cambridge, 1988), pp. 170–3; Brundage, op. cit., p. 512; Kieckhefer, op. cit., pp. 84–5; *Catalogue des Manuscrits de Médecine Médiévale de la Bibliothèque de Bruges*, ed. A. de Pooter (Paris, 1924), no. 470.

28. C. Rawcliffe, 'Consultants, Careerists and Conspirators: Royal Doctors in the Time of Richard III', *The Ricardian*, no. 106 (1989), pp. 250–8; Carey, *Courting Disaster*, pp. 157–8. For Caerleon's involvement with Lady Margaret Beaufort, see below, pp. 118–20.

29. J.D. Comrie, *History of Scottish Medicine* (2 vols, London, 1932), vol. I, pp. 82–3.

30. Ibid., p. 154. The most savage account of Damian's humiliation comes from the acid pen of William Dunbar, who not only mocked him as 'the Antechrist' [sic], but had a low opinion of his medical skills to boot. So low, in fact, that in 'Ane Ballat of the Fenyeit Freir of Tungland' he penned the memorable lines: 'In pottingry he wrocht grit pyne;/ He murdreist mony in medecyne;/ In leichecraft he was homecyd;/ Quhair he leit blude it was no lawchtir;/ Full mony instrument for slawchtir/ Was in his gardevyance' (*The Poems of William Dunbar*, ed. J. Kinsley (Oxford, 1979), pp. 161–4, 341–6).

31. *Thomas Norton's Ordinal of Alchemy*, ed. J. Reidy (Oxford, 1975), p. 50.

32. *Statutes of the Realm*, vol. II, 5 Hen. IV, c. 4; *Calendar of Patent Rolls, 1441–46*, pp. 275, 450, 458; *1446–52*, pp. 547, 583; *1452–61*, pp. 291, 339, 390, 625. Edward IV also issued occasional licences: ibid., *1467–77*, pp. 116, 285, 588.

33. Trinity College Library, Cambridge, Ms. R. 14. 52, f. 53.

34. D. Geoghegan, 'A Licence of Henry VI to Practise Alchemy', *Ambix*, VI (1957/8), pp. 15–16; L.G. Matthews (*The Royal Apothecaries* (London, 1967), p. 48) believes that Henry VI himself 'seems to have developed an interest in the science of the day'. This may well have been so, but the impetus for a royal cure almost certainly came from the queen, Margaret of Anjou, and her adherents at Court, as the membership of the commissions testifies.

35. British Library, Dept of Mss, Sloane 96, ff. 17–17v. For another version among many see Sloane 468, ff. 49v–50; and for the use of such charms in the manufacture of 'cramp' rings see M. Bloch, *The Royal Touch: Sacred Monarchy and Scrofula in England and France*, trans. J.E. Anderson (London, 1973), pp. 95–7.

36. Comprehensive collections of charms, in their various categories, are provided in T. Hunt, *Popular Medicine in Thirteenth-Century England* (Woodbridge, 1990), pp. 78–99, and in T.R. Forbes, 'Verbal Charms in British Folk Medicine', *Proceedings of the American Philosophical Soc.*, CXV (1971), pp. 293–316.

37. *Memorials of London and London Life in the Thirteenth, Fourteenth and Fifteenth Centuries*, ed. H.T. Riley (London, 1868), pp. 464–5.

38. *Johannes de Mirfeld: His Life and Works*, ed. P. Horton-Smith-Hartley and H.R. Aldridge (Cambridge, 1936), pp. 69–71; Kieckhefer, op. cit., pp. 69–75; *Historical Manuscripts Commission, Sixth Report*, p. 551.

39. *The Cyrurgie of Guy de Chauliac*, op. cit., p. 10. It is interesting to note that in the old English tale of the Siege of Jerusalem, when Vespasian's men are wounded and need the care of physicians, 'leches by torche-lizt loken her hurtes, waschen woundes with wyn and with wolle stoppen, with oyle and orisoun ordeyned in charme' (*The Siege of Jerusalem*, ed. E. Kolbing and M. Day (Early English Text Soc., CLXXXVIII, 1932), p. 48).

40. Wellcome Library, Western Ms. 564, f. 76v. This charm calls upon the Trishagion (Holy God, Holy Strong One, Holy Immortal One), customarily invoked during the Good Friday ceremony of creeping to the cross.

41. For examples from the rich literature of dental charms, see B.R. Townend, 'The Story of the Tooth Worm', *Bulletin of the History of Medicine*, XV (1944), pp. 49–54. Reservations about the invocation of saints were, none the less, voiced by

the unimpeachably orthodox Sir Thomas More, who accepted that the practice was open to abuses. See *A Dialogue Concerning Heresies*, ed. T.M.C. Lawler and others (*The Complete Works of St Thomas More*, New Haven, VI, 1981), p. 227.

42. York Minster Library, Ms. XVI. E. 32, f. 47.

43. C.F. Buhler, 'Prayers and Charms in Certain Middle English Scrolls', *Speculum*, XXXIX (1964), pp. 274–5. Girdles were, of course, often associated with enchantment, as in *Sir Gawain and the Green Knight*, ed. B. Stone (pbk, London, 1974), pp. 90, 180.

44. E. Duffy, *The Stripping of the Altars: Traditional Religion in England* c. *1400–1580* (Yale, 1992), pp. 216, 277–84.

45. Flint, op. cit., pp. 400–1.

46. Hunt, op. cit., pp. 79–80; Trinity College Library, Cambridge, Ms. R. 14. 32, f. 135.

47. I. Origo, *The Merchant of Prato* (pbk, London, 1986), p. 302. For English variants of this charm, see Forbes, op. cit., pp. 296–9.

48. *English Medieval Handwriting*, comp. A. Rycraft, Borthwick Wallet, III (York, 1973), no. 10; Kelly, op. cit., pp. 211–12. For later instances of popular magic and medicine, see K. Thomas, *Religion and the Decline of Magic* (pbk, London, 1984), pp. 209–51; and for examples of women using charms and incantations see below, pp. 117–18, 199–200.

49. L.E. Voigts, 'The Latin Verse and Middle English Prose Texts on the Sphere of Life and Death in Harley 3719', *The Chaucer Review*, XXI (1986), pp. 291–305.

50. *Johannes de Mirfeld: His Life and Works*, op. cit., p. 71.

51. S. Skinner, *Terrestrial Astrology: Divination by Geomancy* (London, 1980), p. 37 and chapter V.

52. T. Charmasson, *Recherches sur une Technique Divinatoire: La Géomancie dans L'Occident Médiéval* (Paris, Geneva, 1980), Chapter VIII, *passim*; Carey, *Courting Disaster*, pp. 92–106.

53. Hunt, op. cit., p. 139.

54. As, for example, British Library, Dept of Mss, Sloane 983, ff. 30–30v.

55. H.E. Ussery, *Chaucer's Physician: Medicine and Literature in Fourteenth-Century England* (Tulane, 1971), p. 112; Geoffrey Chaucer, *Works*, ed. F.N. Robinson (Oxford, 1970), p. 21.

CHAPTER FIVE

THE PHYSICIAN

Dethe to the Phisician:
Maistere of phisik, whiche on yowre uryne
So loke and gase and stare a-yenne the sunne,
For al yowre crafte and studie of medicyne,
Al the practik and science that ye cunne,
Yowre lyves cours so ferforthe ys I-runne.
Ayeyne my myght yowre crafte mai not endure
For al the golde that ye ther-bi have wonne;
Good leche is he that can hym self recure.

The Phecissian answereth:
Ful longe a-gon that I un-to phesike
Sette my witte and to my diligence,
In speculatif and also in practike,
To gete a name thrugh myn excellence,
To fynde oute a-yens pestilence,
Preservatifes to staunche hit and to fyne;
But I dare saie shortli in sentence
A-yens dethe is worth no medicyne.

The Dance of Death

By the start of the accounting year, on 1 October 1406, Richard Mitford, Bishop of Salisbury, was already in indifferent health, and may well have been suffering from the illness which finally killed him the following May. A 'certain priest physician' was called in to inspect his urine and provide medicines (at a total cost of 49s.4d.), while another local clergyman supplied fortifying beverages. On at least two occasions, emergency calls were made upon a neighbouring *medicus*, who was summoned by one of the bishop's servants and provided with a spare horse so that he could travel as quickly as possible. Despite their efforts, the bishop got worse, and in early December Master Thomas Thirlwall, *alias* de Reading, *alias* Leech, arrived at the episcopal manor of Potterne in Wiltshire with his two attendants to attempt a cure. He stayed for four days at the beginning of the month, spent eight days in London buying medicines for his patient, and returned to Potterne for a fortnight at the turn of the year. Mitford evidently managed to dispense with professional treatment for the rest of January, but the physician and his staff were again in residence during the first week of February. A few days later Thirlwall visited Oxford to purchase more medical supplies, and on 20 February the bishop received what appears to have been a silver catheter ('*unum instrumentum de argento pro virga virili*'), thoughtfully provided by his friend, Lord Lovell.[1]

Although he needed regular medication throughout March, the bishop did not send for Thirlwall again until April, by which time he had become seriously ill. From the second of the month onwards the physician was either with him at Potterne or busy ordering drugs in Oxford or Salisbury. It was probably at this time that he borrowed a horse from the Abbot of Sherborne in order to hasten to the bishop's bedside, where he was joined, on the 19th, by his distinguished colleague, John Malvern. The arrival, with a retinue of six servants, of one of the country's leading medical practitioners provides a sure indication of Mitford's worsening condition. Both men stayed with him for a week, after which Malvern returned to Oxford, evidently feeling that little more could be done to save the patient. His prognosis proved correct, and the bishop died a few days later, with Thirlwall still in attendance. During these months of illness, medical bills (including fees and travel expenses, but not the cost of board and lodging) came to over £16 10s., a sum well in excess of the net annual income enjoyed by many of the shire knights elected to the 1407 parliament.[2]

Wealthy prelates and the great lords of the realm spared no expense where their health was concerned, seeking out the most highly qualified and fashionable members of a small medical élite largely (but not exclusively) composed of university graduates from England and abroad. Thomas Thirlwall, whom Bishop Mitford seems to have liked and trusted, did not apparently possess a degree, although his colleague, Malvern, had enough for the pair of them: by the time he began treating the future Henry IV, in 1393, he was already a Master of Arts and Doctor of Theology of Oxford University; and he later referred to himself as a *doctor in medicina*, too. Like the bishop, whose background and early career were remarkably similar to his own, he had risen rapidly in the ecclesiastical hierarchy to become a king's clerk and the occupant of many lucrative benefices, so the practice of physic constituted only one part of his busy life.[3]

The idea that preparatory training in the arts was an essential part of a sound medical education may seem strange to modern English readers, accustomed to the highly technological and scientific nature of twentieth-century medical education. They may, indeed, suspect (with good reason) that Bishop Mitford would have fared better at the hands of the local empiric, who successfully cured his kitchen boy's injured skull at this time, albeit without the benefit of any formal tuition in natural philosophy.[4] Contemporaries, however, at least those moving in the social and intellectual circles frequented by Mitford and his kind, saw things very differently. For them, physic impinged on all areas of human life, in health as well as sickness, and made corresponding demands upon their own intellectual resources.

The close connection between art and medicine and the idea that the serious practitioner should cultivate a wide range of scholarly pursuits went back to classical times. In order to understand man's place in the universe, the working of humoral theory and the effects of diet, climate and other natural phenomena upon their patients, Greek physicians believed that it was necessary to extend their field of study far beyond the confines of the human body. '*Vita brevis, ars longa*', the first and most famous of all Hippocrates' *Aphorisms*, well known to every medieval medical student, equated art with science and contrasted the permanence of both with the fragility of life on earth.[5] The structure of the basic syllabus adopted by faculties of medicine throughout Europe in the later Middle Ages reflected this approach by dividing the course of study into 'speculatif' and 'practike' parts, concerned, respectively, with medical theory in the widest possible sense and its practical application. The aim was to produce graduates who were both 'philosophers and technicians', able to utilize their knowledge of the natural world as a means of conserving and restoring health.[6]

As a consequence of this approach almost all the north European universities insisted that prospective medical students not already in possession of a recognized MA should be obliged to spend two or three years acquiring the necessary background before they could graduate. At Oxford candidates for the Doctorate of Medicine who had yet to obtain their first degree were expected, from 1312 onwards, to attend lectures for eight years, a requirement cut to six in the case of suitably accredited individuals.[7] Statutes drawn up in the 1270s for the faculty of medicine at Cambridge had already imposed a far longer period of study for the degree of Bachelor of Medicine upon those without previous qualifications, but did not allow anyone at all to embark upon a doctorate until they had worked their way through the *trivium* (grammar, rhetoric and logic) and *quadrivium* (mathematics, music, geometry and astronomy), which made up the traditional arts course.[8] It was, in fact, taken for granted that a reputable 'maystre and phisicyen' would 'knowe the proporcions of lettres of gramayre, the monemens, the conclusions and sophyms of logique, the gracious speche and utterance of rethorique, the mesures of the houres and dayes, and of the cours and astronomye, the nombre of arsmetryk and the joyous songes of musyque'.[9]

Some of these subjects were considered especially useful in preparing the student for his career. As we have seen in the previous chapter, the practice of medicine demanded a firm grasp of astronomy, while it was believed that a training in rhetoric would not only elucidate many of the figures of speech employed by medical writers, but might also help when dealing with difficult patients. Not everyone was, however, entirely convinced by this line of argument: the oleaginous bedside manner of society physicians led Erasmus of Rotterdam to describe their calling as a degenerate 'subdivision of the art of flattery', far removed from the lofty skill of the rhetorician.[10] Without doubt, the employment of methods originally developed to teach logic resulted in a heavy dependence upon dialectic and the use of syllogistic arguments to expound medical texts in ways never intended by their authors. Candidates for the MD at both Oxford and Cambridge were, for example, supposed to engage in the 'intellectual tournament' of public disputations, defending or opposing questions about the nobility of particular humours or the way the syllabus was divided, just as the logicians did.[11]

Thomas Linacre, who obtained his medical education at Padua in the 1490s, and was thus spared the worst excesses of medieval scholasticism, felt strongly that such exercises should be confined to the faculty of arts. When founding his lecturerships in medicine at Oxford and Cambridge, in 1524, he stipulated that 'the tyme of the sayd redyng' was not to be wasted 'in tretyng of suche questions as Galien calleth logicall, but onely twoche suche questions as be litterall'.[12] Many laymen appear to have shared this view, at least if the following complaint, translated by William Caxton from an earlier French text, is any guide:

> And whan many maysters and phisicyens ben assemblid to fore the pacyent or seke man, they ought not there to argue and dispute one agaynst an other. But they ought to make good and symple colacion to geder, in such wyse as they be not seen in theyr desputynge one agaynst an other, for to encroche and gete more glorye of the world to them self than to trete the salute [well-being] and helthe of the seke man. I mervayll why that, whan they see and knowe that whan the seke man hath grete nede of helthe, wherfore than they make gretter obiection of contraryousnes, for as moche as the lyf of man is demened and put amonge them but hit is be cause that he is reputed most sage and wise that argueth and bryngeth in moste subtyltes. . . . And therfore ought the phisicyens and cyrurgyens leve, whan they be to fore the seke men, all discencione and contrariousnes of wordes, in suche wise that it appere that they studye more for to cure the seke men than for to despute.[13]

Students wishing to incept in medicine at Oxford or Cambridge were required to read and attend lectures on what, by Continental standards, appears to have been a rather narrow and conservative choice of texts (colour plate 14). The 'theoretical' part of the syllabus was devoted to Galen's *Tegni* and the *Aphorisms* of Hippocrates, while the 'practical' half concentrated on the latter's *Regimen Acutarum*. Lecturers at Cambridge worked their way through his *Prognostica* as well, and at Oxford they included Nicholas of Salerno's *Antidotarium* and the *De Febribus* of Isaac Judaeus if time allowed.[14] The striking absence of Avicenna and other eminent writers and encyclopaedists from this list does not mean that English students remained ignorant of their work. On the contrary, college libraries were well stocked with medical textbooks, and we can assume that background reading was expected as a matter of course. The impressive catalogue of ancient and modern masters, from Dioscorides to Bernard Gordon, set out by Chaucer in *The Canterbury Tales* as evidence of the Physician's learning probably gives us a better idea of the sources used by students of the period.[15] Like him, they would certainly have been familiar with John of Gaddesden's *Rosa Anglica*, which was composed during his time as a university lecturer during the early fourteenth century, and cites over forty different authorities. Significantly, however, this, the only work of international renown to be produced in medieval Oxford, already seemed rather outmoded when it appeared. Most continental writers had abandoned the medical compendium in favour of a less derivative approach (Guy de Chauliac was particularly dismissive about Gaddesden's dependence on others), but it obviously met the needs of English readers.[16]

Although medicine aroused considerable general interest at Oxford and Cambridge, and many students reading for the MA probably attended occasional lectures on the subject to broaden their knowledge of natural philosophy, the two faculties remained small and understaffed. Only forty individuals are known either to have read or taught medicine at Oxford during the fourteenth century and fifty-four during the fifteenth, while a mere fifty-nine graduated in it from Cambridge between 1300 and 1499. This rather poor showing, which contrasts dramatically with the flood of medical students emerging from Paris, Montpellier and the major Italian universities during the same period, resulted in part from the dominant position of theology, which took pride of place as a further degree.[17] Early patrons of English university colleges had been particularly anxious to foster theological studies, not only endowing numerous fellowships for that purpose, but also limiting quite strictly the opportunities for training in other areas. Thus, for example, the foundation statutes of Merton College, Oxford, actually forbade the study of medicine, even though some fellows got round the ban by calling it philosophy; at New College only two out of seventy scholars were allowed to take it up; and at Magdalen a maximum of three out of forty had approval to do so.[18] The active encouragement of theology at the expense of other subjects inevitably affected teaching standards, too, by attracting the best lecturers, and this in turn helped to increase student numbers. The practical consequences of this situation may be gauged from the fact that about five hundred Doctorates in Theology were awarded at Oxford in the course of the fifteenth century, while only forty such degrees appear to have been given in medicine.[19]

Although they may also have remained relatively small in relation to their rivals, many continental faculties of medicine enjoyed an influence out of all proportion to their size because of local connexions with the rich and powerful. Lecturers in medicine at Freiburg were frequently castigated for spending too much time in the homes of noble patients when they should have been teaching, but at least such lucrative diversions dissuaded them from moving elsewhere. The obvious lack of a ready market for professional medical services in England's two university towns clearly discouraged able physicians from taking academic posts, and even the newly qualified, who were supposed to stay as regents (lecturers) for two years after incepting as MDs, proved reluctant to do so.[20]

The regency system, adopted by those north European universities which followed the Parisian model, was intended to provide a regular supply of teachers, but could only work well in large cities or centres of patronage where young graduates had the chance to build up a practice at the same time. Moreover, since lecturers were not selected because of their skill or experience, the quality of tuition could be variable, the delivery uninspired. The setting up by heads of state in parts of Italy and Germany of salaried professorships in medicine was one way of circumventing this problem, at least in areas where married laymen studied the subject in significant numbers. Bologna possessed two such chairs (in theory and practice) by 1305; and Padua had no fewer than five before the close of the fourteenth century. But here, too, there were other incentives, besides the prospect of a regular wage, to attract the best minds.[21]

Almost from the start the English university authorities recognized that it would be impossible to enforce the rules about regency where medicine was concerned. A continuous shortage of appropriately qualified lecturers was anticipated in the Oxford statutes of 1312/13, which assumed that masters from the faculty of arts would step in to fill the gap; and in 1450 the congregation actually had to nominate a theologian to act as *scrutator* (assessor) in the faculty of medicine because nobody there possessed a doctorate.[22] The problem was compounded by a general readiness to allow exemptions from lecturing, although in many cases these merely acknowledged a *fait accompli*. Even without grace to discontinue his regency, it is unlikely that James Fryse would have remained a day longer in Cambridge after incepting as an MD in 1461, since he had just been retained at £40 a year as one of Edward IV's physicians. Three years later William Lempster, another able graduate destined to wear the Yorkist livery, left the university under similar circumstances. Not surprisingly, William Skelton's study for an MD was disrupted in 1469 because no resident lecturers could be found to teach him, but matters were hardly improved when he, too, eventually obtained permission to follow suit.[23]

Writing of Oxford in the same period, one historian has recently concluded that 'the small size of the faculty and the haphazard and inconsistent nature of the instruction offered must have been grave deterrents to all but the most enthusiastic students of medicine'; and it is hard to disagree. Matters were altogether different in Vienna, where between 1400 and 1465 a total of forty regents are known to have lectured in medicine to a local audience of students drawn mainly from the city. Here, as in Paris, the presence of a large and splendid court drew practitioners like a magnet, and contributed not a little to the status of those faculty members who found employment there.[24]

Without strong financial inducements, of the kind offered by the smaller, provincial universities of Italy and Germany, it was clearly unrealistic to expect talented and ambitious young men to live in voluntary exile, miles from the fount of wealth and patronage. Riches, promotion and professional recognition were not to be had in the lecture halls of medieval Oxford and Cambridge, but at Court, in the households of great lay and ecclesiastical lords, and in the homes of affluent Londoners. The immediate, tangible profits of medical practice at this social level took the form of fees, ecclesiastical preferment and grants of land on a generous, sometimes lavish, scale.[25] During the later Middle Ages the salaries accorded to leading physicians in attendance upon the king ranged from about £40 to £100 or more a year, topped up with occasional gifts of cash by way of special reward. In addition, they drew expenses of at least a shilling a day while on duty (rising to 2s. on foreign expeditions) and could rely on an allocation of £5 or more each year for furred robes appropriate to their status. In view of the fact that some physicians were paid rather more than knights of the body, appearances were clearly important.[26]

Other members of the royal family followed this example, remunerating their medical advisors at roughly the same rate as senior household staff: both the Black Prince and his younger brother, John of Gaunt, retained physicians at fees of up to £40 a year, over and above a fixed daily wage during foreign campaigns. The prince was a kindly employer, who allowed his 'leech', William Blackwater, an even larger annuity and allowance for robes after his retirement 'for good service rendered so long as he was able to work'.[27] Just as a knight or an esquire might move from the affinity of one lord to another, or take fees from a number of patrons at once, so practitioners at the top of the profession hoped to augment their incomes in this way. Having first contracted to work for the Earl of Salisbury at a salary of £5 a year, payable for life, the physician John Bray entered John of Gaunt's employment in 1372 (earning twice this amount), and probably on his recommendation was engaged at a further £12 a year to attend his elderly and failing father, Edward III. Bray continued to receive the money after Richard II ascended the throne, so by the time of his own death, in 1381, he was drawing at least £27 a year. Since Gaunt had intervened in 1379 to prevent him losing all his goods and going to prison because he had failed to settle a debt of £21, and also presented him with gifts of game from time to time, his patronage and personal protection were clearly invaluable.[28]

By the second quarter of the fifteenth century a handful of married laymen had graduated as physicians, but until then the profession was dominated by clerics, who could easily and conveniently be rewarded with valuable livings. John Arundel, MD, chaplain and physician first to Henry Beauchamp, Earl of Warwick, and then to Henry VI, occupied a series of at least seven rectories, fourteen canonries and prebendaries, the Archdeaconry of Richmond and the wardenship of the hospital of St Mary Bethlehem in London before becoming Bishop of Chichester in 1459. From then onwards he abandoned medicine to concentrate on an administrative and ecclesiastical career, but he had still been treating the king as late as 1456.[29] Pluralism on such a flamboyant scale clearly required papal approval, which, in turn, could more easily be secured with the help of a powerful lay patron. In 1343, for example, the Earl of Surrey petitioned Clement VI on behalf of his clerk, Walter Lyndrigge, MD, who was already dean of the king's free chapel at Hastings and Archdeacon of Lewes. In response to this request Lyndrigge now also became a canon and prebendary of St Paul's in London, being excused the customary examination in Rome one year later because he could not be spared from his duties as 'dear clerk and physician' to another noble patient, William, Earl of Huntingdon, without risk to the latter's health.[30]

The grant of a living was, from the patron's point of view, an ideal way of retaining or rewarding a physician, since it made no direct demands upon the donor's cash income. In 1395, for example, Richard II awarded his 'clerk and leech', John Middleton, MA, an annuity of £40, payable at the Exchequer, until he could be provided with benefices to the value of £100 a year (a figure increased to 200 marks (approximately £133) shortly afterwards).[31] This arrangement clearly worked to their mutual advantage, as the king would eventually be able to divert the money to other uses, while Middleton was assured of a higher income than might otherwise have been available. For a monarch with absolutist tendencies, anxious to strengthen the royalist element in the upper ranks of the Church, the promotion of medical advisors (who surely ranked among the most trusted of retainers) had even more to recommend it. In 1391 King Richard obliged the monks of Beaulieu Abbey in Hampshire to accept his physician, the Cistercian,

Tideman of Winchcomb, as their abbot, promoted him two years later to the Bishopric of Llandaff, and had him translated to the see of Worcester in 1396.[32]

Because of the large amounts of property which constantly came into their hands through confiscation or forfeiture successive Kings of England sometimes chose to allocate rents from this source (or even the land itself) to their physicians and surgeons. Since these revenues did not constitute a charge upon the royal demesne, and the grants rarely extended beyond the life of an individual practitioner, it was once again possible to be open-handed at comparatively little cost. Thus, in the early 1460s, Edward IV conveyed a number of messuages and tenements in London, seized from rebel Lancastrians, to the above-mentioned James Fryse, who clearly needed somewhere to live near the Court.[33] In theory, at least, a firm title to bricks and mortar had notable advantages over a pension, which could easily fall into arrears. By August 1471, for example, the annuity of £40 assigned to Fryse's colleague, Dominic Sergio, had not been paid for over four years: despite peremptory orders to the Exchequer he had yet to receive a penny of it the following May; and at least £100 remained overdue in 1475.[34]

Henry VI's remarkable generosity to his 'doctor in medicine', John Somerset, in allowing him to exchange fees worth £60 a year for a life estate in the manor of Ruislip in 1439 apparently offered just such a guarantee of security, although his readiness to allocate the same property to King's College, Cambridge, a few years later left Somerset a poorer and extremely bitter man (especially as he had played a notable part in founding the college).[35] Since there was no certain way of insuring against royal whims, or triumphing in the face of institutional bureaucracy, the shrewd practitioner naturally sought to collect as many fees, grants and livings as possible to protect himself from loss. An unforeseen political crisis could, even so, upset the best and most careful calculations. Once the wheel of fortune had turned in favour of rival claimants to the throne, as happened uncomfortably often during the Wars of the Roses, royal physicians, just like other courtiers, fell victim to their own success. Henry VII was understandably reluctant to entrust his person to a committed Yorkist such as Fryse, who was promptly evicted from his London properties. It is interesting to note that the previous owner now accused him of obtaining them 'by inordinat, undewe and damnable meanes ayenst the lawes of God and nature', and, implicitly, of exercising a sinister influence upon King Edward. On the other hand, Fryse's professional status and reputation protected him from serious reprisals, and he was allowed to end his days as a pensioner at the London church of Holy Trinity, Aldgate.[36]

It should not, however, be supposed that such potentially rich (albeit sometimes temporary) rewards lay within the grasp of every ambitious physician. As in all other spheres of medieval life, the scramble for patronage was unrelenting and fierce, made far harder in this case by foreign competition. The superiority of medical education on the Continent, most notably in Italy, the arrival in England of practitioners already in the service of the European princesses and noblewomen who married into the royal family, and the growing interest in humanism and astrology shown by leading members of the aristocracy conspired to place native graduates at a disadvantage. The language barrier so painfully encountered in London by the 'aliaunt', Eryke de Vedica, who could 'not speke the langage of thys land' and thus got fleeced by his patients, was unlikely to pose much of a problem in circles frequented by fluent Latinists and French speakers.[37] Pancius de Controne, physician, confidant and financial advisor to both Edward II and Edward III, drew over £150 a year at the peak of his influence; and although his fellow countryman, John Paladyn, had to make do with rather less (100 marks) for professional services, he was given £200 in 1367 to cover the cost of his journey home with a retinue of six servants.[38]

Peter of Florence and the Spaniard, Paul Gabrielis, also attended Edward III and his queen, albeit in return for more modest annuities of £40 and £20 respectively.[39]

During the early years of the fifteenth century foreigners dominated medical practice at Court. Not only did Henry IV retain his father's French physician, Louis Recoches, to whom he offered £40 a year, the wardenship of the hospital of St James, Westminster, and many generous gifts, but he also engaged at least three others from overseas, including the Jewish practitioner, Elias de Sabbato, who demanded a safe-conduct permitting him to travel with ten of his co-religionists. Elias stayed for only a year, but at least one of the four, David Nigarillis from Lucca, was so pleased with his post as warden of the royal mint and his annuity of 80 marks that he took out letters of denization.[40] As the Middle Ages drew to a close a small but steadily growing number of English students decided to improve both their medical training and prospects of promotion by studying abroad. Like Thomas Linacre, who took his MD at Padua in 1496, they were discouraged by the state of the faculties of medicine at Oxford and Cambridge and critical of the outdated scholasticism prevalent there.[41] The social and academic cachet of a foreign degree was, without doubt, important in securing the preferment of men such as William Hattecliffe and John Argentine, who advanced rapidly in the service of the Crown.[42]

The role of the university-trained physician quite often took the form of dietician, spiritual counsellor and general confidant rather than that of medical practitioner in the strict sense of the word. He had, of course, been educated in a tradition which regarded all aspects of human life as the legitimate preserve of medicine, and which, moreover, left the nuts and bolts of surgical procedure to craftsmen rather than academics. This division of labour was not merely a matter of convenience or even snobbery: the Church itself had insisted that senior clergy should have nothing to do with surgery, thus implicitly widening the gulf between theory and practice. A ruling of the fourth Lateran Council of 1215, concerned with clerical involvement in acts likely to cause bloodshed, had forbidden anyone in major orders (subdeacons, deacons or priests) from performing operations likely to require cautery or incision.[43] Exemptions could, as always, be made; but in England, where throughout the Middle Ages the overwhelming proportion of qualified medical students belonged to the priesthood, few sought to question or evade the ban. Nor was there much resistance elsewhere. At the University of Paris all graduates in medicine were required to swear a formal oath, from 1350 onwards, that they would never attempt any kind of 'manual surgery' whatsoever; and fear of the spiritual consequences of accidental homicide, which, as we have seen, weighed heavily with some surgeons, proved a universally powerful deterrent.[44]

Because of these restraints a significant number of physicians were reluctant even to venture beyond the safe confines of preventative medicine. And whatever personal scruples they may have felt about using a cautery or a lancet, those desirous of clerical preferment had little choice but to accept the prohibition, as the incumbent of a living with the cure of souls was expected either to be already in major orders or else to assume them within a short time. Just occasionally it might be possible to postpone this promotion, as Henry V managed to do on behalf of his physician, Nicholas Colnet, who quite probably had to combine surgery with medicine while serving with the royal army in France. Although Colnet occupied a rectory and two canonries worth up to 140 marks a year, he was allowed, in 1414, to remain in minor orders for seven years, during which time he could operate in the field with a clear conscience.[45] In the event, Colnet encountered none of the problems faced by Master Thomas Goldyngton, one of the few clerks in minor orders known to have been employed as a surgeon at the English Court. Perhaps Goldyngton's real mistake was to offer his professional services on the open market in Derby and Carlisle, where Edward III had assigned him the mastership of two hospitals (as well as a third near Alnwick). Having initially encouraged him to become an absentee pluralist, the king became anxious in 1348 about complaints that Goldyngton was conducting a lucrative practice to the detriment of his charges, and ordered formal inquiries to be held into any potential abuses. The return of the commissioners who investigated the situation at Carlisle found, on the contrary, that the surgeon had used money from his patients to rebuild the hospital and improve its finances, although his absences were noted less approvingly.[46]

The Prior of Carlisle, who headed this investigation, seems not to have been unduly concerned about Goldyngton's pastoral commitments, perhaps because he was not in higher orders. Far greater reservations had, however, long been voiced by the ecclesiastical authorities with regard to senior clergy who practised medicine, since it threatened to distract them from their religious obligations. Initially, restrictions were imposed upon regulars, who had taken monastic vows and were thus discouraged from mixing on intimate terms with the laity. (Sometimes these terms were very intimate indeed: the justices who met at York in 1218 heard how Simon, a monk and physician, had first seduced one of his patients and then murdered an informer who threatened to tell her husband.)[47] Secular clergy, too, might be tempted to concentrate upon the physical rather than the spiritual welfare of their flocks. In March 1494, for example, Walter Knyghtley, MD, the Chancellor of St Paul's Cathedral in London, was absolved by the Pope from a sentence of excommunication passed against him for his 'excess' in studying and practising medicine without the appropriate dispensation. A man 'of the greatest renown and most expert expounder of medicines', Knyghtley had discharged his teaching duties at Oxford with unusual zeal, and evidently had many patients. At least Alexander VI now gave him formal permission to treat them, 'short of incision and cauterization'.[48]

It is thus hardly surprising that medical education at Oxford and Cambridge differed so radically from that at some of the Italian universities, where most of the students were laymen. At Padua in the late fifteenth century, for example, there was a separate chair in anatomy and surgery; dissections took place regularly in winter; and it was possible to pursue a three-year course in surgery, covering the treatment of tumours, wounds, ulcers, dislocations and fractures.[49] Nevertheless, given the place of the physician in English society, a more scholastic, 'speculatif' training, concentrating on theory, could prove unexpectedly useful at times. His studies in natural philosophy would certainly have equipped him with all the information necessary to devise the appropriate *regimen* for his patron, most notably with regard to food and drink.

This seems to have been the principal task of Edward IV's medical staff, who fought a determined but doomed struggle to curb his notorious self-indulgence. However polished their rhetorical skills may have been, it is unlikely that they ever managed to exercise the control over his eating habits vested in them by royal ordinance:

> The doctour of physic stondith muche in the presence of the Kynges meles, by the councelyng or answering to the Kinges grace wich dyet is best according, and to the nature and operacion of all the metes. And comynly he shuld talke with the steward, chambrelayn, assewer [sewer] and the master cooke to devyse by counsayle what metes or drinkes is best according with the Kinges dyet; and whan he woll at mete and souper in the Kinges chambre or hall, or in his own chambre, devysyng the Kinges medecens.[50]

Panic about the possible spread of 'leper or pestylence', and the need to ensure that 'no perileous syk man' came near the royal person meant that Edward's physicians also bore a heavy responsibility with regard to the accurate diagnosis and fast removal of anybody suffering from unpleasant or contagious diseases. They were sometimes required to place their expertise in this respect at the service of the community: in 1468, for example, three prominent 'doctors of arts and physicians' then employed by the Crown were commissioned to examine a woman from Brentwood in Essex to see if she had leprosy. Their report, which contains a detailed account of the inspection, suggests that they took their duties seriously, 'considering her person, treating and handling her, and making their discourse of all the symptoms of the disease, whether it was found in her or no'. Having systematically worked their way through an impressive list of 'forty and more distinguishing symptoms', they certified her fit to live in the community.[51] Towards the end of the Middle Ages such assignments became a regular, if not routine, part of the work undertaken by senior members of the medical profession. In fifteenth-century France at least seventy-seven physicians were called upon to pronounce upon suspected cases of 'leprosy', besides being summoned to give evidence at autopsies and in legal proceedings where an expert opinion was needed.[52]

The first duty of the physician in royal, baronial or ecclesiastical service was, however, towards his patron, whose requirements could prove hard to satisfy. English sources have yet to reveal a daunting tale similar to that of the French physician, Seguin de Cohardi, who, in 1454, was commanded by René, Duke of Anjou and King of Naples, to examine a sick lion in his menagerie, but there is no lack of evidence about disputes over conditions of service and the requirement to give more conventional medical advice.[53] Although it offered a welcome degree of financial security, the promise of an annual fee, paid according to the terms of a legally binding contract, had distinct disadvantages. The indentures drawn up in 1449 between Humphrey, Duke of Buckingham, and his physician, Thomas Edmund (who obtained his MD at Oxford in the following year), hardly differed from those used to recruit members of the ducal affinity. In return for an annuity of ten marks a year, Edmund was to serve the duke for life, attending him before all others at home and abroad. This was a heavy commitment, which might require his presence for months at a time, and would obviously prevent him from accepting many other patients. Even so, as a shrewd and ambitious careerist, he clearly felt that his connexion with one of the most powerful men in England made the sacrifice worthwhile. The duke had over fifty-seven profitable livings in his patronage, and was, moreover, half-brother to Thomas Bourgchier, who became Archbishop of Canterbury in 1454. The calculation paid off: at least two of Edmund's benefices lay in Duke Humphrey's gift, and within a short time he had become the archbishop's secretary.[54]

Others found the burden of indentured service harder to bear, and fell out with their employers as a result. Simon Bredon, an eminent writer and collector of medical treatises, sometime fellow of Merton College, Oxford, and physician to Richard, Earl of Arundel, quarrelled spectacularly with the Prior of Lewes over the interpretation of his contract. The prior, who had retained him in 1361 with a generous fee of £20 a year and the promise of free board and lodging, 'for his good and noteworthy service and counsel to us and our monastery, performed and to be performed henceforward', felt that he might justifiably stop the payments after Bredon had not only failed to appear when summoned, but had even refused to send any medicines or offer advice. This view was upheld in court, where one of the judges emphasized the special obligation incumbent upon a practitioner. 'Illness is so privy', he argued, 'that only a physician can diagnose; the physician is bound to counsel and aid his patient; since the patient himself cannot diagnose in order to notify the physician, nor, because of illness travel to him, the physician has to travel to the patient.'[55]

Not surprisingly, then, many practitioners preferred to work on an *ad hoc* basis, taking fees from wealthy patients as and when their services were required, rather than pledging their undivided attention to one particular individual, family or institution. Edward, Duke of Buckingham (great-grandson to Duke Humphrey), favoured this system, and relied upon a small group of medical advisers, including Thomas Bentley, MD, and Henry Hawte, who had been admitted to Oxford University on the recommendation of Elizabeth of York, as being 'young in years, but old in knowledge and learning'. When going on pilgrimage or travelling up to London, the duke might summon Master John Bartlet of Oxford or Stephen Tey, a Canterbury physician, paying them at a daily rate of about 6s.8d., which obviously suited them better than a permanent contract. If his behaviour towards other long-suffering members of his household is any guide, Buckingham (who was still relatively young and fit) can hardly have been an easy patron. Budgets for the ducal entourage allowed for the daily presence of one physician about his person, but prudently assumed that there would be a rapid turnover of personnel.[56]

At all levels of the profession, from humble empiric to royal physician, medical men accepted payment in kind. Plate, jewels or robes could, after all, be converted into hard cash, and had a greater immediate value than the promise of a pension which, as noted previously, might soon fall into arrears. As well as leaving monetary bequests worth well over £100 in his will of 1417, the above-mentioned Nicholas Colnet made numerous legacies of valuable plate and clothing accumulated during a mere four years as 'clerk, serjeant and physician' to Henry V. Whatever the risks to his immortal soul, service with the king in France had certainly proved profitable: from the Duke of Orléans, whom he apparently treated after his capture at Agincourt, he received an elaborately worked silver cup and a ewer, which was by no means the finest piece in his collection.[57] Kings and noblemen were generally happy to place their medical staff at the disposal of relatives and distinguished visitors (or even prisoners), who proved generous in return. A ruby ring, given by the Duchess of Norfolk to Richard III's physician, William Lempster, MD, may well have followed a successful cure, although if the great quantities of money and plate listed in his will are any guide she can only have been one of many satisfied patients.[58]

Medieval satirists never tired of denouncing physicians for their cynical exploitation of the naïve and vulnerable. Without doubt, many people were prepared to pay any price and believe any promises in the hope of recovering their health; and some did indeed fall victim to unscrupulous practitioners. Men and women suffering from unsightly skin diseases, which might easily be taken for leprosy, were particularly susceptible, since the social consequences of a positive diagnosis could be so devastating. In 1408, for example, one John Clotes came before the court of the Mayor of London to complain about his treatment at the hands of a Flemish 'leech' named John Luter. The latter had taken delivery of fifteen semi-precious jewels called 'serpentyns', a gold tablet and a sword, together worth almost £9, in return for curing him of '*le lepre*'. Rigorous interrogation by the mayor revealed a tale of fear and self-deception on the part of the plaintiff and of callous opportunism on that of the leech, who was found guilty of fraud.[59]

Cases of this kind, and no doubt gossip about the massive salaries of up to £100 or more earned by a tiny handful of practitioners at Court provided social commentators with powerful ammunition. The stock image of the grasping, heartless physician (a figure satirized by writers from Martial to Trollope) occupied a prominent place in the medieval rogues' gallery, alongside the crooked lawyer and lecherous monk. Law and medicine were, indeed, often held to corrode the sensibilities and sharpen the appetite for gain in exactly the same way:

Phisiciens and advocates
Gon right by the same yates;
They selle her science for wynnyng,
And haunte her craft for gret getyng.
Her wynnyng is of such swetnesse
That if a man falle in siknesse,
They are full glad, for her encres;
For by her wille, withoute lees,
Everich man shulde be sek,
And though they die, they sette not a lek.
After, whanne they the gold have take,
Full litel care for hem they make.
They wolde that fourty were seke at onys,
Ye, two hundred, in flesh and bonys,
And yit two thousand, as I gesse,
For to encrecen her richesse.
They wole not worchen, in no wise,
But for lucre and coveitise.[60]

Nor could satirists resist a well-aimed gibe at the elegant clothes which distinguished the most successful – and by implication most rapacious – medical men: Chaucer's Physician wears the traditional colours of red and grey favoured by the profession, but his robe is expensively lined 'with taffata and with sendal'. Perhaps the poet was thinking of real-life examples, such as William Tankerville, who received £4 and a fur-trimmed robe worth 26s.8d. each year from the monks of Westminster Abbey until 1368, when his dress allowance went up to 30s. so that he could afford a gown 'lined with three furs'.[61] That fat fees and costly apparel could be earned by men whose advice seemed little more than basic common sense provided another source of grievance. As William Langland pointed out with some asperity, physicians would be largely redundant if people ate and drank in moderation:

And if thow diete thee thus, I dar legge [wager] myn eris
That Phisik shal his furred hood for his fode selle,
And his cloke of Calabre with all the knappes [buttons] of golde,
And be fayn, by my feith, his phisik to lete,
And lerne to laboure with lond lest liflode hym faille.
Ther aren mo lieres than leches – Lord hem amende!
They do men deye thorugh hir drynkes er destynee it wolde.[62]

Langland's great poem, *Piers Plowman*, ends with an apocalyptic vision of the coming of Antichrist, in which medicine plays a small but characteristically inglorious role. Despite the size of his fee, the physician can provide his patient, Life, with nothing more effective than a 'glasen howve' (a glass helmet), which will shatter at the first blow from Death's standard-bearer, Elde (Old Age). Nor is he any better equipped to withstand the onslaught himself:

And Lif fleigh for feere to Phisik after helpe,
And bisoughte hym of socour, and of his salve hadde,
And gaf hym gold, good woon, that gladede his herte -
And thei gyven hym ageyn a glazene howve.
Lyf leeved that lechecrafte lette sholde Elde,
And dryven awey Deeth with dyas [remedies] and drogges.
And Elde auntred hym on Lyf – and at the laste he hitte
A phisicien with a furred hood, that he fel in a palsie,
And there dyed that doctour er thre dayes after.
'Now I se', seide Lif, 'that surgerie ne phisik
May noght a myte availle to medle ayein Elde.'[63]

The confrontation between Death and Physic, as personified in the form of an expensively clothed doctor of medicine carrying a glass urinal, assumed particular poignancy as successive outbreaks of plague swept the country from 1348 onwards (colour plate 15). Paradoxically, however, the powerlessness of conventional medicine to halt the disease did nothing to slacken the demand for professional advice. On the contrary, those who could afford to do so continued to retain their own medical staff, often paying even higher fees than before, while the rest provided a ready market for tracts about the best ways of avoiding infection. Bishop Mitford's physician, John Malvern, was himself the author of such a work, which survives in several copies.[64]

Far from damaging the relationship between doctor and patient, the unpredictable and often painful aspects of medieval medicine tended to bring them closer together. Fear of death, and perhaps even more of protracted suffering could easily upset the balance of power, placing the seriously ill in a dependent, sometimes even subservient, position. A dramatic instance of this reversal of roles, which confirmed onlookers in their worst suspicions about calculating, upstart physicians, occurred during the last months of Louis XI of France (d.1483). His horror of dying was apparently such that he would not allow anyone so much as to mention the subject in his presence, while at the same time he meekly submitted himself to constant humiliation at the hands of the medical profession. The irony of a situation in which the imperious despot, who had ruled his court with a rod of iron, now cringed in terror before a mere leech made a painful impression on one of his advisors:

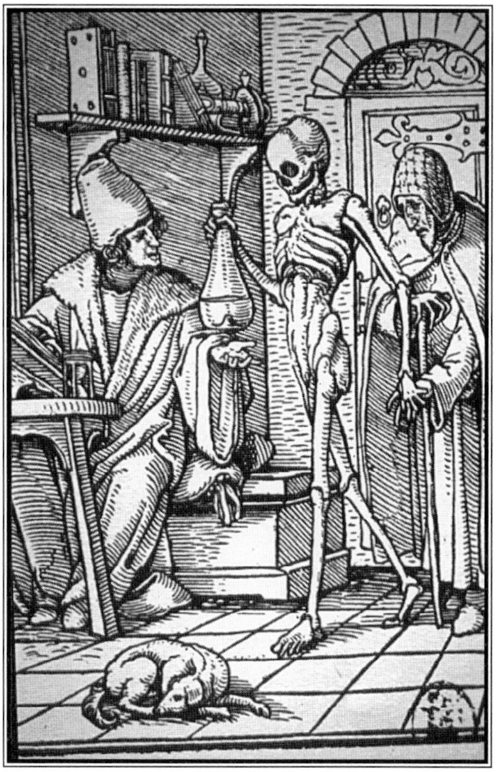

A warning to medical practitioners. Despite his obvious learning and mastery of scientific knowledge, the physician cannot 'heal himself' (Luke 4: 23), and is as susceptible to mortality as his most feeble and elderly patient.

> How wretched it was for this king to endure such fears and such suffering. He had his physician, called Master Jacques Cotier, to whom he gave 55,000 crowns in cash in five months, which is at the rate of 10,000 crowns a month, and the bishopric of Amiens for his nephew, and other offices and lands for him and for his friends. The aforesaid physician was so incredibly rude that one would not say such outrageous and offensive things to a menial servant as he said to him; and the aforesaid Lord King feared him so much that he did not dare to send him away. Even though he complained about him in conversation he simply did not dare replace him, as he had done with all his other servants, because the aforesaid physician audaciously said these words to him: 'I know very well that one morning you'll send me packing, just like the others, but by the ——', here he swore a terrible oath, 'you won't last another eight days afterwards!' These words hung so heavily upon him, that from then on he could only flatter him and ply him with gifts. Which was for him absolute purgatory on earth, given the unquestioning deference shown to him by everybody, including the great.[65]

Whether Cotier had made an astute psychological assessment of a difficult patient, or was merely (as Louis's courtiers supposed) an ambitious opportunist out to line his own pockets, we shall never know. Clearly, however, the royal or baronial physician was uniquely placed to exploit the fears and weaknesses of his patron, and could easily, almost imperceptibly, insinuate himself into a position of political power. This was particularly true of the academically distinguished and able graduates recruited into the service of the English Crown during the fifteenth century: indeed, two such men, John Somerset and William Hatteclіffe, are now better known for their administrative rather than their medical careers. But both possessed doctorates in medicine, and both had originally been engaged as royal physicans. Between 1428 and 1439 Somerset accumulated fees to the value of £140 a year in this capacity, only then taking up office as Chancellor of the Exchequer.[66] Hatteclіffe likewise spent a long period as 'doctour in medicyns and phisicion', first to Henry VI and then to his more robust successor, Edward IV, who made him his secretary and deployed him on a number of diplomatic missions.[67]

The nature of the *regimen sanitatis*, which effectively concerned every aspect of the subject's life, from sexual behaviour to his or her general state of mind, gave the physician *carte blanche* to proffer advice on the most delicate topics. If, as was so often the case, he had taken orders, this advice would undoubtedly concern the spiritual as well as the physical health of his patron. His astrological skills would also be in constant demand, making him the repository of highly confidential and even dangerous information. At some point the medical practitioner became a trusted personal advisor, his position strengthened by the already close relationship which bound him to his employer, his suitability attested by an impressive university background. We can actually observe this moment of transition in the career of Lewis Caerleon, MD, a noted astrologer and mathematician, who attended Lady Margaret Beaufort in the summer of 1483, when she was plotting to put her son on the throne:

> This Margaret for want of health usid th'advyse of a physition namyd Lewys, a Welsheman born, who, because he was a grave man and of no smaule experience, she was wont oftentimes to conferre frely with all, and with him famylyarly to lament her adversitie. And she, being a wyse woman, after the slaughter of king Edwardes children was knowen, began to hope well of hir soones fortune, supposing that that dede wold withowt dowt proove for

> the profyt of the commonwelth, yf yt might chaunce the bloode of King Henry the Sixth and of king Edward to be intermenglyd by affynytie. . . . Wherfor furthwith not neglecting so great oportunytie, as they wer consulting togythers, she utteryd to Lewys that the time was now coom when as king Edwardes eldest dowghter might be geaven in maryage to hir soon Henry, and that king Rycherd, accountyd of all men enemy to his countree, might easyly be dejectyd from all honor and bereft the realme, and therfor prayd him to deale secretly with the quene of suche affayre; for the quene also usyd his head, because he was a very learnyd physytion. Lewys nothing lyngeryng spak with the quene, as yeat remaning in sayntuarie, and declaryd the matter not as delyveryd to him in charge but as devysyd of his owne heade. . . .[68]

Within a short while, Caerleon, whose 'scyence' enabled him to come and go as he pleased without exciting suspicion, had hatched a conspiracy between the two women. From his point of view, at least, the failure of the ensuing rebellion was not an unmitigated disaster, since the

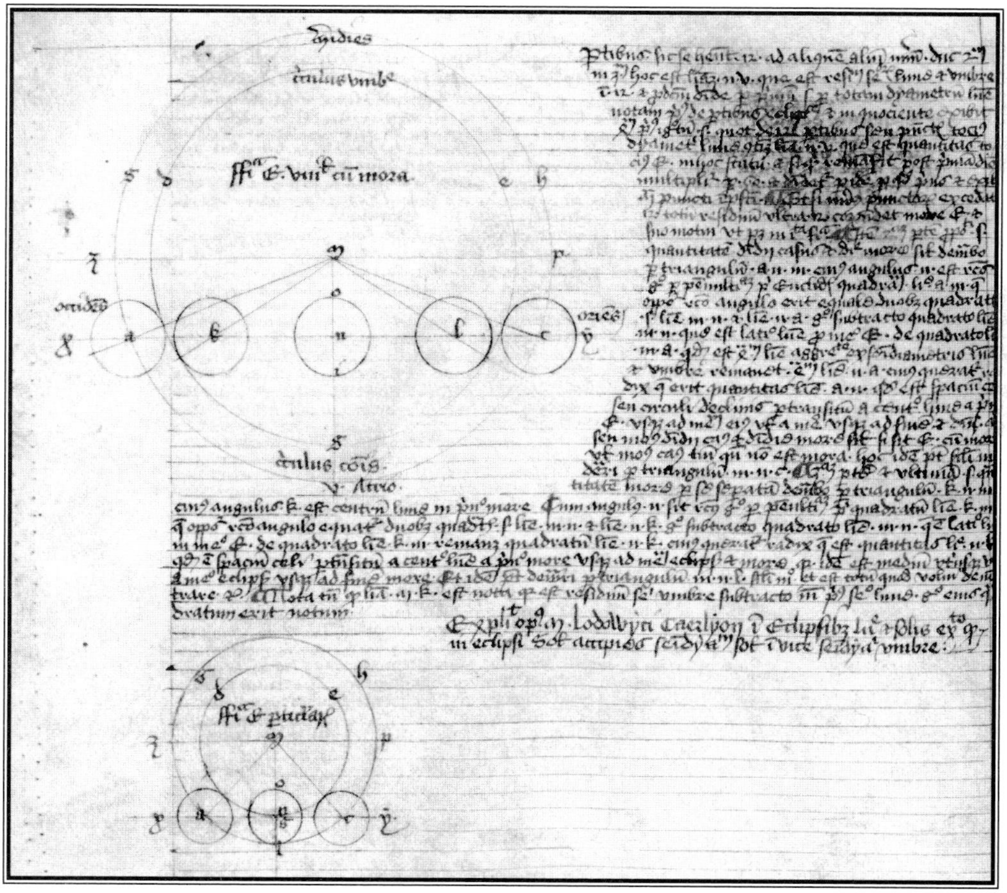

Calculations about solar eclipses from an astronomical treatise compiled by Lady Margaret Beaufort's physician, Lewis Caerleon, during his imprisonment in the Tower of London. He was incarcerated after the failure of the 1483 rebellion, in which he played a notable part.

authorities allowed him to pursue his astrological studies in prison. Perhaps he forecast the eventual triumph of his patron and his promotion to the post of royal physician at a fee of 60 marks a year: appropriately, under the circumstances, he treated the new queen, whose marriage he had helped to bring about.[69]

It is interesting to note that Caerleon had been fined 20s. in 1466 for failing to deliver the lectures in medicine required of him as a regent at Cambridge.[70] His dissatisfaction with the system was probably as much professional as personal, since there was a strong feeling among graduate physicians that the universities should be doing more to control the licensing of medical practitioners throughout England and not simply in Oxford and Cambridge as was then the case. In theory, any leech or physician working in Oxford was supposed to have attended classes in medicine for four years (eight if they did not already possess an MA), and to have undergone an examination before the regents; but the enfeebled faculty of medicine had problems enforcing its authority even on home ground, and could do nothing elsewhere to stop women and other 'unlearned' folk from treating the sick.[71] It was, of course, always difficult to prevent students from taking on patients before they were properly qualified: in France, where the rules were much stricter and the great faculties of medicine at Paris and Montpellier far more powerful, about a third of practitioners known to have attended a university never completed their studies or bothered with a licence. Since, however, these men had received some academic training and often possessed a degree in arts, they did not constitute the threat to professional standards (and professional incomes) posed by 'outsiders', who could expect little quarter.[72]

Encouraged by examples of firm action from across the Channel, and perhaps also heartened by the interest in medicine shown by Henry V and his brothers, senior members of the two university 'scoles of fisyk' begged the parliament of 1421 to introduce a national system of licensing, supported by harsh penalties. Having established that all men were ruled by the three 'sciences' of theology, medicine and law, which ought, in turn, to be 'practised principaly by the most connyng men in the same', they went on to protest that:

> many unconnyng and unapproved in the forsayd science practiseth, and specialy in fysyk, so that in this roialme is every man, be he never so lewed, takyng upon hym practyse, y-suffred [allowed] to use hit, to grete harme and slaughtre of many men. Where if no man practised theryn but al only connynge men and approved sufficeantly y-lerned in art, filosofye and fisyk, as hit is kept in other londes and roialms, ther shulde many man that dyeth, for defaute of help, lyve, and no man perysh by unconnyng. Wherfore pleseth to youre excellent wysdomes that ought, aftre your soule, have mo entendance to your body . . . to ordeine and make statuit, perpetualy to be straytly y-used and kept, that no man, of no maner estate, degre or condicion, practyse in Fisyk from this tyme forward bot he have long tyme y-used the scoles of fisyk withynne som universitee, and be graduated in the same. That is to sey, but he be bacheler or doctour of fisyk, havynge lettres testimonyalx sufficeantz of on of those degrees of the universite in the whiche he toke his degree yn. Undur peyne of long emprisonement, and paynge xl li. [£40] to the Kyng; and that no woman use the practyse of fisyk undre the same payne.[73]

Although it received the royal assent (which accorded similar powers of licensing to masters of surgery within their respective guilds), this petition was clearly doomed to failure. Even had the faculties of medicine at Oxford and Cambridge actually managed to produce a large and regular supply of graduates, the demand for the expensive, often rather esoteric services they were trained to offer would have been strictly limited. The petitioners must soon have realized how impractical such a scheme would be, and elected instead to exploit their obvious influence at Court and in the City by confining their efforts to London.

Detailed plans for a joint college of physicians and surgeons, with absolute control over the licensing and practice of all forms of medicine in the capital, were submitted to the mayor and aldermen just two years later. The authorities pronounced them 'good and honest and accordyng to open reason', but, having given their approval, then proceeded to undermine the college's authority by allowing the London barbers to operate independently (as explained in the next chapter). A permanent regulatory body of this kind would have given a valuable boost to academic medical studies, since the founders clearly envisaged that the 'faculte of physyk' would be composed largely, if not exclusively, of graduates. They may well have been familiar with existing models in Milan, Nimes and Bordeaux, where chartered corporations of physicians remained quite separate from the universities, but accepted only men with medical degrees. The qualifications demanded of the rector, who had to 'be doctour of medicyns, maistre of arte and philosophie, or a bachiler in medicyns of long tyme, in vertue and konnynge approved' set the tone, the first (and only) incumbent being none other than Gilbert Kymer, MD, physician to Henry V, Henry VI and Humphrey, Duke of Gloucester, and future Chancellor of Oxford University.[74]

For the best part of a century after the collapse of the London college the country's leading practitioners resigned themselves to the status quo, doing little, either individually or collectively, to resuscitate the venture. A combination of idealism, drive and (most important) powerful connexions was needed to convince the authorities that such a scheme would indeed be viable, and, moreover, of practical benefit to the community as a whole. Thomas Linacre, who had observed at first hand the impressive scale of medical provision in Italian cities, and was painfully aware of the disorganized and isolated state of the medical profession in England, was ideally suited for this task. His enthusiasm for the 'civic humanism' currently advocated by Thomas More and Erasmus found a ready response at Court, which he eagerly exploited (his first published translation of Galen, made in 1517 from Greek into Latin, was dedicated to Henry VIII). Interest in enlightened schemes for public health and welfare was also strong in the City, where Linacre had many friends with concerns similar to his own. The outbreak there of a particularly severe epidemic of sweating sickness, followed by plague, in 1517, proved an even more urgent incentive for prompt measures to improve medical services, as also did anxiety about the number of quacks and empirics ready to exploit the sick (see Chapter VIII).[75]

Royal letters patent incorporating the new college of physicians were awarded one year later, in response to a petition from Linacre, five associates and his friend and patient, Cardinal Wolsey, whose political star was then firmly in the ascendant. The preamble refers quite openly to the superior standards of health care then available in Italy and other parts of Europe, and the desire to emulate the best continental models.[76] The English had, in fact, to look no further than France (where about 15 per cent of known physicians appear to have been employed under contract by urban communities) for examples of effective organization and the involvement of the medical profession in civic life.[77] As a first move towards this goal, the college was authorized to examine and license practitioners in London, but when its charter was confirmed by parliament, in 1523, these powers were extended to cover the whole country. Henceforward, only graduates might 'exercyse or practyse in physyk through Englond' without being formally approved by the president and three fellows.[78]

Later statutes of the college, drawn up in 1555, suggest that from the start candidates for admission were expected to possess a distinguished academic record, as well as proving their familiarity with the Galenic corpus. Perhaps for this reason, membership remained low: a mere twelve fellows are recorded in 1523, and only six more at the end of the 1530s. Despite the royal favour and support which they enjoyed, it thus seems unlikely that this small group of physicians could have taken more than a few halting steps in the direction mapped out by Linacre, especially where their scrutiny of other practitioners was concerned.[79] In this respect they had much to learn from the surgeons, whose artisan status may have made them socially inferior to graduate physicians but at least provided them with a solid organizational structure, as well as a firm economic and legal base from which to launch their campaign for a craft monopoly.

NOTES

1. For an early depiction of the use of a catheter, see A.S. Lyons and R.J. Petrucelli, *Medicine: An Illustrated History* (New York, 1978), p. 396.
2. *Household Accounts from Medieval England*, ed. C.M. Woolgar (Records of Social and Economic History, new series, XVII, 1992), pp. 261–430.
3. C.H. Talbot and E.A. Hammond, *The Medical Practitioners in Medieval England* (London, 1965), pp. 166–7.
4. *Household Accounts from Medieval England*, op. cit., p. 428.
5. *Hippocratic Writings*, ed. G.E.R. Lloyd (pbk, London, 1983), p. 206.
6. P. Kibre, 'Arts and Medicine in the Universities of the Later Middle Ages', *Mediaevalia Louaniensia*, series one, VI (1978), p. 215.
7. F.M. Getz, 'The Faculty of Medicine before 1500', in *The History of the University of Oxford, Volume II, Late Medieval Oxford*, ed. J.I. Catto and R. Evans (Oxford, 1992), p. 383.
8. D.R. Leader, *A History of the University of Cambridge, Volume I, The University to 1546* (Cambridge, 1988), p. 203.
9. William Caxton, *The Game and Playe of the Chesse*, ed. W.E.A. Axon (London, 1883), p. 119.
10. Kibre, op. cit., pp. 220–1; Erasmus of Rotterdam, *In Praise of Folly*, ed. H. Hopewell Hudson (Princeton, 1970), p. 45.
11. Leader, op. cit., p. 204; Getz, op. cit., p. 383; C.H. Talbot, 'Medical Education in the Middle Ages', in *The History of Medical Education*, ed. C.D. O'Malley (Berkeley, California, 1970), pp. 76, 82.
12. J.M. Fletcher, 'Linacre's Lands and Lecturerships', in *Essays on the Life and Work of Thomas Linacre c. 1460–1524*, ed. F. Maddison, M. Pelling and C. Webster (Oxford, 1977), pp. 128–31, 168.
13. Caxton, op. cit., pp. 120–1.
14. Getz, op. cit., p. 384; Leader, op. cit., p. 203. For details of the Parisian medical syllabus, which included works by Rhazes, Averroes and Avicenna, see P. Kibre, *Studies in Medieval Science: Alchemy, Astrology, Mathematics and Medicine* (London, 1984), article XII, pp. 223–5.
15. Geoffrey Chaucer, *Works*, ed. F.N. Robinson (Oxford, 1970), p. 21. That Chaucer's list of the Physician's professional attributes is in no way satirical should already be apparent from the previous chapter. Certainly, his reading matter is exactly what might have been expected of a serious medical student. See H.E. Ussery, *Chaucer's Physician: Medicine and Literature in Fourteenth-Century England* (Tulane, 1971), pp. 103–4.
16. Getz, op. cit., pp. 390–1. H.P. Cholmeley's study, *John of Gaddesden and the Rosa Medicinae* (Oxford, 1912), is anecdotal rather than scholarly.
17. Getz, op. cit., pp. 382, 394; Leader, op. cit., p. 202. For a discussion of medical education in French universities see D. Jacquart, *Le Milieu Médical en France du XIIe au XVe Siècle* (Haute Études Médiévales et Modernes, series 5, XLVI, 1981), pp. 63–71; and for Italy, N.G. Siraisi, *Medieval and Early Renaissance Medicine* (pbk, Chicago, 1990), pp. 57–64.
18. V.L. Bullough, 'Medical Study at Medieval Oxford', *Speculum*, XXXVI (1961), pp. 600–12.
19. Fletcher, op. cit., p. 119.
20. Ibid., pp. 110–11.
21. Siraisi, op. cit., p. 61; C.B. Schmitt, 'Thomas Linacre and Italy', in *Essays on the Life and Work of Thomas Linacre*, op. cit., p. 58.
22. Leader, op. cit., pp. 202–3; Getz, op. cit., pp. 383–4.
23. A.B. Emden, *Biographical Register of the University of Cambridge* (Cambridge, 1963), pp. 243, 262–3; *Calendar of Patent Rolls, 1461–67*, p. 79; Talbot and Hammond, op. cit., pp. 414–15.
24. Fletcher, op. cit., pp. 110, 120.

25. For a general discussion of remuneration see C. Rawcliffe, 'The Profits of Practice: the Wealth and Status of Medical Men in Later Medieval England', *Social History of Medicine*, I (1988), pp. 61–78.
26. John Faceby, MD, for example, was awarded £100 p.a., with the promise of a pension of £20 a year for his widow, in 1444, plus a daily allowance of 1s. and a gown every year in 1445 (*Calendar of Patent Rolls, 1441–46*, pp. 271, 334); Jordan of Canterbury got only 20 marks a year, in 1338, but his two sons were later paid 6d. a day each, and his daughter 7½d. because of his sterling services (ibid., *1338–40*, p. 194; *1350–54*, pp. 357, 501); Thomas Bemmesley drew £40 a year from 1483 (ibid., *1476–85*, no. 1067), as did Walter Lempster, MD, from 1486 (ibid., *1485–94*, p. 48), and William Hattecliffe, MD, from 1452 (ibid., *1452–61*, p. 26). See also notes 35–7 below.
27. *The Register of Edward the Black Prince*, ed. M.C.B. Dawes (4 vols, London, 1930–3), vol. IV, pp. 94, 208, 454.
28. *John of Gaunt's Register, Part I, 1371–75*, ed. S. Armitage-Smith (Camden Soc., third series, XX, 1911), nos 547–9; *John of Gaunt's Register, 1379–83*, ed. E.C. Lodge and R.S. Somerville (Camden Soc., third series, LVI, 1937), no. 1734; *Calendar of Patent Rolls, 1374–77*, pp. 354–5, 368, 382; *1377–81*, pp. 320, 340.
29. A.B. Emden, *Biographical Register of the University of Oxford to 1500* (3 vols, Oxford, 1957–9), vol. I, pp. 49–50. Arundel was last paid for medical services in 1456 (PRO, E101/410/14, f. 19).
30. *Calendar of Papal Petitions, 1342–1491*, pp. 19, 51. Talbot and Hammond (op. cit., pp. 371–2) imply that Lyndrigge was attending only the Earl of Surrey at this time.
31. *Calendar of Patent Rolls, 1391–96*, pp. 584, 621, 705; *1396–99*, p. 266. Middleton also received a messuage in London, where he might store 'divers goods' (probably medicines) for the king (ibid., p. 41). In 1399 Richard II likewise granted his physician, Geoffrey Melton, 40 marks a year until he could be found a benefice without cure of souls worth £40 p.a., or with cure to the value of 100 marks (ibid., p. 577).
32. Talbot and Hammond, op. cit., p. 362; T.F. Tout, *Chapters in the Administrative History of Medieval England* (6 vols, Manchester, 1920–33), vol. IV, pp. 9, 222. Richard actually attended Tideman's enthronement as Bishop of Worcester.
33. *Calendar of Patent Rolls, 1461–67*, pp. 79, 188, 270. In 1473 Fryse, who came originally from Friesland but must by then have been thoroughly Anglicized, was granted letters of denization (ibid., *1467–77*, p. 396).
34. PRO, E404/74/1/110, 75/1/20; *Calendar of Patent Rolls, 1467–77*, pp. 336, 512.
35. Rawcliffe, op. cit., p. 73; Leader, op. cit., pp. 206–7.
36. See C. Rawcliffe, 'Consultants, Careerists and Conspirators: Royal Doctors in the Time of Richard III', *The Ricardian*, no. 106 (1989), pp. 250–8, for a fuller discussion of the effects of dynastic change on the upper reaches of the medical profession.
37. PRO, C1/64/154.
38. Talbot and Hammond, op. cit., pp. 234–7, 174–5. Siraisi (op. cit., p. 62) points out that although he was no more than 'modestly successful' at home in Lucca, Controne was able by virtue of his foreign training to convert a 'respectable but hardly distinguished record' into a position of great power and influence at the English Court.
39. *Calendar of Patent Rolls, 1367–70*, pp. 42, 103; *1374–77*, pp. 354, 552; Tout, op. cit., vol. IV, p. 182.
40. For Recoches see PRO, DL28/3/2, f. 11; E101/404/21, f. 45; *Calendar of Patent Rolls, 1399–1401*, p. 228; *1401–5*, pp. 9, 170, 345; for de Sabbato, C.H. Talbot, *Medicine in Medieval England* (London, 1967), p. 205; and for Nigarillis, *Calendar of Patent Rolls, 1408–13*, pp. 28, 269, 363, 392. Henry IV's other foreign physician was Peter Dalcobace, from Portugal (Talbot and Hammond, op. cit., pp. 246–7; PRO, E404/34/101).
41. Fletcher, op. cit., p. 118.
42. For Argentine's career see Leader, op. cit., pp. 207–10; and for Hattecliffe's, note 62 below.
43. D.W. Amundsen, 'Medieval Canon Law on Medical and Surgical Practice by the Clergy', *Bulletin of the History of Medicine*, LII (1978), pp. 40–2.
44. Jacquart, op. cit., pp. 56–9.
45. *Calendar of Papal Letters, 1404–15*, p. 507; Talbot and Hammond, op. cit., pp. 220–2.
46. Talbot and Hammond, op. cit., pp. 345–6; *Calendar of Inquisitions Miscellaneous*, vol. II, no. 1456; vol. III, no. 6.
47. Amundsen, op. cit., pp. 28–38; *Rolls of the Justices in Eyre for Yorkshire*, ed. D.M. Stenton (Selden Soc., LVI, 1937), pp. 377–8.
48. *Calendar of Papal Letters, 1492–98*, p. 180. This incident is not noted in the biography of Knyghtley provided by Talbot and Hammond (op. cit., pp. 367–9).
49. Schmitt, op. cit., p. 59.
50. A.R. Myers, *The Household of Edward IV* (Manchester, 1959), pp. 123–4.
51. *Calendar of Close Rolls, 1468–76*, pp. 30–1. P. Richards (*The Medieval Leper and his Northern Heirs* (Cambridge, 1977), pp. 40–1) believes this procedure (with its emphasis upon humoral theory) reflects 'the iron grip of medievalism on medical practice', although it might be argued that the scrupulous care shown by the physicians and their concern for the patient cast contemporary medicine in an extremely favourable light.
52. Jacquart, op. cit., pp. 288–9.
53. E. Wickersheimer, *Dictionnaire Biographique des Médecins en France au Moyen Age* (Paris, 1936), p. 734. His solicitude

for dumb animals was rewarded: in the same year Seguin was retained as civic physician at Angers, at a generous salary; and he eventually acquired the lordship of Atheny in Maine.

54. C. Rawcliffe, *The Staffords, Earls of Stafford and Dukes of Buckingham 1394–1521* (Cambridge, 1978), pp. 83, 239.

55. J.B. Post, 'Doctor Versus Patient: Two Fourteenth Century Law Suits', *Medical History*, XVI (1972), pp. 298–300; Bredon's contribution to medical studies at Oxford is assessed by Getz (op. cit., p. 393).

56. For Bentley see PRO, E36/220, ff. 2v, 15v; Talbot and Hammond, op. cit., p. 334; Emden, *Biographical Register of the University of Oxford*, op. cit., vol. I, p. 170; for Hawte, ibid., vol. II, p. 886; PRO, SP1/22, ff. 64, 72; for Bartlet and Tey, Longleat House (Mss of the Marquess of Bath), Ms. 6415, f.6. Buckingham's household ordinance is PRO, E101/518/5, part 1.

57. *The Register of Henry Chichele*, ed. E.F. Jacob (Canterbury and York Soc., XLII, 1937), pp. 215–16.

58. Talbot and Hammond, op. cit., pp. 396–70.

59. *Calendar of Plea and Memoranda Rolls of London, 1381–1412*, p. 289. Attitudes towards the leper are discussed above, pp. 14–17.

60. Chaucer, op. cit., p. 618. This is from his (or possibly another poet's) translation of *The Romance of the Rose*.

61. Ibid., p. 21; Talbot and Hammond, op. cit., p. 417. The changing status of *medici* employed by the Westminster monks is described in B. Harvey, *Living and Dying in England 1100–1540: The Monastic Experience* (Oxford, 1993), pp. 82–3.

62. William Langland, *The Vision of Piers Plowman*, ed. A.V.C. Schmidt (London, 1978), p. 75 (B passus VI, vv. 268–74).

63. Ibid., pp. 256–7 (B passus XX, vv. 168–79).

64. Talbot and Hammond, op. cit., p. 167.

65. Philippe de Commynes, *Memoires*, ed. J. Calmette (3 vols, Paris, 1924–5), vol. II, p. 319. Cotier was not the first physician to make a personal fortune out of treating a French king. Guillaume Harsley, who cared for Charles VI during his first bout of insanity, was, according to Froissart, paid over 1,000 gold crowns for his efforts. 'It is the object of all medical men to gain large salaries and as much profit as possible', noted the chronicler, adding that Harsley 'died very rich, possessed of 30,000 francs. He was the most niggardly man of his time: his whole pleasure was amassing money, and never spending a farthing at home, but eating and drinking abroad whenever he could' (*Sir John Froissart's Chronicles*, ed. and trans. T. Jones (4 vols, Haford, 1803–5), vol. IV, pp. 367–8).

66. See note 33 above. Somerset was certainly still the king's physician in 1430, when he is described as '*nostre cher bien aime clerc, meistre es medicines et nostre doctour*' (PRO, E404/46/299); and in 1432 he received an additional £60 a year 'for his services about the King's person, both teaching him and preserving his health' (*Calendar of Patent Rolls, 1429–36*, p. 241). For his appointment as chancellor, see ibid., *1436–41*, p. 418.

67. Hattecliffe's career as secretary is examined in J. Otway-Ruthven, *The King's Secretary and the Signet Office in the Fifteenth Century* (Cambridge, 1939), pp. 64–8, 73, 77, 79–80, 85, 103–4, 124, 135, 155. For his medical career, see Talbot and Hammond, op. cit., pp. 398–9.

68. *Polydore Vergil's English History*, ed. H. Ellis (Camden Soc., XXIX, 1845), pp. 195–6.

69. For Caerleon's career see P. Kibre, 'Lewis of Caerleon, Doctor of Medicine, Astronomer and Mathematician', *Isis*, XLIII (1952), pp. 100–8; and Leader, op. cit., p. 154.

70. Emden, *Biographical Register of the University of Cambridge*, op. cit., pp. 116–17.

71. Getz, op. cit., p. 384.

72. Jacquart, op. cit., p. 62.

73. *Rotuli Parliamentorum*, vol. IV, p. 158. Conciliar approval, given in the name of the absent Henry V, is noted on p. 130.

74. T. Beck, *The Cutting Edge: Early History of the Surgeons of London* (London, 1974), pp. 63–7. Although he is now remembered for his association with Humphrey, Duke of Gloucester, and Oxford University (Emden, *Biographical Register of the University of Oxford*, op. cit., vol. II, pp. 1068–9; Talbot and Hammond, op. cit., pp. 60–3; and above p. 90), Kymer was also close to Henry V, who assigned him 40 marks in 1417 (PRO, E404/33/19), and Henry VI, who summoned him when he was 'occupied and laboured as ye know wel with sikenes', to provide expert help (SC1/43/182).

75. C. Webster, 'Thomas Linacre and the Foundation of the College of Physicians', in *Essays on the Life and Work of Thomas Linacre*, op. cit., pp. 198–222.

76. G.N. Clark, *A History of the Royal College of Physicians of London* (2 vols, Oxford, 1964), vol. I, pp. 54–61.

77. Jacquart, op. cit., p. 121.

78. *Statutes of the Realm*, vol. III, 14 and 15 Hen. VIII, c. 5.

79. Webster, op. cit., pp. 210, 217. See also Clark, op. cit., Chapter V, and pp. 376–92 for the text of the 1555 statutes.

CHAPTER SIX

THE SURGEON

Nedeful it is that a surgian be of a complexcioun weel proporciound, and that his complexcioun be temperat. . . . A surgian muste have handis weel schape, longe smale fyngris, and his body not quakynge, and al must ben of sutil witt, for al thing that longith to siurgie may not with lettris ben writen. He muste studie in alle the parties of philofie and in logik, that he mowe undirstonde scripturis; in gramer, that he speke congruliche; in arte, that techith him to prove his proporciouns with good resoun; in retorik that techith him to speke semelich. Be he no glotoun, ne noon envyous, ne a negard; be he trewe, unbeliche [humble] and plesyngliche bere he him-silf to hise pacientis; speke he noon ribawdrie in the sike mannis hous; geve he no counseil but if he be axid; ne speke he with no womman in folie in the sik mannes hous; ne chide not with the sike man ne with noon of his meyne, but curteisli speke to the sijk man, and in almaner sijknes bihote him heele, though thou be of him dispeirid; but never the lattere seie to hise freendis the caas as it stant. Love he noon harde curis, and entermete [meddle] he nought of tho that ben in dispeir. Pore men helpe he bi his myght, and of the riche men axe he good reward. Preise he nought him-silf with his owne mouth, ne blame he nought scharpliche othere lechis; love he alle lechis and clerkis, and bi his myght make he no leche his enemye. So clothe he him with vertues, that of him mai arise good fame and name. . . . So lerne he fisik, that he mowe with good rulis his surgerie defende. . . .

Lanfrank's 'Science of Cirurgie'

In November 1519 Thomas Ross, sometime warden of the fellowship of surgeons of London, ran into trouble with the authorities at Westminster. His efforts to prevent the 'alien' Balthazar Guercio from practising in England had led to his being bound over in unusually heavy securities of £100 not to 'trowbell, vex or inquiet' the Italian, whose position as surgeon to the queen, Katherine of Aragon, made him an extremely powerful opponent, until he had proved his case. This hinged upon the unambiguous argument that, as 'an handy crafte', surgery ought only to be undertaken by those with an appropriate training in manual skills, and Ross was duly instructed to present his evidence. The ensuing petition, which begins by tracing the history of his calling back to the siege of Troy, provides us with one of the best, and certainly most authentic, definitions of late medieval and early Tudor surgery:

> hit restyth most principally in manuall applicacon of medicines: in stanchyng of blod, serchyng of woundes with irons and with other instrumentes, in cuttyng of the sculle in due proporcyon to the pellicules of the brayne with instrumentes of iron, cowchyng of catharactes, takyng owt bonys, sowyng of the flesshe, launchyng of bocchis [lancing boils], cuttyng of apostumes, burnyng of cankers and other lyke, settyng in of joyntes and byndyng of theym with ligatures, lettyng of blod, drawyng of tethe, with other suche lyke, which restyth onely in manuall operacon, princypally with the handes of the werkman. And surgery ys in comparyson to phisik as the crafte of carpentar ys comparyd to geometrie: for

> lyke as the geometer consideryth causis of compasse, quadrangles, triangles and counterpeyses, and as his conyng servyth for buyldyng . . . the carpenter occupyeth hit manually to his owne profyte and of necessite profitable to man, wherfor yt ys callyd *ars mechanica.*[1]

Ross's claim that surgeons had little to do with the inner workings of the human body or with the more arcane reaches of humoral theory, his spirited defence of a medieval tradition 'auctorised by our mother Holy Church', and his attack on presumptuous foreigners with new-fangled ideas about medicine should not necessarily be taken as evidence of a closed mind hostile to scholarship or progress (part of his appeal was, after all, set out in competent Latin, and he may even have translated Henri de Mondeville's surgical writings into English). Rather, he was anxious to defend the hard-won privileges of his craft against those 'entendyng in this reyalme of England custumably to contynewe and dwell withoute lycense, lawe or contradiccyon'.

As we have already seen, the decree of the fourth Lateran Council of 1215, forbidding clergy of the order of subdeacon or above to engage in any activities likely to cause bloodshed, did not prevent those in lesser orders (such as Guy de Chauliac) from wielding the knife, but it became increasingly unusual to find learned clerks with surgical expertise. The ideal, so often reiterated in contemporary textbooks, that the good surgeon should have received a medical education, was certainly respected by those laymen who now hastened to fill the gap, and many continental universities made some formal tuition available to them. Such was not, however, the case in England, where, with a few notable exceptions, surgeons and barbers did not study alongside the clerical élite. They acquired their training through the rigorous system of apprenticeship adopted by all artisan guilds: intellectual pursuits, although encouraged, remained a private matter. There was, for example, no equivalent of the College of Saint-Cosme in Paris, whose members were accepted as students by the faculty of medicine from 1436 onwards, thus inevitably becoming absorbed into the academic establishment.[2]

William Hobbes, principal surgeon to Edward IV, possessed a Cambridge MD, and one or two friars are known to have practised both medicine and surgery in baronial households during the previous century; but, as Ross's deposition clearly reveals, any further developments along these lines were bound to encounter resistance, if only because of the very different ways in which the two disciplines were now perceived and taught.[3] The idea that surgeons might choose, if they wished, between a university education or a more practical course of study, as was the case in Florence (where one common fraternity sufficed for exponents of medicine and surgery alike), must have seemed both impractical and audacious to fifteenth-century Englishmen.[4]

Boys (and sometimes girls) wishing to learn surgery contracted instead to serve for a minimum period of five or six years under a master, who in turn assumed responsibility for their support and education. This obligation was not taken lightly: in Bristol, barbers failing to offer a full seven-year period of training to their charges were fined 40s. from 1439 onwards, but they could be highly selective in return.[5] Because of the intimate and specialized nature of their work, apprentices were supposed to be personable in appearance, with 'clene handes and wele shapen nailes, clensed fro all blaknes and filthe'. Writers on the subject, who traditionally began their textbooks with a homily on the moral and intellectual virtues of the good practitioner, demanded such attributes as keen eyesight, manual dexterity, 'stable handes noght quakynge' and physical strength, although in practice it may have been difficult to find the perfect specimens they envisaged.[6] Certainly, in 1482, the barbers of London undertook to present all new apprentices for a compulsory medical examination to see if they were 'lepur or gowty, maiymed or disfigured in any parties', at least to the extent that they might alarm the patients.[7]

During his five or six years of tutelage an apprentice learned how to perform all, or most, of the surgical techniques listed above, and was also expected to acquire a sound working knowledge of anatomy. Authorities such as Guy de Chauliac placed great importance upon this aspect of the surgeon's craft:

> Every werkman is i-holden to knowe the subiecte in the whiche he wircheth, and ellis he erreth in wirchynge. But a cirurgien is a werkman of the helthe of manis body; therfore he is holden to konne the kynde of composicioun of it. And by this manere resoun, he is holden to konne anothomye. It is confermed by a liknes, for in the same manere wircheth a blynde man in a tre as a cirurgien in the body when he knoweth nought anothomye. But the blynde man kyttynge the tree ofte tymes, forsothe as it wer alwey, he erreth in taking uppon hym more or lasse than he schulde, therfore in the same wise a cirurgien when he can [knows] not anothomye.[8]

Although it is impossible to tell exactly how much instruction about the human body would have been given empirically by dissection, we can be reasonably confident that medieval surgeons had far more opportunities to examine the human cadaver than was once believed. The practice of embalming, which involved the removal of the viscera, sometimes for burial elsewhere, was common among the upper classes. Members of French and English royal and baronial families were generally preserved in this way by their surgeons, who sustained quite heavy expenses as a result: it cost over £15 to embalm Henry VI, and almost as much was spent in 1489 on the murdered Earl of Northumberland. Predictably, the gentry soon followed suit, providing local practitioners with a valuable opportunity to explore the inner workings of their former patients, and perhaps discover what had killed them.[9] Less evidence has survived about the holding of autopsies in cases of violent or otherwise suspicious death, but courts in France and Italy occasionally ordered them, on the obvious assumption that those involved had sufficient experience to offer an informed opinion. Autopsies might also be sanctioned in the interests of the living: efforts were made in 1407 to discover the progress of the disease

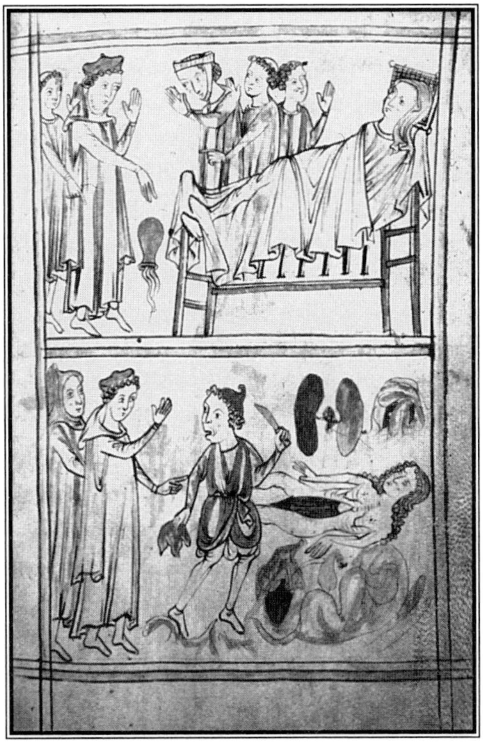

In the top part of this illumination, the physician gives an unfavourable prognosis after examining his patient's urine. Below, he appears to catch a lay practitioner red-handed in the act of dissecting the corpse (perhaps while embalming it), an activity rendered all the more questionable because the body is female. The papal bull, Detestande Feritatis, *appeared in 1299 shortly after this drawing was made.*

which killed the Bishop of Arras so that a fellow-sufferer might be helped; and it was thanks to a post-mortem held on the saintly Cardinal Albergati in 1435 that the Florentine Carthusians acquired their most cherished relic – a bladder stone the size of a goose's egg.[10]

The promulgation in 1299 of the papal bull *Detestande Feritatis*, designed to prevent the 'cruel and profane' dismemberment of corpses for multiple burial and the practice of boiling down the bodies of men and women who had died a long distance from home, has been seen as an attempt by the ecclesiastical authorities to check the burgeoning practice of dissection. Were this the case, however, Boniface VIII would undoubtedly have been far more specific, and in the long term his bull did little more than ensure that medical practitioners disposed of human remains in a decent fashion. Within a few years papal indults permitting the old 'abhorrent' burial practices were readily available to those who could afford them; and by the middle of the fourteenth century de Chauliac (a 'leche and commensale chapeleyne of oure lorde the Pope') was writing quite openly about the different ways of preparing subjects for the anatomist. Although hedged about with restrictions and generally confined to a very few occasions each year during the winter, dissections soon became an accepted part of medical education. They were conducted in universities across Europe with the full consent (and sometimes active encouragement) of the local ruler or civic authority. Indeed, from 1482 onwards the medical students at Tübingen attended them with the blessing of the Pope himself.[11]

At the start of the sixteenth century the surgeons and barbers of Edinburgh successfully petitioned the civic authorities for permission to take annually 'ane condampnit man efter he be deid to mak antomell of, quhairthraw we may haif experience, ilk ane [each one] to instruct utheris', promising to say prayers for the soul of the deceased in return. It was not until 1540 that the newly formed Company of Barber-Surgeons of London obtained a formal allocation of this kind, when they secured the cadavers of four malefactors every year for the purpose of dissection.[12] But the bodies of convicted felons, cut from the gallows, and of unclaimed or unrecognizable accident victims must sometimes have found their way on to the table before then, as medieval English practitioners were urged to exploit this source of supply. Significantly, under the circumstances, the impetus did not come from the small and poorly organized faculties of medicine at Oxford and Cambridge, which did not offer their students the opportunity to observe dissections, but from those engaged in 'manual operacion'. Like many writers with personal experience of conducting 'anathomies', the author of an early fifteenth-century surgical treatise felt that reading about the human body, however valuable, was no substitute for the real thing. Closely following de Chauliac, he distinguished between the two types of instruction:

> Onn ys techynge of bokys, yf at all yt be profytabyll, yet yt ys not allynges so sufficient as ys the othyr maner of anathomie, for the partes of the membyrs may better be sene with eyne in ded [by looking at bodies] than in letters wretyne onn the boke. Never the latter, man ys schorte and slydynge away, ther for yt ys nedfull to have syght of anothomie wretyn in letters. The secund maner of anathomie and experyens is of dede mens bodys, for lechys may be experte throw syght of newly dede mennys bodys, as of them whos heddys have be smetyne of, or hangyne, be the wyche may be made anathomie of membyrs and offyces inwarde of the flesch and brawne and skyne, of many waynys and arterres and senewys, be the wyche dyverese had and many has knowlege. . . .[13]

The idea that dissection might be employed to verify, enlarge upon or even correct received medical theory was, however, quite alien to most physicians or master surgeons, who regarded the exercise largely as a means of tuition rather than discovery.[14] For this reason they were quite prepared to substitute animals, who posed no theological problems and were far easier to come by. There were, moreover, many classical precedents: 'it plesyth to olde lechys and most to Galiene', noted one author, 'that the nobeler of the ynner lymes were i-shewyd be the anathomie of wyld bestys; and a monge wylde bestys summe be lyke to us with oute, as an ape, and summe wyth ynne, as a swynn [pig]; and therfore we ordeynn be the anathomie to be mayd of hem'.[15] If English apprentices were only infrequently able to attend human dissections, autopsies or embalmings, there was certainly no shortage of four-legged subjects on which to practise their craft.

Human anatomy is a difficult subject to master, and the medieval student needed additional assistance in the way of textual commentary, diagrams and pictures to help him understand how the body worked. Naturalism was, however, neither attempted nor required. Instead, the goal appears to have been a generalized representation or reduction of bodily parts, which demanded neither accuracy nor a sense of proportion. Anatomical illustrations were based not upon direct observation of individual cases or dissections, but were usually copied or adapted from existing manuscripts. These drawings certainly do not reflect the state of contemporary knowledge (even the most cloistered monk could hardly have imagined that the human foetus resembled a muscular young man with long hair): rather they served as lists, pointers and clues to the function of bodily parts and their relationships with each other. The use of mnemonic systems or 'memory theatres' based upon sketches of the body was not confined to medicine. In an age before printing, philosophers maintained that a good memory (which flourished best in the cold, dry environment characteristic of a 'melancholy' complexion) could be cultivated through the use of visual images bearing carefully chosen letters and symbols. Thus, a personification of grammar with words and pictures drawn on her head and limbs would serve as a device for the memorization of figures of speech. In a medical context, therefore, the aim was to provide a map with a few signposts to assist the traveller.[16]

A traditional set of five or more squatting figures (of Arab origin), for example, depicted veins, arteries, bones, nerves, muscles, the reproductive system of both sexes and the principal organs (colour plate 4). These were highly schematic, and bore little, if any, relationship to what the physician or surgeon would have observed in the course of his practice. Guido de Vigerano, who produced an influential *Anathomia* in the 1340s, had himself taken part in dissections, although no hint of this can be detected from the elegant figures which accompany his work. Guy de Chauliac expressed some impatience with his teacher, Henri de Mondeville, for using pictures like Vigerano's to illustrate his anatomy classes when he might have employed dissection. Perhaps the London barbers and surgeons who owned a variety of anatomical textbooks likewise employed them as a teaching aid, around which practical demonstrations could be organized whenever a cadaver became available.[17]

After his long period of training, the young barber or surgeon might be obliged, largely for financial reasons, to content himself with a life spent as a journeyman in the employment of others, but his great aspiration would be to set up in business as a master himself. From the fourteenth century onwards (and far earlier in some parts of Europe) this required a licence, the granting of which was strictly controlled not only by his fellow-guildsmen but also by the local authorities, who had a vested interest in maintaining high standards. In France the process was both protracted and daunting: at Montpellier candidates had to work for one week under the constant surveillance of each of the four masters who constituted the examining body, while in

Reims aspirant phlebotomists spent sixteen days demonstrating their grasp of medical theory, their understanding of the human body and their ability to make surgical instruments.[18] Having phlebotomized some twenty different individuals, one of whom he claimed had veins as hard as corns, and spent lavishly on food and drink for the examiners, a candidate named Hostelin was still found 'incapable and insufficient' in 1476 by the Parisian Barbers, who may have accepted free dinners but none the less refused to be suborned.[19]

The right to license practitioners in London remained a controversial issue throughout the later Middle Ages because of the rivalry between barbers and surgeons. Such intense competition almost certainly led both groups to make increasing demands in terms of the skill, experience and general medical knowledge of new masters. An account of the interrogation undergone by Robert Anson, who was examined in 1497, some five years after the warring parties had finally achieved a *modus vivendi*, reveals that permission to practise was not awarded lightly. The task of assessing his competence to perform specific 'manwall operacions' then fell to the physician, John Smyth, MD, 'instructour and examener of the seide feliship, be the same for that intent chosen'. The proceedings took place, with some solemnity, before a 'gret audiens of many ryght well expert men in surgery and other' gathered in their common hall, and resulted in the award of an official diploma. Previously, senior members of each of the two guilds would have been responsible for examining candidates and ensuring that, once accepted, they kept their premises and instruments up to the mark.[20]

That leading exponents of surgery, at least, could hold their own in the company of learned physicians and clerks is apparent from the widespread evidence of book ownership and private study among craft members during the later Middle Ages. Following John of Arderne's advice that 'the excercyse of bokes worshippeth a leche', many sought to improve their knowledge and no doubt also their professional status by reading. Thus, for example, when he died in 1442 the Londoner Henry Asshebourne left his seven 'principal books', including a *parvum Lanfrancum*, an *Anathonomye* listing all known diseases from head to foot, a French surgical text and a treatise by Arderne, to his son, with instructions that they were eventually to revert to the Charterhouse for the use of the monks.[21] In a lengthy will, which testifies to the remarkable wealth of some London surgeons, John Dagville (d.1477) not only disposed of a store of plate which any nobleman might have envied, but promised 'all my bokes belongyng to my crafte of sirurgie and also all my bokes of phisik, as well tho bokes that be written in Englissh as tho that be written in Latyn' to his younger boy, Thomas. Since the latter inherited 'all the medicynes that be in both my shoppes with all the instrumentes of my craft, both silvere, laton and iron', we may assume that he carried on the practice. But his elder brother, John, was a surgeon, too, and on his death ten years later one of these 'grete bokes' passed to his erstwhile master and executor, William Wentwang, another bibliophile fluent in both French and Latin.[22] Quite possibly these works were annotated by the owners: in 1479, the Parisian barber Colin Galerne became involved in litigation with a copyist whom he had commissioned to produce an elegantly written text from Galen, with well-spaced lines and wide margins so that he could interpolate his own gloss.[23]

Both Richard Esty (d.1475/6) and his colleague, Thomas Collard (d.1481), bequeathed books to the library of their own guild, the London Barbers, which must by then have been fairly comprehensive. Gifted apprentices sometimes inherited their masters' most cherished works of reference (as Thomas Morstede did from Thomas Dayron, who left him his two best books of surgery and physic, apparently in Latin), but it took a long while for a young man to build up a substantial collection, and in the meantime the guild could encourage scholarly pursuits. The

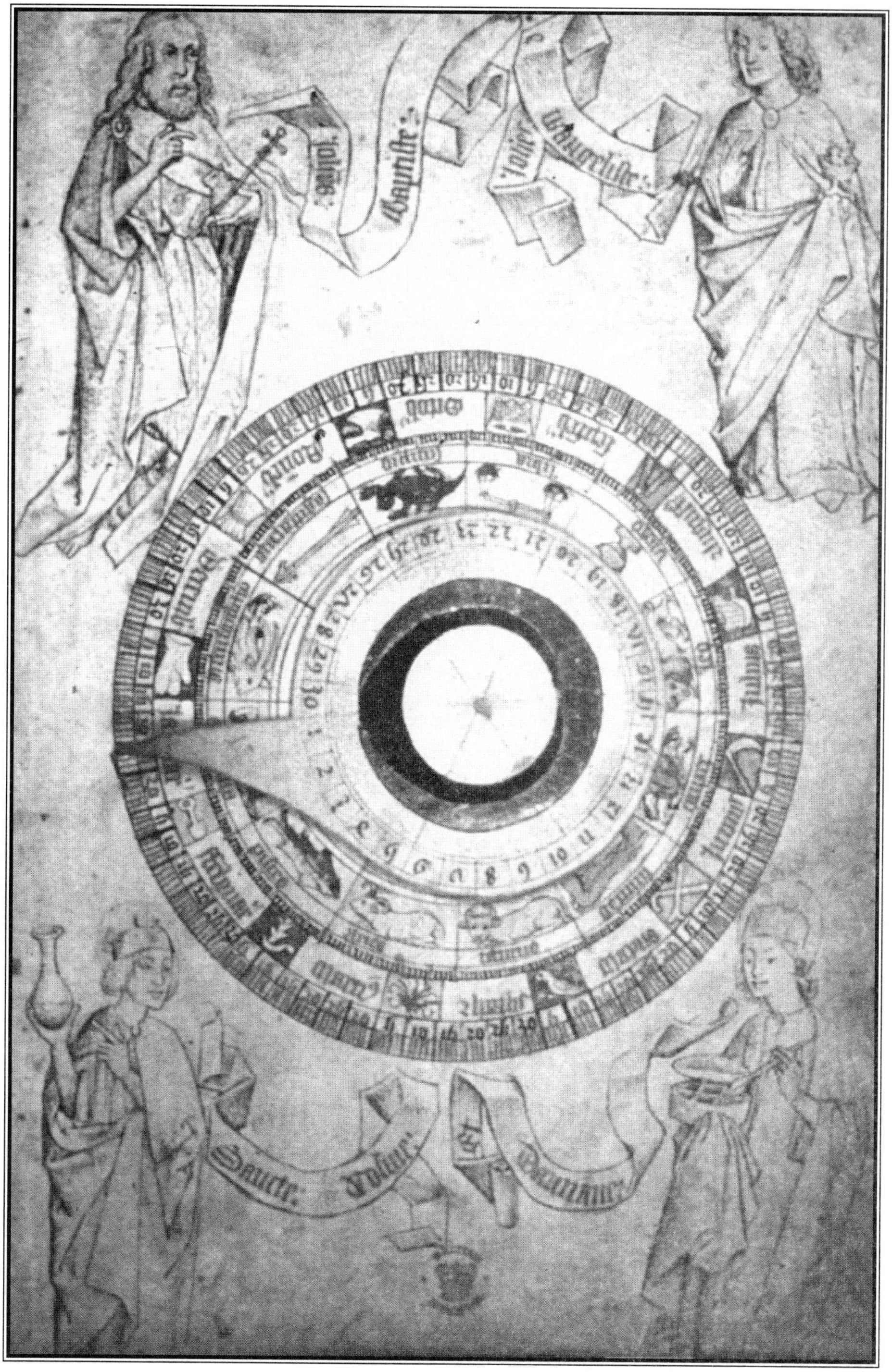

A volvelle from a book belonging to the York Barbers. This movable device could be rotated to establish the position of the sun or moon in relation to the other planets and signs of the zodiac at any hour of the day, and thus to determine if it was wise to proceed with treatment. St John the Baptist and St John the Evangelist, patron saints of the guild, stand at the top, while St Cosmas, the physician, and St Damian, the surgeon, appear at the foot.

training of 'men of good capasite and abill in maners and conyng, sufficiently lerned, enfourmed and labored by long experyens', was a serious matter. It is unlikely that the York Barbers managed to accumulate as many volumes, although one of their books, now in the British Library, suggests that they, too, sought to master the basic tenets of Galenic medicine. From 1505 onwards, if not before, the barbers and surgeons of Edinburgh refused to admit *any* apprentice 'without he can baithe wryte and reid' – a necessary requirement in view of the stringent examination in anatomy, humoral theory, astrology and surgical practice which he would have to take before qualifying as a master.[24]

The easy familiarity with Latin and French enjoyed by some practitioners explains why a significant proportion of surviving medical compilations contain works in both languages, as well as English. But most surgeons and barbers could cope only with material in the vernacular, and examples began to circulate widely from the end of the fourteenth century, often with accompanying diagrams and illustrations to convey potentially difficult information and reduce the amount of written text.[25] Surgeons who would previously have elected to write in Latin (as John of Arderne customarily did), now recognized that clear, basic instruction manuals in English would assist and inform a far wider readership. In 1392, for example, an anonymous Londoner decided to produce just such a treatise based upon his own adaptation of work by Lanfrank of Milan and Henri de Mondeville, interspersed with more personal observations about cures he had attempted himself.[26] The preface reveals an attractive combination of humility and didactic zeal shared by many such authors:

> The Holy Trinite, that is heed and welle of kunnynge, gevere and grauntere of grace to alle tho that by her power traveilen truly aboute science and kunnynge, that is helpe and edifiynge to his peple, graunte you grace that this compilacioun schal have so far to usen and disposen the fruyt of medicyns and of worchinge, in it conteyned, that it turne specialy to the worschipe of God and profight of the peple. The which compilacioun of sirurgie, I have compilid and drawen aftir the discret auctorite of my moost worschipful maistris and predessessouris of the same science, and specialy aftir the noble counseil of my worthi maistir Lamfranke, puttynge therto worchynge that I have assaied and proved in my tyme, and othere expert medicyns y-gaderid of dyvers worcheris that thei also han assaied and proved. . . .[27]

Quite often the original would be abridged and simplified as well as translated, or else the editor might choose to compile a selection of extracts from standard medical and scientific works hitherto only available in Latin. Since the labour involved was, rightly, perceived as a charitable enterprise, intended to help men and women who could not afford the fees charged by members of the professional élite, and to spread valuable knowledge about healing, it was often undertaken by priests. We have already encountered the barber Thomas Plouden, who persuaded a clergyman friend to select, explain and put into English extracts from an academic tract on phlebotomy, which as it stood posed an intellectual as well as a linguistic challenge.[28] Such commendable altruism was not, even so, always enough: a fifteenth-century book once owned by 'Richard Dod de London, Barbor Sorion' contains heavily, but not always accurately, edited translations of medical and surgical works originally in Latin, among which John of Arderne's treatises on anal fistulae and medicaments appear to have suffered particular indignities.[29] Yet, given the problems of vocabulary and comprehension facing the translator of technical material, these efforts bear witness to an important stage in the dissemination of specialist information outside the universities.

However seriously they may have pursued their studies, surgeons still prided themselves above all in their skill at 'manwall operacion'; and, like the other artificers to whom they were often compared (and readily compared themselves), they belonged to urban craft guilds subject to control by municipal authorities. Except in London, where surgeons and barbers split into separate, mutually hostile mysteries, there was no overt demarcation between the two groups, at least for organizational or administrative purposes. In the City, however, the numerically superior guild of barbers (established before 1308) fought off repeated offensives by a small, but select, fellowship of surgeons (in evidence by 1369), and even made sporadic attempts to monopolize the process of examination and licensing.[30] As in other parts of England some barbers practised almost exclusively as surgeons or tooth-drawers, others followed 'both the art of barber and science of surgeon', and an indefinite number concentrated upon shaving and hairdressing. The widespread and constantly growing demand for phlebotomy (which, after 1215, could not be undertaken by any clerk in major orders) meant that blood-letting and other minor operations were increasingly performed by the latter group as well, so that one way or another almost all of them offered some form of rudimentary medical treatment.

Tension and suspicion between well-educated surgeons with important social connexions and those whom, rightly or wrongly, they regarded as little more than rude mechanicals were by no means confined to London, although it was here that they assumed their most acute form. Competition for rich rewards attracted large numbers of practitioners, and a struggle for power as well as profit inevitably ensued. At least the City's surgeons were spared the two-pronged attack faced by their colleagues in Paris, where physicians from the faculty of medicine actively abetted the barbers, whom they astutely considered to be more tractable, in their fight for independence. Having, in 1493, permitted them to attend lectures in Latin and make use of a skeleton for anatomy classes, the faculty actually agreed a few years later that barbers might be accorded wider access to medical training and tuition – a move designed to infuriate the surgeons, who had been fighting a losing battle against their presumptuous subordinates for the best part of two hundred years.[31]

It looks as if some London surgeons, such as Nicholas Bradmore, employed barbers to serve as their assistants, but resented any ideas of professional equality. John of Arderne, who records rather smugly how he saved a patient left at death's door by an incompetent barber, urged his readers to take great precautions when performing difficult surgery, in case knowledge of the techniques used fell into the wrong hands. His concern was not about empirics, but barbers, who 'would usurpe this cure, appropriand it to thamself unto unworschip and not litel harme of maystres'.[32] The Mayor and Corporation of London, who exercised close supervision over all the city guilds, took a rather different view. The fellowship of surgeons rarely numbered more than a dozen or so senior figures, whose patients came largely from the royal Court or the ranks of the aristocracy, whereas their rivals were not only more numerous but also more intimately involved in the life of the community. It was, after all, the barbers who superintended the baths and kept a careful watch for carriers of infectious diseases, as well as treating the great majority of ordinary citizens when they were sick or hurt.[33]

No doubt for this reason the rulers of London, who themselves all belonged to craft or commercial guilds, consistently supported the Barbers in their struggle for autonomy, defending and consolidating their powers of self-regulation. Nor were the Barbers themselves slow to assume a position as guardians of the health and welfare of the commonalty. In response to a petition of 1376, in which they claimed that a horde of unqualified and ignorant opportunists had presumed 'to intermeddle with barbery, surgery and the cure of other maladies', the mayor allowed them to inspect and examine all newcomers practising these crafts, along with their instruments, 'to see they are good and proper for the service of the people'.[34] Some forty years later, much to the annoyance of the surgeons, it was further established that two master barbers, renowned 'as well for their knowledge and probity as for the different kinds of difficult cures that have been sagaciously performed by them', would henceforward be chosen *solely* to oversee the exercise of surgery by fellow guild members, without reference to any higher authority save the mayor.[35]

Plans for a joint college of physicians and surgeons, drawn up in 1423 by the City's most distinguished practitioners, were effectively sabotaged by the corporation's refusal to abandon this arrangement. The physicians involved might have countenanced a 'limited association' with surgeons of the better sort, but clearly expected the Barbers to come to heel and take direction from their social and professional superiors. Any idea of collaboration between such a diverse group of individuals, ranging from court physicians to phlebotomists and bone-setters, was clearly unthinkable, at least to members of the professional élite.[36] Having survived this threat, the Barbers went from strength to strength: they obtained a royal charter of incorporation in 1462, and finally obliged the surgeons to accept the inevitability of compromise at the end of the century.[37] It was not until 1518 that the physicians of London began to make up for lost time by establishing an organization of their own; the confident performance of the artisans they affected to despise may, indeed, have taught them some useful lessons.

There was far less confrontation in other English towns, where physicians were relatively thin on the ground, and ambitious, highly qualified surgeons too few in number to warrant the formation of a separate fellowship or group. Even men such as Nicholas Woodhill of York, who was retained for life in 1436 to serve as the Countess of Westmorland's surgeon, did not scorn to associate with the city's barbers: on the contrary, he was actually imprisoned for conspiring with one of them to abduct a servant.[38] In most major urban centres the local barbers' guild routinely supervised all forms of medical activity without encountering much in the way of professional rivalry. At Beverley, for instance, any surgeons, physicians or tooth-drawers intending to practise for a year or more were required, from 1416 onwards, to contribute to the guild at the same rate as the brethren. A new scale of fees, this time leviable upon even the most transitory 'foreign' practitioners, including blood-letters, tightened their grip even further as the century drew to a close and more stringent licensing became the norm.[39]

Part of the money thus raised at Beverley was earmarked for the cost of the play mounted every April by the town's barbers, and for the upkeep of 'lights' or candles maintained by them in memory of the souls of departed colleagues. At York, too, a similar charge was made upon surgeons and leeches working independently in the city, again to help finance a guild pageant and discharge various spiritual obligations. Here, as at Beverley, the barbers customarily enacted the scene of Christ's baptism in the River Jordan, an appropriate choice in view of the especial devotion shown by medical men towards St John the Baptist. One of the most common charms employed in late medieval England (with the hope of staunching blood) invoked the image of the fast-flowing water brought to a standstill at this sacred moment, so the river itself assumed a symbolic part in the drama. A contemporary audience would be familiar with the Old Testament story of Naaman the Syrian, whose leprosy vanished after he had bathed seven times in the Jordan (2 Kings, 1–27); they would know, too, that the sacrament of baptism brought physical as well as spiritual healing; and many would themselves have obtained a rare moment of relief from chronic pain by taking medicinal baths. The play had a comic aspect as well: after enduring more than their fair share of discomfort at the hands of barbers and leeches, the spectators could enjoy a few ribald jokes at their expense, since the urinal, that ubiquitous badge of their profession, was also known as a jordan and sometimes served to pour the holy water over Christ's head[40] (colour plate 7).

The religious, ceremonial and social aspects of guild life loomed large in the consciousness of members, and figure prominently in most sets of regulations. Concern for the welfare of the souls of departed brethren, whose time in purgatory might be shortened by the provision of candles, obits and prayers, may have been particularly strong among surgeons, because of the Church's strict interpretation of culpability for homicide: devout practitioners could at least reassure themselves that everything possible would be done by their successors to mitigate the coming ordeal. The fraternity of the Norwich Barbers (dedicated to God, the Virgin and John the Baptist) undertook, shortly before 1388, to donate two wax candles weighing forty pounds every year at midsummer, for daily use at high mass at one of the cathedral altars; and in London elaborate provisions were then in place to ensure that every member of the barbers' guild was buried and remembered with due reverence. Practitioners in Bristol had some trouble in raising the funds to support 'here light brennyng in the fest of Corporis Christi in the generall processione in the honoure of the blessed sacrament', but a new scale of fines, introduced in 1439, solved the problem.[41]

By the end of the Middle Ages the distinctly secular question of licensing and the enforcement of craft monopolies had begun to dominate guild deliberations. In most places the right to practise was restricted to freemen, who themselves constituted a privileged group within the ranks of the urban male population. In Bristol the rules were sufficiently relaxed to allow any barbers who might be passing through the port to ply their trade on the premises of an established master, but the latter had, without exception, to be fully enfranchised. Ordinances of the mid-fifteenth century, instructing all of them to work openly in shops 'and not in chambres, halles nor in non other prive places' (on pain of a 12s.4d. fine for each offence) enabled the authorities to keep a check on newcomers, as well as encouraging the others to avoid dangerous or uncertain cures.[42]

Since 'no man or woman whatsoever' was permitted to practise surgery, tooth-drawing or anything else of a remotely medical nature in fifteenth-century York unless they were either working under the direction of a master barber or otherwise sanctioned by the guild, the latter also exercised, in theory if not in fact, what we today would describe as a closed shop. A levy was even imposed upon physicians and leeches, who might not otherwise treat patients in the city.[43] If the evidence of rapidly increasing guild membership is any guide, this attempt to corner the market seems to have been remarkably successful. Some two hundred barbers (the designation 'surgeon' or 'barber-surgeon' was never used in contemporary local records) obtained the freedom of the city between 1272 and 1499, the great majority being enfranchised from 1350 onwards: sixty between then and 1399, seventy between 1400 and 1449, and fifty-five between 1450 and the end of the period. A far smaller number of leeches and *medici* also became free, and were presumably attached to the guild in some way. On the other hand, at least fifty other practitioners, mostly barbers, are known to have been active in York at various times without enjoying this privilege, and consequently without being eligible for full guild brotherhood. Some of them may have escaped the watchful eye of the authorities, but the majority probably paid for short-term permits or worked in one of the city's exempt liberties.[44]

Statistics from Canterbury suggest that licensed freemen represented the tip of the iceberg. Here unenfranchised individuals were allowed to trade as *intrantes* upon payment of a modest annual fine. No fewer than sixty-five barbers, a surgeon and one *medicus* seized this opportunity between 1390 and 1449, although only fourteen of them, all barbers, went on to become free. Since eight other barbers, three surgeons and one physician took up the freedom during the first half of the century, this gives us a total of seventy-seven approved medical practitioners. Between 1450 and the end of the century, at least thirty-three more barbers, a surgeon and a *medicus* appear among the *intrantes*, a third of whom (again all barbers) eventually paid for the franchise. Six more barbers can be identified from the roll of freemen, so it looks as if Canterbury authorized a minimum of forty-one new persons to give medical or surgical treatment during this period. Some would have concentrated on hairdressing, while others did not stay for very long. But the impression is one of steady growth, notably in the second quarter of the century.[45] A similar pattern emerges in Norwich, where the barbers' guild originally foresaw problems in keeping membership above a dozen. Between 1350 and 1399 only fourteen barbers and one leech were enfranchised, but over the next fifty years at least forty-one barbers and four leeches are named in the registers of freemen (nine of them in 1445/6), and a further twenty-five barbers took the oath between 1450 and 1499.[46] Allowing for the respective sizes of York and Norwich, and the increased demand for practitioners generated by sick pilgrims visiting York Minster and Canterbury Cathedral, these trends appear remarkably similar.

Besides documenting the struggle against outsiders, guild ordinances, such as those approved by the rulers of York in the late fourteenth or early fifteenth centuries, give us a valuable insight into the practice of surgery in provincial England, and thus merit detailed examination. The city fathers, commendably anxious to protect the health and safety of the populace, had already decreed, in 1301, that practitioners were to be properly trained in the treatment of 'wounds and hurts', and should inform the mayor, under oath, of any potentially dangerous cases in their care (as we have seen, such an arrangement could benefit the surgeon as well as the patient). More specifically, they insisted that old (*sic*) bandages were to be bought in the open market, in full view of the general public; vendors of 'ripped or bloodstained' dressings were to be brought before the bailiffs; and, as a final deterrent, any leech engaging in this unsavoury trade was 'to be taken just like a felon, murderer or red-handed thief, and sent to prison at the King's will'. In this instance, however, the authorities were probably more concerned to prevent the secret disposal of evidence of violent crime and the clandestine treatment of suspects than they were to encourage hygiene, since their pronouncement follows closely the parliamentary act of 1276 defining the duties of a coroner.[47]

Evidently in response to the dramatic expansion of surgical practice in York and the growing sophistication of the guild system, the new ordinances now vested far stricter disciplinary and supervisory powers in a warden and searchers elected annually by the barbers themselves. They were to insist upon fair but firm behaviour towards apprentices, who were not to be lured away by one master from the service of another, diligently to examine the premises of all recently admitted masters and assess their capacity as practitioners, prevent the leasing out of such premises to unapproved persons, and impose a heavy scale of financial penalties upon any guild member, employee or 'foreigner' who broke the rules. In this they were fully supported by the civic authorities, to whom, in return, they paid a share of the fines:

> And if the searchers do not find the new master acceptable, he shall be warned by them to stop his practice as a master until such time that he is found fully qualified in his art to

practise as such, and is approved as competent. And if he refuses to stop at the first warning, then on the second warning he shall be fined 6s.8d., payable to the chamber [of the city] and the guild in equal portions. If, however, he refuses to stop after the third warning, then his basins and other signs which he has displayed in the highway to advertise his craft shall be seized by the searchers then in office and taken to the chamber on Ouse Bridge in the presence of the mayor without impediment . . . and then he shall be fined by the mayor and searchers as they see fit. . . .[48]

The question of shop signs could itself prove highly contentious: in London the barbers were warned by the mayor, in 1307, to adopt a less offensive form of publicity. The display of bowls or phials of blood 'in their windows, openly in view of folks' was henceforth banned (on pain of a 2s. fine), and they were ordered to pour their waste products discreetly into the Thames. In Paris, too, there was concern about the prompt disposal of blood, which had to be thrown away within a matter of hours and never stored overnight.[49] Sunday trading caused even more problems. Thomas Arundel, Archbishop of Canterbury, censored the London Barbers for ignoring the laws of God and repeatedly breaking the Sabbath: in 1413 he complained to the mayor that 'temporal punishment is held in more dread than clerical, and that which touches the body or the purse more than that which kills the soul', instructing him to discipline the offenders in an appropriate fashion. A ban was then imposed throughout the southern province, probably to little effect. In Beverley the rules were modified to allow shaving (but not surgery) on Sundays throughout August and September, while the converse held good in York, where barbers treating the sick with medicine or phlebotomy were free to ply their trade every day of the year. The Corporation of Bristol made limited concessions on the understanding that a fixed share of any proceeds from Sunday trading would go to 'the needy and poor'.[50]

Almost without exception, the members of English guilds were anxious to establish procedures which would easily and quickly settle internal disputes or quarrels arising between craftsmen and private citizens. With regard to surgery, the issue was particularly sensitive, partly because mistakes could easily result in death or mutilation, but also as a result of genuine differences of opinion about methods of treatment. The London Barbers, for example, were forbidden to sue each other at common law without leave of the masters or wardens, and then only after all attempts at amicable agreement had failed. Similar restrictions were introduced by the fellowship of surgeons in 1435, supported by the threat of a draconian fine of 20s. for each offence. The masters were urged from the start to take each dispute 'into her hand, and thei dueli and truli to examine and redresse it rigtwysli and consciensli for bothe parties'. Anxiety that 'maters and causis aperteynynge to the secretis of the same seid craft' might become public knowledge, and even pass into the hands of their rivals, if they were aired in court, was a powerful incentive to compromise. Some acrimonious disagreements must, however, have been expected, since the scale of penalties included a noble (6s.8d.) 'if ony of the seid felowschip drawe ony wepene in violence or unlawfulli menace ony persoone of the seid crafte', and 20s. 'if ony of hem smite anothir'. At least there would have been no shortage of trained medical help in the event of bloodshed.[51]

Lawsuits about malpractice were frequently submitted to the arbitration of experienced practitioners; and, although laymen and -women understandably nursed some reservations about the latter's impartiality, incompetence or overt venality seem rarely to have been tolerated. The four distinguished barbers from York who undertook to investigate a charge of incompetence made against one of their number, in 1392, found unreservedly for the female plaintiff, to whom they awarded damages of £10 (then considered sufficient to maintain a gentleman for one year).[52] Even less sympathy was shown towards empirics or interlopers operating without official licence or approval. In 1377, for example, three London surgeons testified before the mayor's court that 'lack of care and knowledge' on the part of one Richard Cheyndut had almost cost his patient a leg. Being no less anxious to drive unqualified empirics off the streets, the authorities duly committed Cheyndut to prison, as well as ordering him to pay 50s. to the victim's father.[53]

Some years earlier all the surgeons and physicians of London had been required to give evidence in a case, surely unique in legal history, concerning the illicit shipment from abroad of a cask containing four putrid wolves. Their owner, the vicar of St Margaret's Lothbury, protested that they were a recognized cure for '*le lou*' ('the wolf'), but was handed over for trial in the ecclesiastical courts once the assembled experts had denied all knowledge of the disease and denounced him as an impostor. It is hard to believe that none of these learned men, who claimed to have searched assiduously through all their medical and surgical textbooks for information, knew that 'devouring' skin diseases, such as erysipelas (actually called '*le loup*' in medieval France) or ulcerated cancers, were frequently compared to wild animals, or that folk wisdom maintained that they should be 'fed' with meat to prevent them consuming human flesh. Could the surgeons, who were responsible for treating skin diseases, just possibly have feared the economic as well as the medical consequences of competition from this quarter?[54]

As is evident from a second set of ordinances, composed in English at the close of the fifteenth century, and added at the 'grete instance and labours' of the York Barbers to their existing regulations, the threat posed by unlicensed practitioners was viewed with increasing alarm throughout the country. The guild now claimed the right to examine all those purporting 'to exercise any poynt of surgerie' within five days of their first attempted cure, to investigate and evaluate individually 'all maner cures of surgerie which the said aliens and straungers shal have in hand', and, inevitably, to exact money from the latter.[55] One of the most pressing considerations leading to the amalgamation of the surgeons and barbers of London in 1493, after years of conflict, was unquestionably the need to present a united front against these outsiders. The profession's campaign against unqualified empirics and healers will be examined in Chapter VIII, but it is worth emphasizing here that, along with a genuine commitment to maintain and improve standards, there went a less altruistic desire to corner the profits of practice.

Although none of their number ever rose to occupy high civic office, there can be little doubt that many members of the York guild ranked among the more affluent pillars of the community. On his death in 1392, Richard Dalton, who had been practising in the city for the best part of forty years, was in a position to bequeath quantities of silver plate, a substantial amount of cash for pious works, the contents of a comfortably furnished house, an impressive battery of kitchen utensils (which went, along with several items of bedding, to his cook, Agnes) and, of course, the tools of his trade. Richard Wasdale (d.*c.* 1480–2) evidently nursed some pretensions to gentility, at least if his ownership of two fine doublets (one '*de roebukskynnys*'), a sword, some armour and a dagger is any guide. It is, however, unlikely that he could match the sartorial elegance of his contemporary, John Foster, whose wardrobe contained at least four gowns, including one red, one green and one striped. Their colleague, William Hodgeson (d.1477) also lived well, having accumulated the customary collection of plate, some elegant furnishings (notably a set of bed-hangings of green tapestry) and over £10 in cash.[56]

It might be supposed that, since quite undistinguished practitioners often charged in excess of 20s. or 40s. for an individual course of treatment, most surgeons would have grown very rich indeed. After all, a successful lawyer could not expect to receive much more in annual retainers from each of his wealthier clients, and an auditor or steward would rarely be paid above 60s. a year, even on a great estate. Within a fortnight of being 'hurte wyth an arow on hys ryght arme be-nethe the elbow' at the Battle of Barnet in 1471, John Paston spent more than £5 on 'lechecraft and fesyk and rewardys', being driven to borrow money in order to meet the demands of his surgeon. Only a small part of this fee constituted a net profit, however, since insurance cover had always to be provided for the future. One perfectly legitimate reason for high costs lay in the fact that, like physicians, surgeons and barbers attended many of their patients at home and could be preoccupied for weeks with a few time-consuming cases. Moreover, whereas the physician customarily relied upon apothecaries to make up his prescriptions for him, the surgeon took 'stonys, herbes, rootes, seedes, frutes, gummys, barkes, flowres and suche other' to prepare his own medicines 'manually with handes', thus adding appreciably to his final bill.[57]

Although it had obvious drawbacks for careerists with a string of wealthy patients, the prospect of salaried employment offered welcome security, as well as the promise of useful social connexions. The surgeon William Holm was undoubtedly glad to receive a life annuity of £10 with a fur-trimmed robe in 1361 from his new mistress, Princess Isabella, and to know that all future expenses would be lavishly reimbursed; but his chief cause of satisfaction with the arrangement must surely have been the easy access which it gave him to Edward III's Court. Holm evidently needed no lessons in self-advancement, for within ten years he had been retained by the old king himself, at a similar fee.[58] Membership of the royal entourage was a goal towards which most ambitious surgeons aimed, partly because of the profits to be made and the influence to be exploited, but also for the professional recognition bestowed on those considered fit for the task of lancing, probing or 'kerving' the king's person. Edward IV's household ordinances provided for one resident master surgeon (who ranked below his physician in status but none the less took the rank and livery of an esquire), one yeoman surgeon and an 'honest child' to serve them both. Since at least two or three masters and yeomen were on the payroll at any given time, we may assume that, like other courtiers, they operated a rota system, which left them free to attend other patients. In keeping with Edward's desire for stringent domestic economies, they were urged to recycle 'the old broken meteclothes and towelles perusyd in the ewry' as bandages. No expense was spared, however, on the 'small cofer with playsters and medycens' kept for the king's use, and several royal surgeons ran up large bills as a result.[59]

Traditionally, surgeons at Court drew a fairly modest allowance of 40s. a year with robes, but in practice there was no limit to what they might earn. None were, of course, eligible for ecclesiastical preferment, but they could be provided with stewardships, keeperships of castles, posts as royal messengers, collectors of customs or other lucrative sinecures. On top of substantial annuities, higher than those enjoyed by some household knights, they received grants of land, pardons for offences committed by themselves or their friends and, in the case of foreigners, letters of denization. When old, blind or feeble they were given pensions and comfortable places to live, their widows and children were generously supported, and even in death they were allowed to share in the spiritual benefits purchased at great expense by their employers.[60] Ailing monarchs with weak health, such as the elderly Edward III or Henry VI, could be relied upon to be bountiful patrons, while those of a martial disposition were obviously welcome when warfare offered such alluring prospects of advancement. As well as presenting the surgeon with a valuable opportunity to refine and develop his craft, service in the field enabled those with luck and talent to further their careers by leaps and bounds. There were always risks: practitioners could be shot at, killed or ransomed in just the same way as ordinary combatants, but the potential gains generally outweighed the dangers.[61] One Master Gerard was, for example, paid £10 by Edward IV in 1464 as a reward for 'attending and helyng by our special comaundement certayn our men of our houshold and many othir late hurt in our werress in the north contree'. This left him rather better off than the eight surgeons who accompanied the future Richard III on his expedition against the Scots, in 1482, at a standard fee of 1s. per day, although being under contract and thus in constant proximity to the commanding officers, they were ideally placed to exploit the patronage system effectively.[62]

Monarchs, magnates and wealthy knights rarely went into battle without their own medical attendants, whose terms of employment usually made provision for additional military wages. John of Gaunt's surgeon, Piers Bray, was expected to go wherever he might be needed 'well and suitably arrayed for war', in return for extra pay and equipment, together with full permission to keep whatever booty or prisoners fell into his hands.[63] His conditions of service, identical in most points to those binding the duke's senior retainers, reflected his important position, which may have been enhanced by his kinship with Gaunt's physician, John Bray. Younger, less well-established practitioners could take to the field in other ways. During the fifteenth century small companies of suitably qualified barbers and surgeons from London and the suburbs were recruited in wartime to minister to the general needs of combatants. In 1436 John Harwe, a prominent member of the fellowship of surgeons, undertook to provide a detachment of six to accompany an expeditionary force to Calais; and at the time of Edward IV's projected invasion of France, in 1475, the King's own surgeons were accompanied by a band of twelve Londoners, charged with the welfare of the army as a whole.[64]

Most of the material rewards, as well as the glory, inevitably went to a small cadre of senior practitioners, busy about the royal person. John Bradmore, whose successful treatment of the wounded Prince Henry has been noted in Chapter III, was fortunate in both the place and time of the operation, which was performed in the safety of Kenilworth Castle, but his skill appears beyond question. Already a surgeon to the prince's father, Henry IV, he was subsequently rewarded with the post of searcher of ships in the port of London, which brought him a fee of £10 p.a., several times this amount in bribes and perquisites, and a valuable *entrée* into the ranks of the merchant élite. Bradmore died, in 1412, a wealthy and influential man, although he was soon overshadowed by two colleagues, William Bradwardyne and Thomas Morstede (his successor as searcher), who raised, equipped and led a company of surgeons during the Agincourt campaign of 1415.[65] By then Bradwardyne could look back on a long career spent in the royal livery, during which his expertise as a practitioner had enabled him effortlessly to move from the Court of Richard II (whom he twice accompanied to Ireland, and who increased his fee, in 1398, from ten marks to over £30 a year) to that of Henry IV.[66] So anxious was the usurper to retain him that he actually honoured a debt of £130 still outstanding on medicaments supplied by Bradwardyne to the late King Richard, and also permitted him to farm certain Crown property in Herefordshire. On the outbreak of war along the Welsh border, in 1403, Bradwardyne naturally joined the army of Prince Henry, along with a retinue of six archers for his own protection. Although he may have been obliged to recognize the superiority of Bradmore's technique in treating the prince after the Battle of Shrewsbury, a supplementary pension of £20 a year eventually came his way on the latter's recommendation; by 1410 he had assumed the rank of a serjeant-at-arms; and four years later, when Prince Henry had succeeded his father, he enjoyed another windfall in the form of confiscated bonds worth 40 marks.[67]

It would be interesting to know exactly who masterminded the detailed and hitherto unprecedented arrangements for providing the invasion force of 1415 with general medical support. Both Bradwardyne and the king brought years of practical experience to bear on such matters, but the initial impetus seems to have come from Thomas Morstede, who was to share command of the unit of six archers and eighteen surgeons (at first ten, then twelve had been considered enough, but Henry evidently wanted more). Morstede may have spent less time in the field than Bradwardyne, although the award to him of £40 a year as a royal surgeon, in 1410, testifies eloquently to his abilities. Both men were present at Agincourt with a slightly larger contingent of twenty-one surgeons, and both escaped the ravages of dysentery, which proved a far worse enemy than the French, to do battle at the Exchequer for the settlement of their wages. Like most other English commanders, they had been obliged to accept jewels and plate as a pledge of future payment, and were thus effectively owed over a quarter (£30) of the money due.[68] None the less, the two were soon back in action: in 1416 they received a commission to recruit surgeons and other craftsmen capable of making surgical instruments for the next campaign; and within two years Bradwardyne had joined King Henry in Normandy. The wording of a general pardon issued to Morstede many years later, in 1445, suggests that he either still retained, or had only just relinquished, Henry V's securities, and was thus never fully reimbursed for all his efforts. Even so, he is unlikely to have borne too much resentment towards the late king, who had smiled on him in so many other ways.[69]

By and large, practitioners in royal or baronial service accepted that bills would be left unpaid and expenses forgotten. Such losses could soon be offset by a myriad of intangible benefits, especially as close connexions with great and powerful men counted for more than hard cash in the eyes of the world. We shall, for example, never know how much money William Bradwardyne really made out of his post as keeper of the Marshalsea (the prison of the court of King's Bench), but can confidently assume that only a particular favourite would have emerged unscathed from a scandal involving the mass escape of twelve prisoners.[70] Thomas Morstede's position as one of the richest men in London, with an income of £154 p.a. from land alone, was in part due to his marriage into the ranks of the ruling oligarchy, yet no City merchant would have allowed his daughter to marry a mere surgeon. One who enjoyed the king's good graces, and had a string of offices and commissions to prove it, was, needless to say, a bird of a different feather.[71]

It is, however, important to recognize that far more evidence survives about a small percentage of prosperous and successful surgeons such as those discussed above than about the ones who had trouble in making ends meet. It was one thing for men with powerful patrons to offer limitless credit, secure in the knowledge that they could line their pockets through the workings of 'good lordship', but quite another for ordinary barbers or surgeons, who relied solely upon their daily earnings. Some of them faced ruin through litigation, either because they were sued for malpractice or had themselves to take duplicitous patients to law. The London jurors who found Nicholas Bradmore guilty of negligence in treating an injured thumb, in 1405, awarded the plaintiff damages of 60s., which were raised to £4 by the court, perhaps on the mistaken assumption that he earned as much as his kinsman, the royal surgeon, John Bradmore. Since the aggrieved victim had initially demanded compensation of £40 matters could have been much worse, although the sum still represented a sizeable proportion of Nicholas's annual income.[72]

Grossly inflated claims for damages were a standard feature of legal life, but sometimes juries felt such sympathy for those who had experienced pain and mutilation that they recommended generous settlements. In 1320, for example, one Alice Stockynge recovered over £30 after winning her case against a surgeon who had carried off belongings worth 20s. from her home in order to make good his fee. Under normal circumstances damages would have been minimal, but Alice's account of the sufferings she had endured at his hands appears to have been unusually harrowing.[73]

Because of the dangers involved in even simple operations and the unpredictable effects of many drugs in common use, the medieval surgeon ran a constant risk of being sued. It is hard not to feel sympathy for Nicholas Sax, a German living in London, who almost killed his patient when 'cutting' a fistula, or for Matthew Rillesford, whose use of corrosives went badly wrong. Rillesford seems to have been particularly unfortunate, as he was also taken to court for incompetence in dealing with a case of '*le stone*', which, short of lithotomy, would have been almost impossible to cure at the time (although Lady Lisle, who is discussed in Chapter VIII, evidently contrived to do so). Moreover, some litigants, dissatisfied with their treatment, or just downright dishonest, were always prepared to blacken a practitioner's reputation in order to avoid paying their bills. Quite possibly John West of Wigston in Leicestershire fell into this category: his claim that a local surgeon had been bribed by his enemies to cause irreparable damage to a broken arm was implausible, although he freely volunteered to accept the judgement of a panel of experts.[74]

Practitioners did not need to be reminded that they should reach a clear understanding about fees and expenses *before* commencing treatment; and many seem to have asked more than they ever reasonably hoped to receive. The prudent among them also took bonds or securities from their patients as a further guarantee of payment, since these could be recovered at common law if anything went wrong. Thus, the fee of £10 demanded by the London surgeon John Brown from a priest whom he undertook to cure of 'palsy' (probably a stroke) was underwritten by pledges worth twice this sum, which he called in when the cash failed to materialize. In this instance there seems to have been genuine disagreement over the terms of the original contract, a common enough experience when the parties could not see eye to eye over what precisely constituted a 'cure'. Clearly, the priest's expectation that he would be able to walk with a stick and say mass had not been fulfilled, so he felt justified in withholding payment.[75]

John of Arderne's advice on the subject of money, which often finds its way into books on medieval medicine, may have worked well enough for one of the leading practitioners of the age, who moved in exalted social circles and had a formidable reputation for proficiency as well as learning, but his complacent tone is likely to have proved more of an irritant than an inspiration to some of his contemporaries:

> Ever be warre of scarse askyngis, for over scarse askyngis setteth at not both the markette and the thing. Therefore, for the cure of fistula in ano, when it is curable, aske he competently, of a worthi man and a gret, an hundred marke or fourty pounde, with robez and feez of an hundred shillyng terme of lyfe by yere. Of lesse men fourty pounde, or fourty marke aske he wiyhout feez. And take he noght lesse than an hundred shillyngis, for never in all my lyf toke I lesse than an hundred shillyng for cure of that sekenes.[76]

William Barber of Nottingham was, for example, not only obliged to accept payment in kind from one of his patients, a tankard-maker who promised him three pots of different sizes worth

1s. in return for treatment of an injured arm, but actually had to take the man to court when he failed to honour the agreement.[77] A moving appeal to the Chancellor of England, submitted at the turn of the fourteenth century by the widow of a York barber named John Berham, reminds us that practitioners and their dependants could endure dire poverty. Claiming to have been left heavily in debt by her husband, and to have supported a bedridden and aged mother, as well as four children since his death, she begged for help in paying off their creditors before the whole family starved. Although due allowance should be made for the exaggeration common to such petitions, the contrast with Arderne's buoyant optimism could hardly be greater.[78] Even in London, where opportunities for making money abounded, the guild of barbers found it necessary to provide at this time for brethren 'falling by chance into trouble or poverty', albeit only after they had belonged to the guild for at least seven years. Likewise, their rivals insisted, in 1435, that 'everi cirurgian' should donate 2d. each quarter 'to the profit and worschip of the craft in helping and relevyng the nede of pore men of the same felowschip'. The wealthy barbers John Wilkinson and Roland Frankyssh, both of whom died in the early 1470s, left specific sums of money to help colleagues beset by hardship or illness.[79]

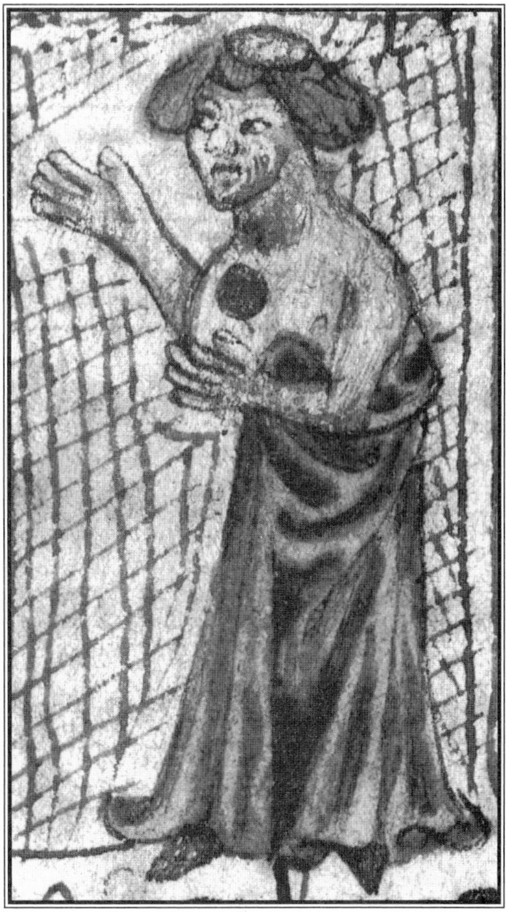

John of Arderne drew heavily on his own experience when writing about surgery. Here he records the successful cure of a chaplain from Colston with a growth on his chest the size of a hen's egg.

For many practitioners concern for the unfortunate went far beyond the confines of guild or fellowship. Not even John of Arderne was immune to fears about the afterlife, urging the successful surgeon to 'visite of his wynnyngis poure men aftir his might, that thai by thair prayers may gete him grace of the holy goste'.[80] Free or cut-price treatment constituted a more immediate and specific form of charity, which medical men were traditionally expected to give the poor, either at their own expense with no hope of recompense on earth (but the promise of a reward in heaven) or, more realistically, under the auspices of a wealthy philanthropist or institution. In fifteenth-century France, where most towns and cities engaged highly qualified physicians and surgeons to serve the community, this aspect of public health assumed particular importance during epidemics, although commendable efforts were made at other times as well.

Over 15 per cent of the surgeons known to have practised in France during the Middle Ages and about 9 per cent of the barbers either worked directly for municipal authorities or were paid by great lords to provide a similar service. It is hard to tell how much of their time would have been devoted specifically to the poor, but we can be reasonably certain that the 7 per cent of surgeons and 10 per cent of barbers associated with hospitals had protracted dealings with the most vulnerable members of society. Some of these men were remarkably distinguished: in Paris, for example, the king's sworn surgeons were required to attend the patients in the Hôtel Dieu, who thus received expert treatment far beyond the means of most citizens. As a general principle, moreover, it was understood that licensed practitioners would 'tend the poor for the love of God'.[81]

No formal arrangements of this kind appear to have been made in medieval England, where the organization of medical help for the poor remained a matter for individual institutions and benefactors, and hospitals rarely offered much in the way of conventional treatment. Occasional acts of royal generosity, such as Henry IV's award of a substantial pension to one Matthew Flynt, 'tothdrawer' of London, so he could provide free dental care for paupers, come to light, but whatever their munificence as almsgivers, English monarchs showed little interest in such matters.[82] Medical practitioners, on the other hand, were acutely aware of their responsibilities. Had it ever been set up, the ill-fated London college of 1423 would have provided free treatment for anyone who had 'fallen in such poverte that he sufficeth nat to make good for the labours of his phisician or of his cirurgean', and would, furthermore, have monitored the fees charged by its members to prevent rapacity or extortion.[83]

We have no means of telling how many barbers and surgeons freely gave their services to charitable causes. That some were prepared to work for little or no remuneration is evident from the will of the wealthy mercer, John Don (d.1479), who had no time for the 'commyn beggeres' and vagrants of London, but profound sympathy for the deserving poor. He was particularly anxious that the surgeon, Thomas Thornton, might

> contynewe in his daily besynes and comfort of the poure, sore and seke peple lakkyng helpe and money to pay for their lechecrafte in London and the subarbes of the same. In especiall, in the hospitalles of Seint Mary, Saint Bartholomewe, Saint Thomas, Newgate, Ludgate and in other places whereas peple shal have nede. And thus to contynnewe by this grace by the space of v [five] yere next ensuyng my decesse. For the which attendaunce and cost in medesines I wolle ther be paied for every yere of the v yere v li. in money. . . . And if it shall fortune him to be slouthfull and not diligent to attende the pour peple, or and it shall fortune him to departe this life . . . thenne my wille is that anothere able persone be provided.[84]

Despite the activities of men such as Thornton, it seems as if a large proportion of the urban poor, and most of the peasantry, were born, grew up, lived their lives and died without ever receiving professional medical help. They looked instead to members of their own community, many of whom were women, skilled in herbal lore and folk medicine. The need for an alternative, cheaper source of treatment was all the more pressing in view of the fact that the nostrums, ointments and tonics prescribed by qualified practitioners added appreciably to the already high cost of their services. Although they belonged, like barbers and surgeons, to guilds rather than universities, the apothecaries of England enjoyed a remarkable degree of influence, largely by virtue of their great wealth. For however expensive their wares might be, and however exclusive the market they supplied, there was always a demand for rare and exotic drugs.

NOTES

1. PRO, SP1/19, ff. 88–9. Ross's defence was hardly original: his account of the craft's classical antecedents appears in *Lanfrank's 'Science of Cirurgie'*, ed. R. von Fleischhacker (Early English Text Soc., CII, 1894), pp. 7–8.
2. *Les Metiers et Corporations de la Ville de Paris*, ed. R. de Lespinasse (3 vols, Paris, 1886–97), vol. III, p. 624.
3. No doubt because of his MD, Hobbes was made keeper of the London hospital of St Mary Bethlehem, a type of appointment rarely accorded to surgeons. Indeed, he is sometimes described as the king's physician (A.B. Emden, *Biographical Register of the University of Oxford to 1500* (3 vols, Oxford, 1957–9), vol. II, p. 938; *Calendar of Patent Rolls, 1461–67*, pp. 182–3; *1467–77*, p. 211; *1476–85*, p. 166). William de Appilton, friar, was surgeon and physician to John of Gaunt, at a fee of 40 marks p.a., in 1373 (*John of Gaunt's Register, Part I, 1371–75*, ed. S. Armitage-Smith (Camden Soc., third series, XX, 1911), no. 836); and Piers Bray was his '*mire et surgien*' a decade later (*John of Gaunt's Register, 1379–83*, ed. E.C. Lodge and R.S. Somerville (Camden Soc., third series, LVI, 1937), nos. 48, 691, and above, p. 140).
4. K. Park, *Doctors and Medicine in Early Renaissance Florence* (Princeton, 1985), pp. 25–6.
5. *The Little Red Book of Bristol*, ed. F.B. Bickley (2 vols, Bristol, 1900), vol. II, p. 154.
6. Besides the quotation at the head of this chapter, see also John of Arderne, *Treatises of Fistula in Ano*, ed. D. Power (Early English Text Soc., CXXXIX, 1910), pp. 4–8, and *The Cyrurgie of Guy de Chauliac*, ed. M.S. Ogden (Early English Text Soc., CCLXV, 1971), pp. 12–14, for lists of qualities desirable in a surgeon.
7. *Annals of the Barber Surgeons of London*, ed. S. Young (London, 1890), p. 62.
8. *The Cyrurgie of Guy de Chauliac*, op. cit., p. 27.
9. The practice of embalming and dismembering the corpse for multiple burial was first explored by C.A. Bradford in *Heart Burial* (London, 1933). E.A.R. Brown, in 'Death and the Human Body in the Later Middle Ages', *Viator*, XII (1981), pp. 221–70, embellishes (but does not adequately acknowledge) this study.
10. M. Alston, 'The Attitude of the Church Towards Dissection before 1500', *Bulletin of the History of Medicine*, XVI (1944), p. 230; M. Vale, 'Cardinal Henry Beaufort and the "Albergati" Portrait', *English Historical Review*, CV (1990), pp. 342–3. For an autopsy performed on the orders of a bereaved father, see above, p. 36.
11. Alston, op. cit., pp. 221–38; K.B. Roberts and J.D.W. Tomlinson, *The Fabric of the Body: European Traditions of Anatomical Illustration* (Oxford, 1992), p. 4. Brown (op. cit.) suggests that as well as having strong personal feelings on the subject, Boniface VIII was motivated by animosity towards the French and a distrust of the friars (who encouraged multiple burials).
12. *Extracts from the Records of the Burgh of Edinburgh, 1403–1528* (Scottish Burgh Records Soc., 1869), p. 103; *Annals of the Barber Surgeons*, op. cit., p. 80.
13. British Library, Dept of Mss, Harley 1736, ff. 9–9v (quoted in T. Beck, *The Cutting Edge: Early History of the Surgeons of London* (London, 1974), p. 109); S.J. Lang, 'John Bradmore and his Book Philomena', *Social History of Medicine*, V (1992), pp. 121–30. This passage provides a virtual paraphrase of de Chauliac on dissection (*The Cyrurgie*, op. cit., p. 28).
14. N.G. Siraisi, *Medieval and Early Renaissance Medicine* (pbk, Chicago, 1990), p. 89. For an example of this, see above, pp. 20–21.
15. Wellcome Library, Western Ms. 290, f. 42.
16. Siraisi, op. cit., p. 90; F.A. Yates, *The Art of Memory* (pbk, London, 1969), pp. 80, 127–8, figure 7A.
17. Roberts and Tomlinson, op. cit., pp. 6–38. P.M. Jones provides a useful survey of anatomical illustrations up to the 1540s (*Medieval Medical Miniatures* (London, 1984), Chapter II).
18. D. Jacquart, *Le Milieu Médical en France du XIIe au XVe Siècle* (Hautes Études Médiévales et Modernes, series 5, XLVI, 1981), p. 81.
19. E. Wickersheimer, *Dictionnaire Biographique des Médecins en France au Moyen Age* (Paris, 1936), p. 299.
20. *Annals of the Barber Surgeons,* op. cit., pp. 69–70; C.H. Talbot and E.A. Hammond, *The Medical Practitioners in Medieval England* (London, 1965), p. 183.
21. John of Arderne, op. cit., p. 4; Talbot and Hammond, op. cit., pp. 74–5.
22. Beck, op. cit., pp. 138–42.
23. Wickersheimer, op. cit., p. 104. Colin Galerne was a neighbour of the poet François Villon and as such figures in the latter's *Grand Testament.* He can hardly have been pleased by Villon's rather dismissive reference to him as a mere barber, nor by the imputation that he was likely to roast in hell (*Le Testament Villon*, ed. J. Rychner and A. Henry (2 vols, Geneva, 1974), vol. I, p. 128; vol. II, p. 231).
24. Beck, op. cit., pp. 165–6; Talbot and Hammond, op. cit., p. 338; *Annals of the Barber Surgeons*, op. cit., p. 70; British Library, Dept of Mss, Egerton 2572, ff. 50–70; *Extracts from the Records of the Burgh of Edinburgh*, op. cit., pp. 99–105.
25. See L.E. Voigts, 'Scientific and Medical Books', in *Book Production and Publishing in Britain, 1375–1475*, ed. J. Griffiths and D. Pearsall (Cambridge, 1984), pp. 345–402, for detailed examples. As she argues, the wide-scale transmission of scientific material by scribes did not automatically result in a general deterioration in standards. Some drawings (as of zodiac or vein men) actually became clearer and more informative.
26. Wellcome Library, Western Ms. 564. (This has been edited by R. Grothe in his 1982 University of Montreal Ph.D. thesis, 'Le Ms. Wellcome 564: Deux Traites de Chirurgie en Moyen-Anglais'.)

27. Ibid., f. 10.
28. F.M. Getz, 'Charity, Translation and the Language of Medical Learning in Medieval England', *Bulletin of the History of Medicine*, LXIV (1990), pp. 1–17; and above, pp. 66–7.
29. P.M. Jones, 'Four Middle English Translations of John of Arderne', in *Latin and Vernacular: Studies in Late Medieval Texts and Manuscripts*, ed. A.J. Minnis (Woodbridge, 1989), pp. 73–4.
30. The history of this struggle is fully recounted in Beck, op. cit., pp. 120–9, and *Annals of the Barber Surgeons*, op. cit., pp. 35–68.
31. *Les Metiers et Corporations de la Ville de Paris*, op. cit., vol. III, pp. 622–9.
32. Talbot and Hammond, op. cit., p. 219; John of Arderne, op. cit., p. 71.
33. *Annals of the Barber Surgeons*, op. cit., p. 25.
34. *Memorials of London and London Life in the Thirteenth, Fourteenth and Fifteenth Centuries*, ed. H.T. Riley (London, 1868), p. 394. This ordinance was confirmed in 1410 (*Calendar of the Letter Books of the City of London, I*, p. 85).
35. *Memorials of London and London Life*, op. cit., pp. 606–9.
36. *Calendar of the Letter Books of the City of London, K*, p. 36; Beck, op. cit., p. 70.
37. *Annals of the Barber Surgeons*, op. cit., pp. 52–68; Beck, op. cit., pp. 148–50.
38. *Calendar of Patent Rolls, 1452–61*, p. 597; PRO, C88/128/34.
39. *Beverley Town Documents*, ed. A.F. Leach (Selden Soc., XIV, 1900), pp. 111, 113.
40. For a charm invoking the curative powers of the Jordan see York Minster Library, Ms. XVI. E. 32, f. 47; and for the symbolism of the river see A. Hayum, *The Isenheim Altarpiece: God's Medicine and the Painter's Vision* (Princeton, 1989), pp. 39–40.
41. *English Gilds*, ed. T. Smith, L.T. Smith and L. Brentano (Early English Text Soc., XL, 1890), p. 27; *Annals of the Barber Surgeons*, op. cit., p. 33; Beck, op. cit., pp. 43–6; *The Little Red Book of Bristol*, op. cit., vol. II, pp. 155–6.
42. *The Little Red Book of Bristol*, op. cit., vol. II, pp. 135–41, 152–7.
43. *York Memorandum Book 1376–1419*, ed. M. Sellars (Surtees Soc., CXX, 1911), pp. 207–10.
44. Figures for enfranchised barbers have been taken from *The Freemen of the City of York, 1272–1558*, ed. F. Collins (Surtees Soc., XCVI, 1896) and analysed by Professor P.M. Stell, who has also kindly supplied the statistics for other practitioners active in the city.
45. *Intrates: A List of Persons Admitted to Live and Trade within the City of Canterbury 1392–1592*, ed. J. Meadows Cowper (Canterbury, 1904) and *The Roll of the Freemen of the City of Canterbury, 1392–1800*, ed. *idem* (Canterbury, 1903), *passim*.
46. *English Gilds*, op. cit., p. 27; *Calendar of the Freemen of Norwich, 1317–1603*, ed. W. Rye (London, 1888), *passim*. During the fourteenth century the guild of barbers of Bristol numbered at least twelve, their names being given in the preamble to the 1395 ordinances (*The Little Red Book of Bristol*, op. cit., vol. II, pp. 69–71).
47. *York Civic Ordinances 1301*, ed. M. Prestwich (University of York, Borthwick Paper, XLIX, 1976), pp. 17–18.
48. *York Memorandum Book 1376–1419*, op. cit., p. 209.
49. *Annals of the Barber Surgeons*, op. cit., p. 23; *Les Métiers et Corporations de Paris*, op. cit., vol. III, pp. 647–8.
50. *Memorials of London and London Life*, op. cit., pp. 593–4; *Beverley Town Documents*, op. cit., p. 111; *The Little Red Book of Bristol*, op. cit., vol. II, p. 70.
51. *Annals of the Barber Surgeons*, op. cit., p. 33; Beck, op. cit., pp. 132–4.
52. *York Memorandum Book 1388–1493*, ed. M. Sellars (Surtees Soc., CXXV, 1914), pp. 25–7.
53. *Calendar of Plea and Memoranda Rolls of London, 1364–81*, p. 236.
54. *Calendar of Early Mayor's Court Rolls of the City of London, 1298–1307*, ed. A.H. Thomas (Cambridge, 1925), p. 51. For '*le lou*' see M.C. Pouchelle, *The Body and Surgery in the Middle Ages*, trans. R. Morris (Oxford, 1990), pp. 168–9.
55. *York Memorandum Book 1376–1419*, op. cit., p. 211.
56. Borthwick Institute, York, York Registry Wills, vol. I, f. 64v (Dalton); II, ff. 20–20v (Hodgeson), 71–71v (Wasdale).
57. *Paston Letters and Papers of the Fifteenth Century*, ed. N. Davis (2 vols, Oxford, 1971–6), vol. I, pp. 437–8, 565; PRO, SP1/19, ff. 88–9.
58. *Calendar of Patent Rolls, 1370–74*, p. 140; *1374–77*, p. 392.
59. A.R. Myers, *The Household of Edward IV* (Manchester, 1959), pp. 124–5.
60. The emoluments of service are discussed at length in C. Rawcliffe, 'The Profits of Practice: the Wealth and Status of Medical Men in Later Medieval England', *Social History of Medicine*, I (1988), pp. 61–78.
61. For example, the French surgeon, Jean de la Roche, was taken prisoner when serving the Duke of Brittany (Wickersheimer, op. cit., p. 430); and Jean le Mire, surgeon to the King of France, had a horse killed in battle (ibid., p. 435).
62. PRO, E404/72/4/54; *Issues of the Exchequer*, ed. F. Devon (London, 1847), pp. 503–4.
63. See note 3, above.
64. *Calendar of Close Rolls, 1435–41*, p. 27; *Foedera, Conventiones, Litterae et cuiuscunque Generis Acta Publica*, ed. T. Rymer (20 vols, The Hague, 1704–35), vol. V, part 3, p. 58.
65. J.H. Wylie, *History of England under Henry IV* (4 vols, London, 1898), vol. IV, pp. 153, 204; PRO, E101/404/21,

f. 45. *Calendar of Patent Rolls, 1405–8*, p. 454. Bradmore belonged to the prestigious City fraternity of the Trinity and SS Fabian and Sebastian, in whose register a copy of his will survives (*Parish Fraternity Register: Fraternity of the Holy Trinity and SS Fabian and Sebastian in the Parish of St. Botolph without Aldersgate*, ed. P. Basing (London Record Soc., XVIII, 1982), pp. 42–3). For details of his career see Lang, op. cit., pp. 121–30.

66. *Calendar of Patent Rolls, 1391–96*, p. 473; *1396–99*, pp. 204, 407, 471, 525; *1399–1401*, p. 49.

67. PRO, E101/404/24, f. 6v; E404/16/399; *Calendar of Patent Rolls, 1401–5*, p. 215; *1408–13*, pp. 94, 224–5; *1413–16*, p. 190.

68. *Society at War*, ed. C.T. Allmand (Edinburgh, 1973), pp. 64–5; *Calendar of Patent Rolls, 1408–13*, p. 233; *1413–16*, p. 100; PRO, E101/45/5, 48/3, 69/4/409; E404/31/420. G.E. Gask, 'The Medical Services of Henry the Fifth's Campaign of the Somme in 1415', in his *Essays on the History of Medicine* (London, 1950), pp. 94–102, provides an overview of the expedition.

69. *Calendar of Patent Rolls, 1416–22*, p. 31; *1441–46*, p. 394; *Report of the Deputy Keeper of the Public Records*, vol. XLI, pp. 697, 798.

70. *Calendar of Close Rolls, 1422–29*, pp. 133–4. Bradwardyne surrendered his post in 1423, but not because of his, or his deputy's, negligence (ibid., p. 83).

71. For Morstede's great wealth see S. Thrupp, *The Merchant Class of Medieval London* (pbk, Ann Arbor, 1962), pp. 246, 260, and Beck, op. cit., pp. 79–86, 92–7.

72. *Select Cases in the Court of King's Bench under Richard II, Henry IV and Henry V*, ed. G.O. Sayles (Selden Soc., LXXXVIII, 1971), pp. 162–3.

73. Talbot and Hammond, op. cit., p. 137.

74. For Sax, who paid the poll tax levied on 'aliens' in London in 1483, see PRO, C1/42/108 and E179/242/25, m. 8v (I am grateful to Miss Anne Sutton for the latter reference); for Rollesford, Talbot and Hammond, op. cit., p. 213; and for West, PRO, C1/68/44.

75. PRO, C1/131/8.

76. John of Arderne, op. cit., pp. 5–6.

77. *Records of the Borough of Nottingham*, ed. W.H. Stevenson (3 vols, Nottingham, 1882), vol. II, pp. 174–7.

78. PRO, SC8/304/15189.

79. Beck, op. cit., pp. 45, 131, 164; *Annals of the Barber Surgeons*, op. cit., p. 33.

80. John of Arderne, op. cit., p. 4. In his will of 1450 Thomas Morstede made generous provision for the poor in areas where he owned land, as well as leaving £100 for pious uses and works of charity (Beck, op. cit., pp. 79–86).

81. Jacquart, op. cit., pp. 120–8. For individual examples of French barbers and surgeons treating the poor see Wickersheimer, op. cit., pp. 149 (Firmin Broullart), 197 (Gilles des Moulins), 248 (Guillaume Yvoire), 299 (Hubert), 395 (Jean de Dury), 422 (Jean de Yperman), 432 (Jean le Conte), 485 (Gilles de Soubzlefour), 543 (Martinette), 597 (Perronet de Chastel), 599 (Philippe).

82. *Calendar of Patent Rolls, 1399–1401*, p. 255. For royal almsgiving to the poor see H. Johnstone, 'Poor Relief in the Royal Households of Thirteenth-Century England', *Speculum*, IV (1929), pp. 149–67.

83. Beck, op. cit., pp. 65–6.

84. PRO, Probate Court of Canterbury, 2 Logge.

CHAPTER SEVEN

THE APOTHECARY

For that I am not
Spycier ne apotecarie
I can not name
All maneres of spyces;
But I shall name a partie:
Gynger, galingale,
Cubibes, saffran,
Pepre, comyne,
Sugar white and broun,
Flour of camelle,
Anyse, graynes of paradys;
Of thise thinges be made confections
And good poudres
Wherof is made
Good sausses
And electuaries for medicines.

William Caxton, Dialogues in French and English

This potecarys crafte is most fullyst of deseyte of all craftys in the worlde, for thies potecarys lake no deseyte in weynge their spice, for other the balance be not like or ellys the beame is not equall or elles they wyll holde the tonge of the balance styll in the holow with their fyngar when they be in weynge. They care nothynge for the welth of ther soule so they may be ryche.

A Fifteenth-Century School Book

The emphasis placed by late medieval physicians upon the need to maintain a humoral balance within the body, and their resort to a growing variety of medicaments to preserve or restore this state of equilibrium generated a widespread demand for sophisticated drugs and potions not readily available in the domestic herb garden or kitchen. As in other areas of scientific endeavour, a major contribution to existing Greek pharmaceutical knowledge had been made by the Arabs, who had greatly expanded and developed the work of such classical authors as Dioscorides and Galen, and whose writings were rapidly disseminated throughout Europe from the eleventh century onwards. The simultaneous expansion of international markets and trading contacts between East and West meant that a wide range of exotic new ingredients became available for wealthy patients anxious to purchase rare, expensive and therefore to them unquestionably more effective forms of treatment. Whether or not physicians themselves were reluctant to prepare and sell the remedies which they prescribed because commercial activities would have undermined their professional status, or simply because it made sense for some tradesmen to specialize as pharmacists in large urban communities, the business of supplying medical and restorative preparations was from quite early on undertaken by spicer-apothecaries. Indeed, the word *apotheke* initially denoted a storehouse in which general goods and not just *materia medica* were kept for sale.[1]

Satirists found a rich vein of material in the symbiotic relationship between doctor and apothecary, which was, at best, seen as an unholy alliance designed to hoodwink the public into buying over-priced, adulterated and largely useless decoctions. Given the need for close collaboration, especially at Court, allegations of fraud and collusion were unavoidable (and probably sometimes true); but the physician, jealous of his superior social and professional position, had no intention of letting his subordinate overstep the mark. Attempts throughout Europe from the twelfth century onwards to control the nascent drug trade reveal a wide range of problems, not least with regard to presumptuous apothecaries who wanted to prescribe and practise on their own account. The proper regulation and licensing of pharmacies, and the need to monitor sales of potentially lethal drugs preoccupied civic and medical authorities alike throughout the late Middle Ages, and the ensuing ordinances provide a valuable insight into this aspect of medieval life.

In an understandable attempt to avoid illness and keep the physician at bay those who could afford to do so dosed and massaged themselves regularly with potions and unguents, consumed quantities of spices, drank aromatic wines and purged themselves of evil humours. Once lost, that rare prize, a sound constitution, was all too often gone for ever, with the result that even the fittest men and women spared neither time nor money where their health was concerned. Only a few were wealthy enough to follow the example of the Italian merchant, Francesco di Marco Datini (d.1410), whose physician urged him to take saffron every day as a general prophylactic, or budget for the annual consumption of medicinal spices weighing over a hundred pounds by their households, as the first Duke of Buckingham (d.1460) did; but there was still a great (and growing) demand for apothecaries' wares.[2] This was fuelled by popular advice manuals, such as the *Secretum Secretorum*, which offered the reader useful suggestions for keeping in good shape:

> Anoynt the som tyme with swete smellynge oyntementes as the tyme requyreth for in suche swetenesse thy hert taketh grete pleasure and is nourysshed therby. And the spyryt of lyfe taketh refeccyon in good odoures: and the blode renneth meryly thrugh the vaynes of the body. After that take somtyme an electuary of a wood called Aloes and of Rubarbe, whiche is a precyous thynge, to the pryce of iiij pens [4d.] . . . and this shall do the moche good for it voydeth the heate of the mouth of the stomake and warmeth the body and wasteth wyndes and maketh good taste and sauoure.[3]

Although the bulk of the population had to make do with home-made remedies culled from the herb garden and kitchen, England still provided a ready market for exotic drugs and spices, which were avidly consumed by layfolk and religious alike. Whereas in Anglo-Saxon times most medicaments had required only rudimentary pharmaceutical knowledge, developments in the Arab world and the ensuing spread of new ideas from southern Europe meant that even quite routine cures became increasingly elaborate. During the 1350s, for example, when the twenty-five or so monks who had survived the Black Death were treating themselves with potions designed to ward off further outbreaks of pestilence, the infirmarer of Westminster Abbey spent an average of £5 a year on medicines. Already, at the start of the decade, unpaid debts due to the monastery's principal apothecary, Thomas Walden, stood at £30, equivalent to the cost of annual board and lodging for three monks; and the bills continued to mount. An account for 1351 alone records the purchase of gum arabic, tragacanth, three types of sandalwood, powdered gold, rhubarb (then, as the quotation above reveals, an expensive luxury), cummin, various kinds of pepper, senna, wormwood, musk and turpentine, which would have been supplemented with simples grown locally for medicinal purposes.[4]

Most of these supplies were imported from overseas, along with the large quantities of sugar which the infirmarer bought, not only to make his potions more palatable but also as a medicine in its own right: being temperately warm and moist, it seemed particularly beneficial for the chest complaints rife in any monastic community. The use of sugar in pharmacy had been pioneered by the Arabs, who were thus able to extend the Greek pharmacopoeia by mixing different combinations of herbs, spices and animal products with a sweet-tasting powder or syrup base.[5] Purchases of sugar, in particular, accounted for a substantial proportion of the money spent by successive royal apothecaries, and made the Italian factors who traded in England extremely rich. No doubt some of the 10,000 lb of sugar and 1,000 lb of candy which the Venetian, Thomas Lauredano, sent to England in 1319 was destined for the royal household, where toothache may have exacerbated an already tense political atmosphere.[6] Earlier, in 1286, a sum of £1,775 had been spent by Edward I on delicacies, medicinal spices, 677 cakes of sugar and over 2,199 lb of flavoured sugar, most of which went towards the making of electuaries, syrups and other nostrums.[7]

As we have already seen in Chapter II, diet, 'the fyrste instrument of medicyne', played a fundamental part in medieval therapeutics: treatment was, of course, prescribed for particular ailments, but in addition each individual regularly consumed cordials and specially prepared food, often on medical advice, either to stimulate or soothe the body. Electuaries, for instance, were thick, heavily sweetened confections of herbs and spices designed to improve the digestion, tempt jaded appetites and provide a general tonic. The Arab writer, Masawaih al-Mardini, *alias* Mesue the younger (d.1015), who was hailed in the West as 'the evangelist of pharmacy', had devoted twelve chapters of his medical formulary to the production of electuaries and similar compounds.[8] Known as the *Grabaddin*, this section was widely used by medieval apothecaries in truncated Latin or vernacular texts, along with the *Antidotarium* of Nicholas of Salerno, which appeared at some point before 1244, and contained 175 receipts of various kinds in its later versions. Nicholas's work had originally been composed as a guide for students confused by the existing sources and measurements: because of its systematic and relatively straightforward approach, it soon became 'the essential pharmacopoeia of the Middle Ages', translations being undertaken for the benefit of those lacking a classical education.[9]

As new information spread throughout Europe from Salerno, so the use of electuaries and other *composita* became a staple of medical practice. In his *Testament of Cresseid*, the poet Robert Henryson depicted Mercury as a wise and solemn 'doctour in phisick', carrying boxes 'with fine electuairis, and sugerit syropis for digestioun, spycis belangand to the pothecairis, with mony hailsum sweit confectioun'.[10] Recipes varied considerably, depending upon the wealth of the customer, the doctor's prescription and the supplies available. At Court it was possible to produce them in bulk using the very best ingredients regardless of price: on one occasion alone in the 1280s Edward I's apothecary made 271 lb of rose, sandalwood and ginger electuaries at a cost of almost £5; and when the king lay dying over £164 was spent on the production of a staggering 2,196 lb of medicinal syrups (incorporating some extremely expensive drugs).[11]

Although those lower down the social scale had to buy their tonics and cordials over the counter, there were still plenty of rare and wonderful concoctions on sale, in the major commercial centres at least. A list of the 'gross spice' and medicaments shipped into London on Venetian galleys at the close of the fifteenth century names some forty or so different pharmaceutical commodities, including all those already mentioned.[12] In addition, cloves, ginger, cinnamon, galinga and nutmeg were widely used; and there was also an enthusiastic, if limited, market for such exotica as elephants' tusks, seed pearls and ambergris, whose cost and rarity amounted, in the minds of the gullible, to a certain guarantee of satisfaction. Coming from as far afield as the East Indies, Ceylon, India, Persia and Egypt, these goods were destined for the shelves of grocers' and apothecaries' shops, where they were either sold direct to the customer (in the case of grocers) or made up on the premises into electuaries, comfits and medicines.[13]

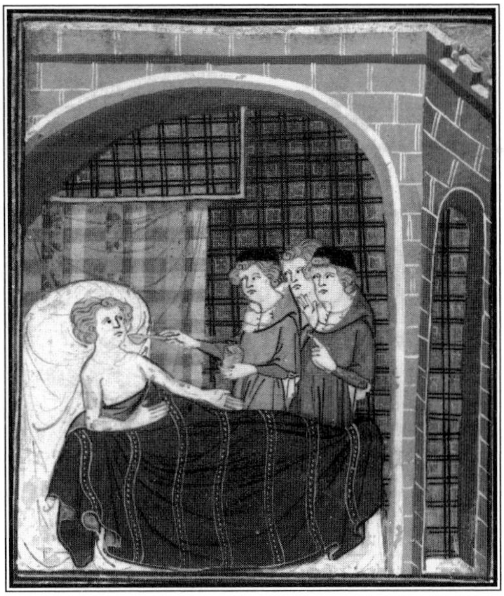

The range of medicaments available to the wealthy was almost limitless. As this French chronicle records, when Louis le Gros was sick 'he drank so many kinds of potions and powders . . . it was a miracle the way he endured it'.

Not everyone approved of the fashion for newfangled forms of treatment, especially as they put money into the coffers of unwelcome foreigners. *The Libelle of Englyshe Polycye*, a tract composed in about 1436 in support of a more aggressive and protectionist use of sea power by the English government, made no bones about the superiority of honest-to-goodness native remedies, although the author did allow a significant, if grudging, exception in the case of sugar:

And that I wene as for infirmities
In oure Englonde are suche comoditees
Wythowten helpe of any other londe,
Whych ben by wytte and prattike bothe i-founde,
That all ill humors myght be voyded sure,
Whych that we garde wyth owre Englysh cure,
That wee shulde have no nede to skamonye,
Turbit, euforbe, correct, diagredie,
Rubarbe, sene, and yet they bene to nedefulle.
But I knowe wele thynges also spedefull
That growene here as these thynges forseyde.
Lett of this matere no mane be dysmayde,
But that a man may voyde infirmytee
Wythoute drugges fet fro beyonde the see.
And yf there shulde excepte be ony thynge,
It were but sugre, trustee to my seyinge.[14]

Despite this spirited defence of home-grown purgatives (all the drugs listed above were believed to eliminate evil humours), the market for foreign imports proved almost insatiable. Every year, for example, large consignments of ginger (which reputedly kept the kidneys in good working order, helped the digestion and strengthened the memory) were dispatched to Norwich Cathedral Priory for distribution among the monks; while just across the road the brethren (but not the patients) of St Giles's Hospital consumed regular supplies of cinnamon – a champion specific against the windy colic and cold stomachs they must have suffered as a result of eating so much salt fish. In some of the larger religious communities the infirmarer himself was responsible for making and dispensing whatever drugs might be prescribed by an attendant physician (at the Cathedral Priory, for example, he regularly purchased phials, flasks and other equipment for distillation on the premises); but in others apothecaries undertook this work, even carrying out routine aspects of treatment, such as the giving of enemas, under medical direction.[15]

It is impossible to generalize about the techniques employed by English apothecaries, although the majority would have possessed the necessary skill and equipment for filtering, distilling, powdering and blending the various commodities on their shelves. Some of the more ancient methods used derived from cooking and dyeing, while others were acquired as a result of developments in alchemy and metalwork. A list of the goods confiscated from John Hexham, a London apothecary convicted and hanged for counterfeiting in 1415, records a still, eighteen bottles containing 'divers waters' which had presumably been produced on it, twenty-five simples from vegetable drugs, fifteen different oils and a handful of animal products, together with various lozenges, pills and ointments. Curiously, in view of the nature of his crime (which presupposes some knowledge of metallurgy), he owned none of the basic tools, such as pestle and mortar or sugar scales, commonly associated with the apothecary's craft, and thus may have operated as no more than a retailer, buying his goods wholesale from one of the richer and more successful members of his guild.[16]

These last were the men who dealt in theriac, the most highly prized and celebrated drug on sale in late medieval Europe, hailed as a universal panacea and commonly believed to possess almost limitless medicinal powers. According to one fifteenth-century English source, 'treacle', as it was known, could prevent swellings or distension, unblock intestinal stoppages, clear the skin of pustules or other blemishes, cure fevers, heart trouble, dropsy, epilepsy and palsy, induce sleep, improve the digestion, restore lost speech, strengthen enfeebled limbs, remove a dead child from its mother's womb, heal wounds and counteract the effects of venomous bites or poison on the body. It was also recommended specifically for use in vaginal suppositories to induce menstrual bleeding and as part of the treatment for a prolapsed uterus, not to mention more generally as a prophylactic against the plague and other infectious diseases.[17] During epidemics, people were advised that

> it is proufitable as wel for hole and seke folkes to drynke tryacle. Therfore take it ij tymes a daye with clere wyn . . . or with clere rose water or with clere ale. Take a quantite of tryacle and ij sponefull of clere wyn or rosewater or ale, dissolve the tryacle in the cuppe and drynke it; and dyne not tyl the myddes of the daye so that the triacle maye have his operacion. . . .[18]

Because of its remarkable qualities, theriac often figured metaphorically in devotional literature concerned with the cure of the soul. In Thomas More's treatise on *The Four Last Things*, for instance, contemplation of death, judgement, heaven and hell is seen as the spiritual equivalent of a dose of 'tryacle' taken to protect the body against contagion.[19] Henry, Duke of Lancaster, on the other hand, chose to compare it with the good example set to a man by improving literature, sermons and advice intended to help him overcome temptation. Unfortunately, however, the 'venom of the devil' used to make this brand of theriac might actually infect rather than cure a weak and vulnerable delinquent who lacked the strength to resist evil. 'Treacle', he writes, 'is the medicine rightly prescribed to make a man reject the poisonous sin which has entered into his soul. And the treacle is made of poison so it can destroy the other poison.'[20] Understandably, then, some people regarded it in an almost mystical light ('Crist, which that is to every harm triacle'), while others turned to it as a source of more immediate comfort ('I have triacle or elles a draughte of moyste and corny ale'), but anyone with money to spend bought supplies shipped in at considerable expense from Italy and marketed by the better sort of apothecary.[21]

A few dealers in major urban centres specialized as 'treacle mongers': between 1412 and 1422 no fewer than six 'treaclers' (one of whom doubled as a 'tuth dragher' or dentist as well) were admitted to the freedom of York; and in the same period Henry Kirton and his friend, William Norwich, were trading as such in, respectively, Westminster and London.[22] Visitors to the capital were clearly expected to stock up on purchases for friends and relatives. In 1451, for example, Margaret Paston begged her husband 'hartyley that ye woll send me a potte wyth triacle in hast, for I have ben rygth evyll att ese, and yowr dowghtere bothe'. John Paston must have had a long shopping list, as Margaret's uncle also relied upon him to dispatch supplies back to Norfolk. Perhaps, like Henry, Earl of Derby (the future Henry IV), Margaret kept her theriac in a silver box commissioned for the purpose: she certainly consumed enough to warrant such an expenditure.[23] Almost thirty years later the family was still dosing itself with large quantities, as this message from one of Margaret's sons reveals:

> Please it yow to weete that I sende yow by Barkere, the berere heroff, iij triacle pottes of Geane [Genoa], as my potecarie swerytht on-to me, and mooreouyre that they weer neuer ondoo syns that they come from Geane; wheroff ye shalle take as many as pleasyth yow. Neuerthe lesse my brother John sente to me for ij; therfore I most beseche yowe that he maye have at the leste on. There is on potte that is morkyn ondre the bottome ij tymes wyth thyes letteris 'M.P.', whyche potte I have best truste on-too.[24]

The reverence accorded to theriac was partly due to its appeal as a costly foreign import and partly to the range of unusual and rare ingredients used by the continental pharmacists who made it under a strict system of licensing. But the fifteenth-century consumer was most likely to be impressed by the drug's long and esoteric history, which, given contemporary attitudes to tradition, provided the most convincing recommendation. The ancient Greeks had produced a variety of theriacs, initially as antidotes to snake bites (the word '*therion*' means a venomous animal), and later for routine prophylactic and therapeutic purposes. One, called Galene, which was the prototype of the medieval version, contained some sixty-four different constituents, most notably the flesh of skinned and roasted vipers. This was supposed to combat the effects of poison ('tryacle made of venym to destroy venym'), although the great medical authority, Galen, had prescribed it for other disorders, too, while stressing the need for extreme caution at every stage of production and treatment. Since it took forty days actually to make Galene, and up to twelve years before the maturing process was fully complete, those involved were often tempted to cut corners or dilute their product.[25]

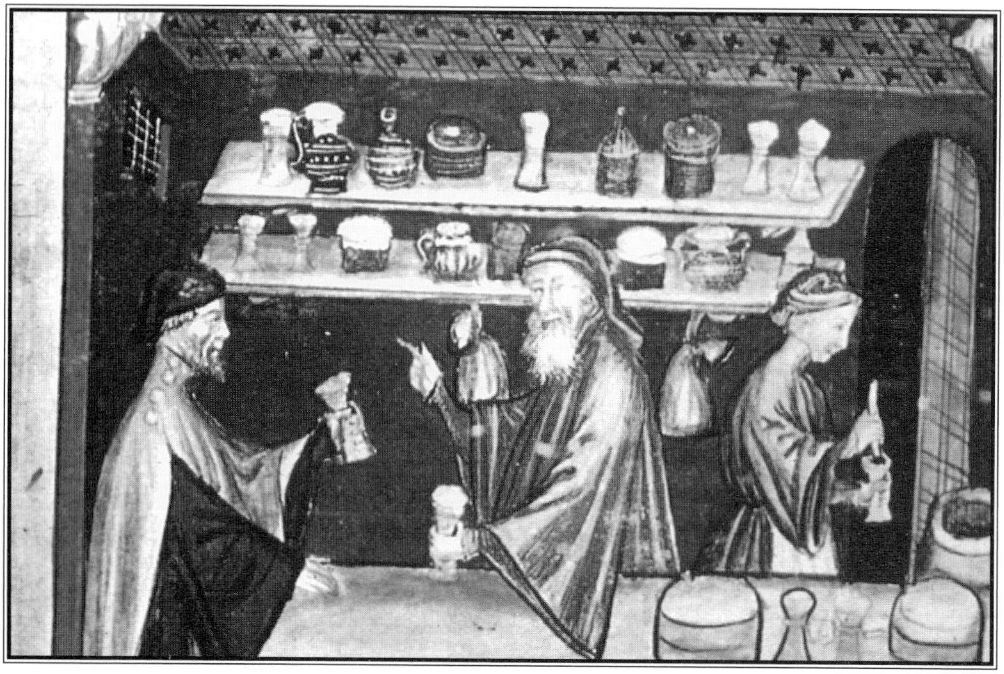

An apothecary selling theriac, which is displayed in large, decorated jars. The accompanying text notes that the drug is warm and dry by nature, and records some of its uses: as an antidote to poison, as a cure for both 'hot' and 'cold' diseases, and as a tonic for people who either lack natural heat or live in chilly climates.

Medieval physicians learnt about theriac from a miscellany of classical and Arabic sources, of which the most influential was a late thirteenth-century translation of Averroes' *Tractatus de Tyriaca*. They were excited, not just by the drug's potential as an antidote to man-made poisons, and, by extension, as a means of eliminating phlegmatic or melancholy humours from the body, but also because of certain wider philosophical issues arising from the contemporary debate about 'universals'. Besides the primary qualities of heat and dryness derived from its numerous ingredients, it was held to possess a 'special form' or unique property wherein lay the secret of its power. The appearance of learned, often arcane, texts on the subject added in no small measure to the mystique surrounding what was already perceived to be a magical elixir, and stimulated the growing demand.[26]

There was, however, nothing mysterious about the manufacture of theriac, which from quite early on was minutely regulated by the civic and medical authorities in the main centres of production. The cost of the drug, the difficult, time-consuming and potentially fatal procedures involved, and the possibility of deceit or incompetence on the part of the pharmacist all demanded constant vigilance, especially as so many commercial and professional reputations were at stake. The apothecaries of Venice were, for example, ordered in 1268 to prepare all supplies of theriac in the presence of *three* leading physicians and to store them for at least six months before putting them on sale. Failure to comply with these and other rigid codes of practice brought imprisonment and heavy fines, the worst cases of fraud incurring corporal punishment as well.[27]

The apothecaries and spicers who imported theriac into England were, in turn, held responsible for the quality of their merchandise. As we shall see, the Grocers' Company kept a careful eye on its members, some of whom appear to have been careless, if not actually dishonest, about the freshness and authenticity of their supplies. In 1432 Robert Sewale was fined 40s. for a repeat offence involving the sale of 'fals triacle' and was warned that next time he would be 'put owt of the craft for alle dayes', a serious penalty which would have deprived him of all trading privileges in London. The civic authorities, too, made a point of inspecting shipments as they were unloaded from incoming galleys. Certain 'bands and pots of treacle' were seized in 1471 on the orders of the mayor and examined by a group of experts, comprising two physicians and seventeen apothecaries, who pronounced them unwholesome. The offending goods were then solemnly burnt at three public bonfires (one of which, significantly, took place in Cheapside, where many apothecaries lived) as a warning to any other shipowners or dealers with low standards.[28]

Concern over the adulteration of expensive drugs or the substitution of cheap, possibly harmful, ones by dishonest apothecaries was as old as the history of pharmacy itself, and gave rise to some predictable complaints. Robert Burton's quip about 'old obsolete doses, adulterine drugs and bad mixtures' dispensed by 'the physitians hangmen, *carnifices* and common executioners' was characteristically astringent but hardly original. In his discussion of medical ethics, the ninth-century Arab writer, Al-Ruhawi, had warned against tricksters who mixed opium with barley flour, ambergris with salt, and camphor with powdered marble or rice in an attempt to defraud physician and patient alike.[29] Five hundred years later Sir John Mandeville drew attention to the way Egyptian traders passed off turpentine and other dubious commodities as a rare type of balm:

> And summe destyllen clowes of gylofre and of spykenard of Spayne and of othere spices that ben wel smellynge and the lykour that goth out therof thei clepe it bawme. And thus ben many grete lordes and othere disceyued. And thei wenen that thei han bawme and thei haue non. For the Sarazines countrefeten it be sotyltee of craft for to disceyuen the cristene men as I haue seen full many a tyme. And after hem the marchauntes and the apotecaries countrefeten it eftsones and thanne it is lasse worth and a gret del worse.[30]

French poets and satirists, from Rutebeuf to Rabelais, likewise made remorseless fun of the easy patter and underhand methods employed by apothecaries and herbalists. On rainy days in Paris, for example, the student Gargantua and his tutor entertain themselves by visiting the apothecaries' shops and observing how the roots, gums, seeds and foreign ointments are doctored to make a greater profit.[31] Yet France was one of the first European countries to introduce both national and regional regulations, which sought to establish adequate levels of training, proper supervision of staff and premises (by physicians as well as senior members of the appropriate craft guild), a uniform standard of weights and measures and clear rules as to what might legitimately be sold over the counter with or without a doctor's prescription. As was also the case in various parts of Italy, particular attention was paid to the importance of keeping properly annotated pharmaceutical textbooks, notably a copy of Nicholas's *Antidotarium* (herbalists were likewise expected to consult the *Circa Instans* attributed to Matthew Platearius), and a *Quid pro Quo*, or list of herbs and plants which might safely be substituted for others.[32]

Since there was no rigidly enforced system for the training and licensing of medical practitioners in later medieval England, it is hardly surprising that neither the state nor the profession managed to impose such firm controls upon the growing number of apothecaries who set up shop from the thirteenth century onwards. They were, of course, obliged, like all other

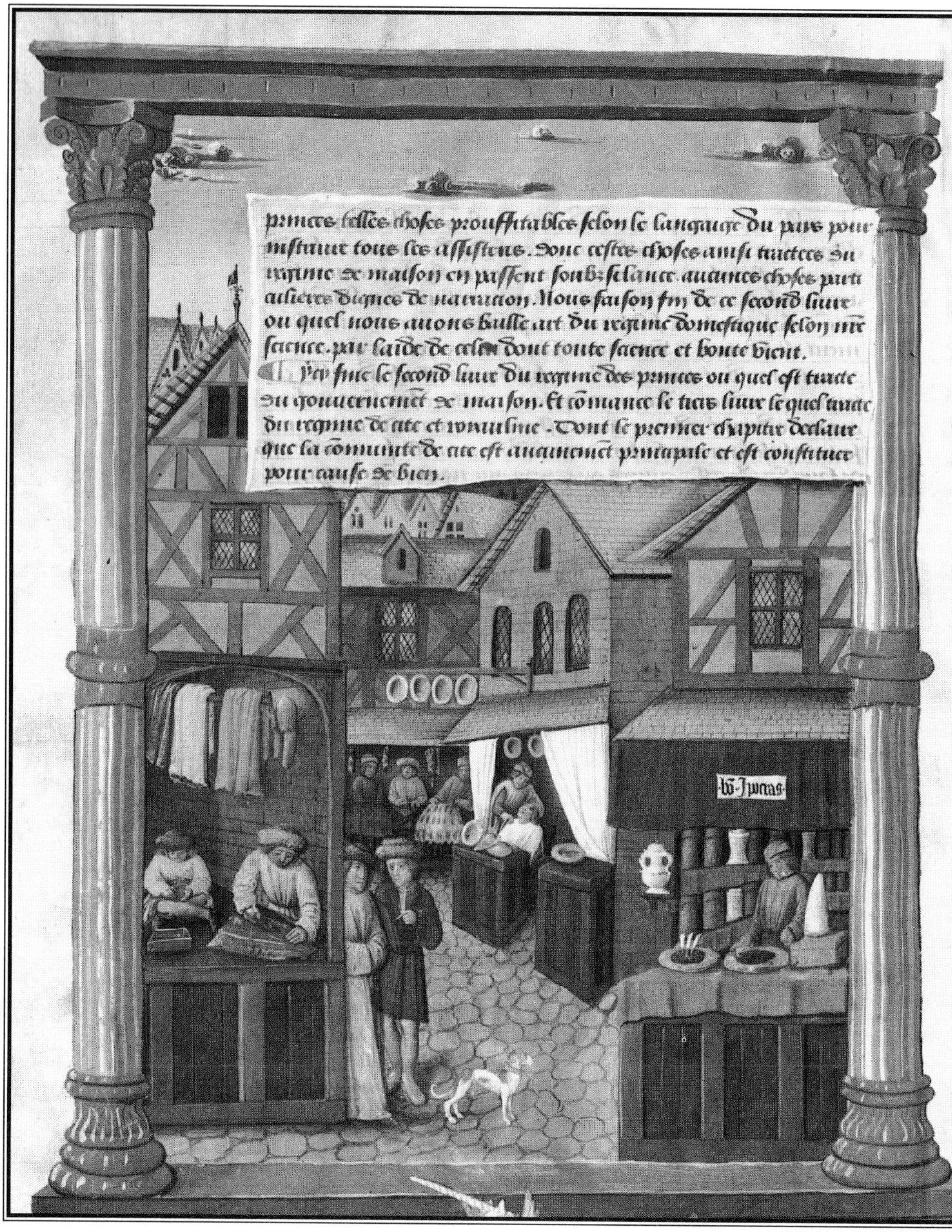

In this French street scene, an apothecary's shop is easily identified by the jars of theriac and other drugs on display, the owner's mixing plates, a large cone of sugar and the sign 'Bon Ipocras' hanging above the counter. Ipocras was a restorative drink, named after the Greek physician.

tradesmen, to obey the law with regard to the correct use of weights and measures, although misunderstandings arose throughout the country at even this elementary level. The 'Troy' or 'apothecaries' weight' of 12 oz to the pound (373.42g) derived from a Roman unit of measurement, and is known to have been employed well before the Norman Conquest. To avoid confusion with the 'London' pound or '*liber mercatoria*' of 15 oz (466.6g), Edward I codified established custom in 1302 by decreeing that Troy weight should henceforth be applied exclusively to 'confections as of electuaries', spices and bullion, while all other commodities would be weighed on the heavier, commercial scale. The raising of the 'London' pound from 15 oz to 16 oz in the next century caused further difficulties, not least because of its rapid replacement by the 'haberty-poie' or '*avoirdupois*' pound (453.59g), which was widely, but mistakenly, believed to contain 16 Troy oz.[33] In 1395 a bemused Nottingham jury complained that the town's apothecaries sold goods 'by unusual and unfaithful weights, not adhering to the standard', yet it was often quite hard to establish exactly how this 'standard' worked, or if one existed at all outside the pages of the statute book.[34]

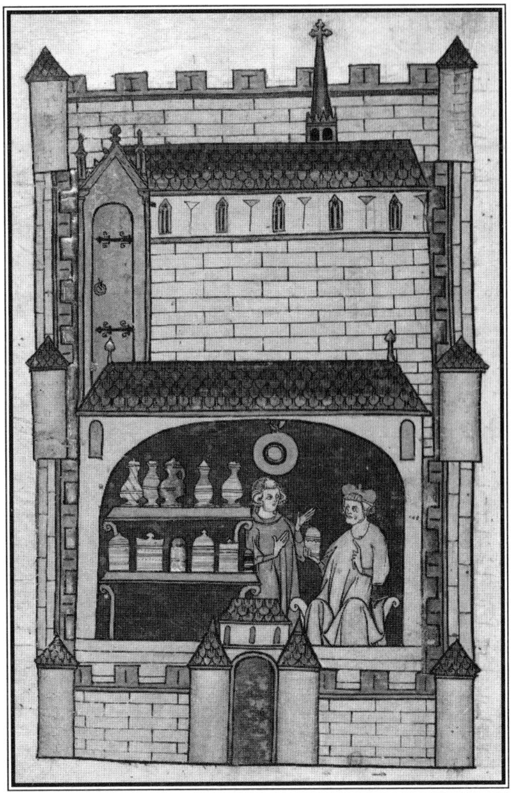

The opening page of an early fourteenth-century French translation of Matthew Platearius's famous herbal, the Circa Instans, *shows an apothecary's shop. A physician in academic robes is either dispensing drugs to his patient or, more probably, instructing the apothecary himself, whose mixing dish hangs from the ceiling.*

The problem was further compounded by the vexed question of whether drugs and spices should be assayed before or after they were cleansed of impurities (and thus made lighter), and who should stamp and measure them as they entered the kingdom. From the late thirteenth century onwards the posts of garbler and keeper of the king's lesser and greater beams (or balances), who were responsible, respectively, for supervising the removal of impurities from spices and weighing the appropriately stamped bundles at the major ports, tended to be the preserve of apothecaries and grocers. This made it easy for the Crown to reward men who supplied the royal household with expensive medicaments on long-term credit, while effectively freeing them from external constraints with regard to the marketing of foreign merchandise. On the other hand, the spicer-apothecaries involved came under pressure 'well and honestly to weigh as well for the poor as the rich', and are unlikely to have abused the system unduly, if only because self-interest dictated otherwise.[35]

All medieval urban guilds were anxious to avoid intervention on the part of either the local authorities or, far worse, the government itself, and tried as hard as possible to retain their independence by imposing strict internal discipline. From the close of the thirteenth century, if not earlier, the London apothecaries had formed a separate mystery, or guild, with their own brokers and wardens, who were sworn before the mayor to uphold commercial standards and ensure that their fellow-traders dealt fairly with the public. A full-scale merger in the 1340s, whereby the grocers, spicers and apothecaries combined into one large company (that of the grocers) with duly augmented financial and administrative resources, led to organizational improvements and the introduction of closer supervisory measures.[36] Many of these simply concerned the freshness, quality and honest weighing of spices, but at the beginning of the next century the company became more anxious about the way compound medicines were prepared and sold.

Starting in 1417 with a search throughout the mystery for old or contaminated ointments, which were to be confiscated and destroyed, the governors went on to order regular inspections, at least once a year, of all 'weyghtys, powdrez, confescriouns, plasters, oynementz and all othyr thyngys that longyth to the same craft'.[37] Their insistence upon collective responsibility by the entire 'felischyp' for fines imposed upon negligent or dishonest dealers was a shrewd move, although it evidently failed to satisfy the leading physicians and surgeons who gave thought at about this time to the setting up of the joint college in the City discussed earlier. According to proposals drafted by them in 1423, every apothecary in London was to be placed under the direct surveillance of a panel comprising the rector of the college, the two surgeons and two physicians currently acting as wardens, and two apothecaries 'assigned therto'.[38] Armed with the power to refer all vendors of 'false medicyns or sophisticate' to the mayor and aldermen for punishment, these expert searchers would have operated on the continental model, and would have undermined, if not completely destroyed, the authority of the Grocers' Company over many of its members. For almost a century the apothecaries of Paris had, for instance, been subjected to biannual searches by members of the faculty of medicine, while those of Breslau were similarly placed under the control of licensed physicians.[39] Relief at the failure of the scheme must therefore have been profound, and may well have led to the introduction by the guild of further self-regulatory measures designed to reassure consumers. Certainly, by 1425 they had accepted the need to impose controls on the trade between London and the provinces. In view of the great quantities of drugs and other medical supplies which passed through the capital each year, the new ordinance had far-reaching consequences, and came quite near, in the event, to the code of practice envisaged by the reformers:

> For as moche as the maystrez have the serche off weytez, poudrez, plastrez, conffits and all other wares with in the craffte, and tho that thei fynde deffectyve to destroye, or amende be avyse off the aldyrmen and the brethyrn off the craffte, where for there schalle no mane bere ne sende to sell pouderes ne no sotil ware in to the countre with owten leve in to the tyme the maystrez . . . may have serche up on hem, up on the peyne [fine] that the maystrez with the Felechyppe woll set there in.[40]

The medical profession did not give up the struggle for control over the licensing and inspection of apothecaries, although it was not until after the foundation of the Royal College of Physicians of London, in the early sixteenth century, that any real progress occurred. Seven years later, in 1525, the Common Council of the City passed an act in support of the college's new monopoly, which placed serious restrictions upon pharmacists. Despite a ruling that physicians were henceforth forbidden to sell any drugs already available from apothecaries, the latter can hardly have welcomed the loss of trade following a ban on commercial dealings with non-registered practitioners, or always have been anxious to keep a careful record of every substance dispensed on their premises.[41]

Other English towns and cities had, meanwhile, been left to monitor their apothecaries as they saw fit, meeting the challenge in a variety of ways. In York, for instance, the mayor and corporation contented themselves with a fairly broad ruling, incorporated into the city ordinances of 1301, that, like physicians, apothecaries should 'know their calling well'. But their stipulation that any harmful concoctions unsuitable for human use should be burned and the culprit banned from trading for life gave them a powerful weapon for use against crooks or charlatans.[42] From the medical point of view the most satisfactory state of affairs obtained in Oxford, where the university's physicians were able to exploit their position to gain effective control over the local apothecaries. Since the right to admit and approve them lay with the chancellor of the university, a rigorous system of licensing evolved. The oath taken by David Styles, in 1526, may perhaps have been influenced by developments in London, although it imposed far greater restrictions than any currently in force there:

> I swear that I will always have in my shop all medicines, species of medicines and confections which concern the art and mystery of apothecary and are necessary for the health of man. . . . That I shall be contented once a year (at least) that certain physicians practising in the University shall visit my shop upon the account of good and bad medicines, in the month of November, or any other time if occasion shall require it . . . and these searchers and tryers of medicines, being of the Vice Chancellor's and Proctors' appointment, shall have power to destroy and throw away all bad and unprofitable medicines and drugs. . . . That I will sell all things appertaining to my trade at a low and reasonable price, and as sold in other places in England. . . . That I will not make up any compound medicines without the presence and advice of some physician admitted to practice, who shall judge these samples fit to be made up into compositions.[43]

The passage, in 1540, of a statute empowering four of 'the best larned, wisest and mooste discrete' members of the London College of Physicians to examine the premises of all City apothecaries and remove any 'defective corruptid' medicines indicates clearly enough that the college was still fighting an uphill battle.[44] As was eventually recognized two decades later, any successful attempt to regulate the drug trade would have to take a firm stand against chicanery on the part of doctors as well as apothecaries, since other abuses, besides the sale of unwholesome or counterfeit medicines, were widespread. Efforts, in 1563, to prevent physicians from prescribing over-priced remedies and then taking a cut of the profits, or entering other dubious arrangements with their apothecaries, probably seemed long overdue to the average Englishman, who, like Geoffrey Chaucer almost two centuries earlier, may have come to suspect that 'ech of hem made oother for to wynne'.[45]

Without doubt, considerable amounts of money could be earned by a successful apothecary, especially one with access to the fashionable London market or, better still, an official appointment at Court. Just as favoured royal physicians and surgeons were able to exploit a rich source of patronage, so apothecaries also used their influence to acquire all manner of perquisites. In 1499, for example, James IV of Scotland gave 'oure lovit familiare servitoure and potingare, William Fowlare, for his gude, trew and thankfull service to be done to ws in his craft and science of pottingary' an annual pension of 20 marks; and a few years later he ordered that a house and shop in Edinburgh which had previously been used by one of the city's pharmacists should be assigned to 'Master Stephane, ypothegar, sa that he may be fundin thair redy to do ws seruice'. Scottish monarchs were traditionally liberal to their medical staff: John, the apothecary charged with providing medicine for Robert the Bruce (and eventually enbalming his body), was paid almost £40, including fees of £18, during and after the king's last illness, in 1329; and his successors drew a more than respectable annuity of £10 for their work.[46]

Apothecaries employed by the English royal household could expect similar rewards. In addition to his regular stipend of £10 a year, John Gryce was made sergeant of the confectionary by Henry VII and given a life interest in a number of valuable London properties, of which 'Le Signe de Le Dolphyn', 'Le Lambe', 'Le Belle' and 'The Rose on the Hoop' were evidently hostelries.[47] Henry Tudor's notorious parsimony made him extremely cautious in the matter of gifts (Gryce's windfall had been confiscated from other people and did not belong to the Crown), but Henry VI had no such inhibitions and offered his apothecaries what, on the face of things, seemed to be lavish, even excessive, preferment. Richard Hakedy, 'our appotecarye and sergeant of oure chaundelerye', suffered from the jealousy and resentment of his colleagues, not least because his basic fee of 40 marks p.a. was alone larger than the annual income of many belted knights.[48] His appointment, in 1442, as garbler of spices in London, Sandwich and Southampton caused an uproar in the City, for despite his long connexion with the Grocers' Company the authorities still regarded him as a royal placeman and claimed the ancient right to choose a nominee of their own.[49]

Although new letters patent of 1448 prudently exempted the port of London from an award which otherwise made Hakedy garbler throughout England, his successor, William Godfrey, was placed in authority there. Indeed, as well as serving as 'yeoman of the chamber and apothecary to the King's person', Godfrey became porter of Exeter Castle for life.[50] Henry VI's poor health and long periods of incapacitating illness ought, in theory, to have lined his apothecaries' pockets, but the equally parlous state of his finances and the interminable delays faced by anyone with business at the Exchequer meant that Hakedy and his associates had to supply large quantities of expensive medicines on credit. In 1443, for example, he submitted a bill for over £81, claiming that he could 'gete no peny unto his greet hurte and hinderance', and asking to be assigned the money from customs duties at Southampton. As garbler, he was in a strong position to recover at least part of this debt, so in the event much of Henry's apparent largesse was no more than a means of settling his accounts.[51]

Even so, rich rewards were always to be had from grateful royal patients, whose generosity to their medical staff naturally included the men who made unpleasant remedies taste so agreeable. In 1321, for example, Edward II confirmed a grant of two houses in Boston, Lincolnshire, presented by his kinsman, John de Bretagne, Earl of Richmond, to his apothecary. After recovering from a serious illness contracted while on a campaign in Scotland, in 1345, Edward III bestowed a life pension of 6d. a day upon the apothecary who had attended him; and some fifteen years later his prisoner, King John of France, included both his physician and his apothecary among the recipients of cash shared out among the employees of his London household at Christmas.[52]

Since the royal apothecary was personally responsible for perfuming and fumigating all the monarch's clothes and bedding, as well as making up whatever preparations might be prescribed by the medical staff, he inevitably moved in close proximity to the royal person. A gift of £20 assigned to William Godfrey notes 'the daily laboures and attendaunces that our welbeloved servaunt hath aboute us'; and it was no doubt as a result of private conversations with Henry VII's queen that John Gryce's servant received 16s. from her privy purse towards the cost of his 'wedding gowne'.[53] The demands of military campaigns, at home or abroad, gave him further opportunities for advancement: not only was he expected to supply the King with a substantial medicine chest for use in the field (such as the two great panniers of 'drogueries and implasta' sent overland from London to Newcastle upon Tyne for Edward II's Scottish expedition of 1322), but often to attend him in person. While still Prince of Wales, in May 1303 Edward summoned his apothecary, Peter Montpellier, to join him at Roxburgh with a quantity of electuaries and spices, and kept him on hand for the next six months, at a fee of 4½d. per day. Peter again accompanied his royal master to Scotland in 1310, thereby achieving a degree of intimacy which many courtiers had reason to envy.[54]

Many other apothecaries established connexions with royal and baronial households indirectly, through their contacts with members of the medical profession. Two of Richard II's physicians and at least one of his surgeons bought 'dragettes and medicin' from the London apothecary, William Wandsworth, who regularly supplied them with oils, distilled water, flavoured sugar, ointments and a wide range of drugs.[55] So far as we know, he was paid reasonably promptly, but the Italian apothecary Bartholomew Thomassyn faced considerable problems in recovering the 'great sum' owed to him for spices by Edward III. A series of complicated negotiations in the summer and autumn of 1342 finally secured a promise of repayment out of the wool and tin subsidies due from Devon, although it is by no means clear that he was ever fully satisfied.[56] Less influential figures, such as Nicholas Abourne of Exeter, found it even harder to collect debts from disobliging customers. Nicholas, who claimed to have provided a member of the powerful Courtenay family with 'certayne potticary stuffe' worth over £14 over a period of thirty years without ever being paid, actually died while litigation was in progress, leaving his widow to continue a valiant but ultimately hopeless fight for compensation.[57]

By and large, however, we need not feel too much sympathy for the more successful practitioners of the apothecary's craft. With their shops and houses in the crowded thoroughfares of England's largest towns and cities they were assured a competent livelihood, and many grew very wealthy indeed. Despite, or possibly even because of, the huge bills run up by his customers at Westminster Abbey, Thomas Walden retained sufficient faith in the efficacy of their prayers to found a chantry worth £100 there. John Adam, one of the most prominent Italian apothecaries resident in fourteenth-century London, was able to leave a similar sum to his brother in his will of 1358; and at about the same time his near neighbour, John Bonydon, made bequests of vestments, plate and books to his parish church, while ensuring that his wife retained a quantity of valuable silver.[58] John Maryns (d.1384) evidently had some regard for a female friend to whom he left £5 and a covered silver cup with gilt lions at the base, but his extensive city properties went, as custom required, to his widow.[59] The contents of John Offham's London household suggest that he too lived in style, for besides the usual quantities of plate, he owned a sword and various pieces of armour, which passed, in 1361, to his favourite apprentice.[60]

Although they were less ostentatiously rich, apothecaries in other parts of England likewise assumed a place among the mercantile élite. As early as 1273, John *le especier aut apothecarius* became Mayor of York, the second city in the kingdom, and not long afterwards an apothecary named Michael is known to have accumulated several houses in Berwick-upon-Tweed. William Hancock (d.1485), who owned land and tenements in York and its suburbs, instructed his executors to hand over £20 in cash to various beneficiaries; and John Weston of Exeter had no trouble in raising securities to the value of £24 from his own store of handsomely decorated silver plate when called upon to underwrite a bond in the early 1490s.[61] Most tradesmen of substance invested in precious metal, which served as a useful reserve to be sold or melted down in times of hardship, but it may well be that some of our men had been given their prize pieces by grateful customers, perhaps sharing them with the society doctors who put business their way. Such largesse was certainly common at the top of the social scale: in 1374, for example, the Duke of Burgundy presented a generous gift of silver to the royal physician and apothecary sent by the King of France to treat him while he lay ill at Ghent.[62]

Medieval satirists enjoyed ridiculing greedy practitioners and unscrupulous pharmacists who schemed together to fleece the credulous and line their own pockets, although few were quite as vitriolic as Chaucer's sometime friend, John Gower. Perhaps he bore a personal grudge against some incompetent or dishonest Southwark apothecary: with its riverside brothels and taverns of dubious repute, the borough, where he lived, would have supplied a ready market for the bizarre cosmetics and aphrodisiacs, weighed on a balance rigged in the shopkeeper's favour, about which he wrote. But to Gower the exploitation of human vanity and lust was a minor peccadillo compared with the lethal deception perpetrated by an apothecary in partnership with a doctor:

> A crooked apothecary can deceive folk well enough on his own at home, but once he's teamed up with a physician then he can trick them a hundred times over! One writes out the prescription and the other makes it up, yet it costs a florin to buy what's not worth a button. . . . The physician and the crooked apothecary really know how to scratch each other's backs: one empties your stomach as often as he can, and the other is an expert at cleaning out your purse, which simply melts away! If your stomach feels heavy, one of them says he'll lighten it by removing all the excess humours; and if your wallet seems full the apothecary and his master will well and truly purge it. The healthiest digestion anyone could wish for is not proof against medicines, and no purse is so long that it cannot be drained by an apothecary.[63]

Because of their close relationship doctors and apothecaries could hardly avoid charges of collusion. For those with enough money, a visit from the physician meant one hefty bill for medical services and several more for the drugs and potions prescribed. Accounts compiled by the executors of Sir Ralph Verney in the 1490s record a total of £9 paid out to 'phesicians' and a further 51s.8d. spent in vain on medicines supplied by two apothecaries, the sums involved far exceeding what had been set aside for masses and obits for the deceased's soul.[64] The potential for fraud was thus considerable, and in many parts of Europe steps were taken at an early stage to prevent it. One of the very first surviving ordinances for the regulation of apothecaries, issued at Arles in the late twelfth century, warned against taking bribes from practitioners, protecting their interests or otherwise according them favours at odds with the welfare of the sick. At Marseilles in 1211, Avignon in 1242 and Venice in 1258 the authorities tackled the problem from a different angle: pharmacists rather than physicians were told not to give expensive presents or embark on mutually beneficial business deals.[65]

Some attempt was made to justify these practices on the ground that patients (especially female ones) would have little confidence in cheap drugs or common remedies no different from those available at home. Writing in the early fifteenth century, the Italian physician Anthonius

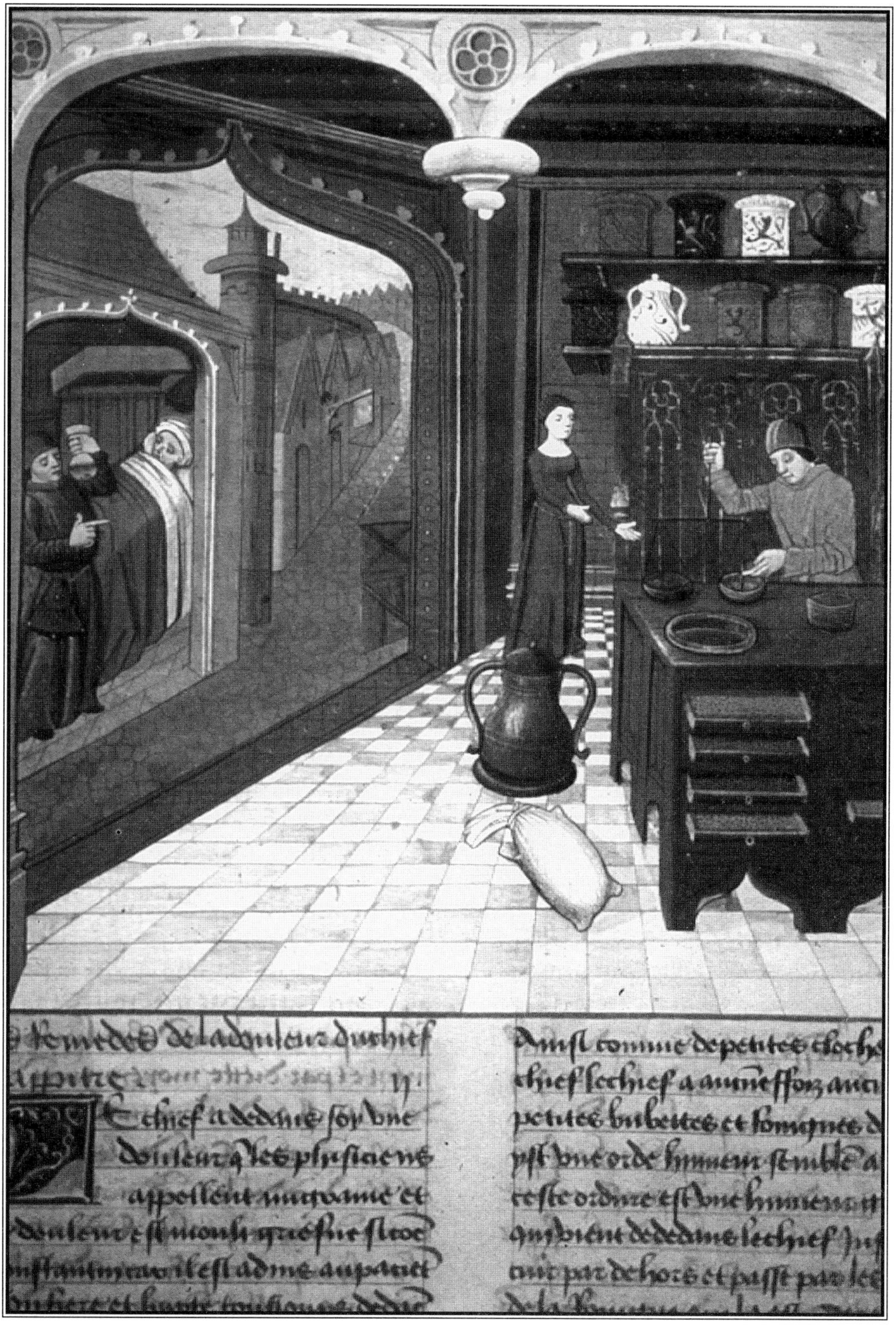

The physician, on the left, examines a patient's urine before prescribing. The medicine is made up for him by the apothecary, whose well-appointed shop, complete with jars of theriac, confirms that their arrangement is mutually beneficial. The large purse around the practitioner's waist speaks for itself.

Guainerius unashamedly recommended deceit in certain cases: 'have a trustworthy apothecary', he urged, 'who will affirm that this syrup has been made from conjugal substances, and see to it that he sells it at a high price so that it commands greater faith'. His suggestion that the practitioner should 'make up for his sin in another way' may have been little more than an empty platitude, however, since he was by no means the only doctor to believe in the psychological value of rare and highly priced medicines.[66]

Whereas in Florence a young physician often started out by contracting to treat patients at an apothecary's shop in return for a fixed salary (and sometimes accommodation as well), and might later strengthen these bonds through a commercial partnership or marriage, a much wider professional and social divide separated the English practitioner and his apothecary.[67] Far from belonging to a common guild and enjoying a roughly similar status, they were associated, respectively, with the world of learning and the bustle of the market-place, and, in theory at least, their relationship was perceived in conventionally hierarchical terms. At the Court of Edward IV, for example, the 'potycary' ranked as a yeoman of the chamber after the master surgeon but before the royal barber, and was strictly accountable to the king's physician for all his expenses.[68] There was, even so, a remarkable degree of collaboration and mutual dependence among the medical staff of the royal household, where apothecaries such as John Clark and Richard Hakedy worked closely with their superiors.

Clark (who was owed over £40 for drugs supplied to the Court in 1462, almost £89 in 1464 and the remarkable sum of £283 in 1475) struck up a personal friendship with Roger Marshall, one of Edward IV's senior medical advisors, whose children were named as beneficiaries of his will. No doubt he felt it only right that they should inherit some of the silver plate he had accumulated as a result of Marshall's readiness to let him share in the profits to be made from his royal and baronial patients, even if they proved slow in settling their accounts.[69] When, in 1465, the first wife of John Howard, the future Duke of Norfolk, lay dying, 'Master Roger', her physician, received four marks 'for his costes and reward in likenge to my lady', while his associate, Clark, was paid slightly less as a fee, together with almost £2 for medicines. Clearly, if not of the sort lampooned by Gower, their partnership was extremely lucrative.[70] As we have already seen, Richard Hakedy likewise did extremely well for himself in the service of the ailing Henry VI, providing a wide range of medicines, some of which were prescribed by the king's physician and chancellor, John Somerset. The latter numbered Hakedy among his most favoured intimates: his ambitious project for the foundation of an almshouse at Brentford involved the apothecary not only as a trustee but also as one of the original patrons for whom prayers were to be said in perpetuity.[71]

If few other apothecaries contrived to benefit their immortal souls through contact with the medical profession, many made useful and profitable connexions which could burgeon into far more than a mere working relationship. In 1480, for example, the physician William Goldwyn wrote from the country to ask his apothecary, John Berell the elder, to superintend personally the making up of three prescriptions for his 'specyall mastres', Lady Stonor. 'And with the grace of God hit schall not be longe or I see yow, and then I purpose for to tary with yow', he added, with a degree of warmth which suggests that the two were old friends. Such indeed was the attachment between them that Goldwyn relied upon the apothecary (or perhaps his son and namesake) to execute his will. Since the task involved litigation for the recovery of at least £114 in unpaid debts due to the deceased, we may assume that Berell was already familiar with, if not a party to, his financial affairs.[72]

Quite a number of the ordinances regulating apothecaries on the Continent demanded a basic level of medical knowledge as well as evidence of proper training in pharmaceutical skills. At Basle, for instance, no one was allowed to set up in business unless they knew how to analyse urine samples; and at Toulouse apothecaries actually studied alongside physicians, with whom for a time they shared the same guild. Even where no such requirements existed, apothecaries obviously learned a good deal about diagnosis and treatment, either by reason of their association with doctors, through private study or, *faute de mieux*, because professional help was not otherwise locally available.[73] It is interesting to note that, in 1468, the Duke of Clarence's apothecary received no fee but was allowed to take 'books of chirurgery' as well as empty pots and boxes instead.[74] Plans by Henry VIII for the foundation of a hospital in London for sixty-six sick paupers assumed that an 'expert appoticaire' would 'alweys be redy and attendaunte upon the . . . ffesycian and surgeon to prepayre suche thinges as they shall devise'; and it looks as if the apothecaries who supplied medicines to his father's foundation at the Savoy would likewise have done the rounds with the resident medical staff, acquiring useful experience as they did so.[75]

Testamentary evidence reveals that many English apothecaries owned books, and would, by the fifteenth century at least, have had little trouble in adapting to the Parisian statute of 1322 which insisted upon the presence of a literate person in every pharmacist's shop. Besides an array of drugs and equipment, including a still, mortars of various sizes, flasks, scales and a pewter spice-plate, together worth £5, the York apothecary Constantine Damme (d.1398) left a portable breviary and two volumes of 'antidotes'. One of his successors in the city, William Ruckshaw (d.1474), bequeathed a book to each of his apprentices; and Laurence Swattock of Hull (d.1492) specified that 'my ij bookes of ffesik called Nicholesse [the *Antidotarium* of Nicholas of Salerno]' were to go to his assistant, albeit on the understanding that he would henceforth show a more 'luffing disposicion to Jenet my wife'.[76] Two lawsuits fought in the court of Chancery towards the end of the medieval period cast a less favourable light upon relations between masters and their apprentices, although both indicate clearly enough that the latter expected to receive a long period of tuition (ten years in both cases) and be given a sound education, if necessary at grammar school.[77] It is thus hardly surprising that many apothecaries felt themselves to be quite capable of undertaking minor surgical operations or prescribing medicine to the sick; and some were evidently acknowledged as experts. Another York apothecary, Robert Bolton, was even appointed, in 1432, to arbitrate in a dispute over medical negligence, undertaking personally to supervise the treatment of the plaintiff and monitor his progress.[78]

Generally speaking, however, physicians were reluctant to encourage any steps in this direction. In the mid-fourteenth century, the *medici* of Valencia complained about an apothecary who had begun to provide free health care for the poor, despite the fact that he could boast years of experience 'on account of long practice and many conversations with masters and other practitioners of medicine'. And those who actually charged for their services caused even more resentment, as the ordinances made in Paris, Venice and other European cities attest.[79] In medieval England the medical profession was neither large enough nor sufficiently powerful to establish, let alone maintain, such a monopoly: competition from quacks, wise women and other empirics made it particularly wary of men who could offer advice over the counter in a reassuringly authoritative fashion. In public this unease found expression in attacks upon the competence of apothecaries to treat the sick, sometimes, it must be said, with ample justification. In 1354 three London surgeons testified before the mayor's court that 'a certain enormous and horrible hurt' on the jaw of one Thomas de Shene had been rendered incurable because of the ignorance of the spicer-apothecary who had applied medication without seeking proper advice. But it was not until the start of the sixteenth century that the corporation took active steps to prevent apothecaries such as Roger Smyth from treating patients simply because they had 'no manner speculacion and cunnyng that to do'.[80]

The passage of legislation early in the reign of Henry VIII (discussed in the next chapter), restricting medical practice to those with approved licences, made it technically illegal for apothecaries to offer more than drugs to their customers. A few prosecutions followed, notably in cases involving injury to the patient, such as that brought in 1539 against George Hill, 'potycarye' of Norwich, who was committed to prison 'ffor that he hath used the science off Surgerye, he nat beyng expert theryn nor yet admytted therunto according to the lawe, and mynystred to dyvers persons within this citie'. Having agreed damages with a woman whom he had reputedly harmed, Hill was banished from Norwich and warned 'atte his perell' to cease peddling his cures until he had acquired the right credentials.[81] But the profession found it extremely difficult to move against rivals who were so well placed to dispense and prescribe, and seemed at times to be almost overwhelmed by the competition. During the early eighteenth century (a 'golden age' for the practice of pharmacy) Robert Pitt was to complain that London stood on the point of being colonized by apothecaries, whose gaudy shop-signs hung in every alley-way and passage.[82] Nor were apothecaries the only threat to the beleaguered army of physicians and surgeons fighting to establish a professional and commercial monopoly in medieval England: on the contrary, a great army of herbalists, midwives and freelance practitioners caused far more concern, not least because so many of them were women.

NOTES

1. For the historical background to this chapter, see G.E. Trease, *Pharmacy in History* (London, 1964), chapters I–VIII, *passim*.
2. I. Origo, *The Merchant of Prato* (pbk, London, 1986), pp. 294, 377; C. Dyer, *Standards of Living in the Later Middle Ages* (pbk, Cambridge, 1989), p. 63 (where no mention is made of the fact that spices were consumed as much for medicinal as culinary reasons).
3. *Secretum Secretorum*, ed. M.A. Manzalaoui (Early English Text Soc., CCLXXVI, 1977), p. 339.
4. B. Harvey, *Living and Dying in England 1100–1540: The Monastic Experience* (Oxford, 1993), pp. 84–5, 96; E.A. Hammond, 'The Westminster Abbey Infirmarers' Rolls as a Source for Medical History', *Bulletin of the History of Medicine*, XXXIX (1965), pp. 268–72.
5. M. Levey, *Early Arab Pharmacology* (Leiden, 1973), pp. 52–3; G.E. Trease, 'The Spicers and Apothecaries of the Royal Household in the Reigns of Henry III, Edward I and Edward II', *Nottingham Medieval Studies*, III (1959), p. 22.
6. *Calendar of State Papers Venetian, 1202–1509*, ed. R. Brown (London, 1864), p. 3.
7. *Records of the Wardrobe and Household 1285–1286*, ed. B.F. Byerly and C.R. Byerly (London, 1977), no. 2349. Most members of the English royal family in the Middle Ages had a sweet tooth: see also L.G. Matthews, *The Royal Apothecaries* (London, 1967), p. 11.
8. Levey, op. cit., pp. 72–3.
9. T. Hunt, *Popular Medicine in Thirteenth-Century England* (Woodbridge, 1990), pp. 14–15.
10. *The Poems and Fables of Robert Henryson*, ed. H.H. Wood (Edinburgh and London, 1958), p. 113.
11. *Records of the Wardrobe and Household 1286–1289*, ed. B.F. Byerly and C.R. Byerly (London, 1986), no. 64; Trease, 'The Spicers and Apothecaries of the Royal Household', op. cit., Appendix D.
12. *Calendar of State Papers Venetian*, op. cit., pp. cxxxvii–cxxxviii.
13. The Arabs had developed their *materia medica* to number about four thousand simple and compound remedies in all, but only a fraction of these were regularly used in England (Levey, op. cit., p. 173). A *Tarif des Gabelles* drawn up at Avignon in 1397 lists some 145 therapeutic substances then on sale, however, including dried mummy and other exotica (L. Reutter de Rosemont, *Histoire de la Pharmacie a travers les Ages* (2 vols, Paris, 1931), vol. I, pp. 196–7).
14. *The Libelle of Englyshe Polycye*, ed. G. Warner (Oxford, 1926), p. 19.

15. For purchases by the infirmarers of Norwich Cathedral Priory, see Norfolk County RO, DCN1/10/1–38; for spices bought by St Giles's Hospital, ibid., press G, case 24, shelf A, general accounts 1465–1501, 1485–1508, 1509–27. The work of apothecaries attached to Westminster Abbey is explored in Harvey, op. cit., pp. 83–5.
16. PRO, E153/1066/1–2. This document is discussed in detail by Trease (*Pharmacy in History*, op. cit., pp. 71–2), who suggests that Hexham was probably no more than a retailer. It is interesting to compare this very modest inventory with one drawn up in March 1453 on the sale of a pharmacy in Avignon belonging to Philippe Felix. Besides some highly sophisticated equipment, the latter had acquired a remarkable quantity of rare and costly drugs, precious stones noted for their medicinal properties and powdered gold (Reutter de Rosemont, op. cit., vol. I, p. 197). The contents of Constantine Damme's shop in York were also considerably more impressive (above, p. 165).
17. British Library, Dept of Mss, Sloane 96, f. 39; *The 'Sekenesse of Wymmen'*, ed. M.R. Hallaert (Brussels, 1982), pp. 35, 57; G. Wilson, *Theriac and Mithridatum, A Study in Therapeutics* (London, 1966), p. 100; Wellcome Library, Western Ms. 564, ff. 86, 108.
18. *A Litil Boke the Whiche Trayted and Reherced Many Gode Thinges Necessaries for the . . . Pestilence* (John Rylands Facsimiles, III, 1910), p. 5.
19. *The Workes of Sir Thomas More, Knyght* (London, 1557), p. 73.
20. Henry of Lancaster, *Le Livre de Seyntz Médicines*, ed. E.J. Arnould (Oxford, 1940), pp. 56–9.
21. Geoffrey Chaucer, *Works*, ed. F.N. Robinson (Oxford, 1970), pp. 67, 148.
22. *Freemen of the City of York, 1272–1558*, ed. F. Collins (Surtees Soc., XCVI, 1896), pp. 117, 127, 129, 133; *Calendar of Close Rolls, 1413–19*, p. 63; *1419–22*, p. 130.
23. *Paston Letters and Papers of the Fifteenth Century*, ed. N. Davis (2 vols, Oxford, 1971–6), vol. I, p. 243; *Expeditions to Prussia and the Holy Land Made by Henry, Earl of Derby*, ed. L. Toulmin Smith (Camden Soc., new series, LII, 1894), p. 12. Henry's Queen, Joan of Navarre, also used theriac. In 1419 her effects included 'j pynte de treacle', as well as a variety of other drugs (A.R. Myers, *Crown, Household and Parliament in the Fifteenth Century* (London, 1985), p. 124). See too PRO, E101/402/18, for purchases by Queen Isabella in 1394.
24. *Paston Letters and Papers*, op. cit., vol. I, pp. 512–13.
25. Wilson, op. cit., pp. 47–82.
26. Arnald de Villanova, *De Dosi Tyriacalium Medicinarum*, in *Opera Medica Omnia*, vol. III, ed. M.R. McVaugh (Barcelona, 1985), pp. 57–73. Bernard Gordon, one of Arnald's successors at Montpellier and author of a more simplified treatise, *De Tyriaca* (*c.* 1305), describes a near-fatality caused by an excessive dose of theriac. He emerges as the saviour of the negligent apothecary who had swallowed too much of the drug in an attempt to counteract an accidental intake of poison (L. Demaitre, *Doctor Bernard de Gordon: Professor and Practitioner* (Toronto, 1980), p. 76).
27. *Documentazioni Cronologiche per la Storia della Medicina, Chirurgia e Farmacia in Venezia 1258–1382*, ed. V. Stefanutti (Venice, 1961), pp. 43–8; L. Reutter de Rosemont, op. cit., vol. I, pp. 309–11. As late as 1645 the diarist John Evelyn noted 'the extraordinary degree of ceremony' surrounding the public preparation of theriac (Wilson, op. cit., p. 104), which was by then highly ritualized.
28. *Manuscript Archives of the Worshipful Company of Grocers of the City of London 1345–1463*, ed. J.A. Kingdon (2 vols, London, 1886), vol. II, p. 225; *Calendar of the Letter Books of the City of London, L*, p. 103.
29. Robert Burton, *The Anatomy of Melancholy*, ed. T.C. Faulkener and others (2 vols, Oxford, 1989–90), vol. II, p. 210; Levey, op. cit., p. 167.
30. *Mandeville's Travels*, ed. P. Hamelius (Early English Text Soc., CLIII, 1919), pp. 32–3.
31. François Rabelais, *The Histories of Gargantua and Pantagruel*, trans. J.M. Cohen (pbk, London, 1969), pp. 92–3. For Rutebeuf on sellers of weird and wonderful medicines see his *Oeuvres Complètes*, ed. M. Zink (2 vols, Paris 1989–90), vol. II, pp. 239–47, and below, p. 176
32. *Les Statuts et Règlements des Apothicaires*, ed. F. Prevet (15 vols, Paris, 1950), vol. I, pp. 6–59; Hunt, op. cit., p. 15. Although, as N.G. Siraisi points out, in *Medieval and Early Renaissance Medicine* (pbk, Chicago, 1990), pp. 141–7, the availability of so many reference books was not necessarily a guarantee of either accuracy or reliability.
33. R.D. Connor, *The Weights and Measures of England* (London, 1987), pp. 117–30.
34. *Records of the Borough of Nottingham*, ed. W.H. Stevenson (3 vols, Nottingham, 1882), vol. I, p. 281.
35. *Calendar of the Letter Books of the City of London, D*, pp. 296–7; Trease, *Pharmacy in History*, chapter IX, *passim*; Matthews, op. cit., pp. 26, 33.
36. Matthews, op. cit., p. 26; *Calendar of the Letter Books of the City of London, C*, p. 17; *E*, p. 232. Sometimes, as in 1365, the company was still known as 'the mystery of grocers, spicers and apothecaries' (ibid., *G*, p. 204).
37. *Manuscript Archives of the Worshipful Company of Grocers*, op. cit., vol. I, pp. 111, 120.
38. T. Beck, *The Cutting Edge: Early History of the Surgeons of London* (London, 1974), p. 66.
39. *Les Statuts et Règlements des Apothicaires*, op. cit., vol. I, pp. 29–33; Reutter de Rosemont, op. cit., vol. I, p. 211.
40. *Manuscript Archives of the Worshipful Company of Grocers*, op. cit., vol. I, p. 154.
41. G.N. Clark, *A History of the Royal College of Physicians of London* (2 vols, Oxford, 1964), vol. I, p. 79.
42. *York Civic Ordinances 1301*, ed. M. Prestwich (University of York, Borthwick Paper, XLIX, 1976), p. 18.

43. R.T. Gunther, *Early Science in Oxford* (14 vols, Oxford, 1925–45), vol. III, pp. 7–8. The idea of fixing the price of drugs was popular throughout Europe, as regulations from various parts of Italy, France and the Holy Roman Empire reveal (Reutter de Rosemont, op. cit., vol. I, p. 271).
44. *Statutes of the Realm*, vol. III, 32 Hen. VIII, c. 40.
45. Clark, op. cit., vol. I, p. 96; Chaucer, op. cit., p. 21.
46. *The Exchequer Rolls of Scotland, 1264–1359*, p. 213; *1488–96*, pp. 59, 62, 143, 228, 298, 356, 389, 460, 534, 613; *1497–1510*, pp. 54, 122, 233, 274, 376–7; J.D. Comrie, *History of Scottish Medicine* (2 vols, London, 1932), vol. I, p. 145.
47. PRO, E159/282, ff. 3–4v; *Calendar of Patent Rolls, 1485–94*, pp. 251, 366, 469; *1494–1509*, pp. 115, 136, 164, 203, 505. Gryce's near-contemporary, John Pykenham, who had previously served Edward IV's queen, was assigned a similar fee of £10 p.a. as apothecary to Elizabeth of York in 1488 (Myers, op. cit., p. 314 and note).
48. *Calendar of Patent Rolls, 1436–41*, p. 525; *Rotuli Parliamentorum*, vol. V, p. 191. Hakedy's career is outlined by Matthews (op. cit., pp. 45–8), who discusses the work of the late medieval royal apothecary at length in the first three chapters of his book.
49. *Calendar of Patent Rolls, 1441–46*, p. 128; *1446–52*, p. 107. Hakedy's term as warden of the Grocers' Company, in 1446/7, was marred by a dispute with one of his fellow-governors (*Manuscript Archives of the Worshipful Company of Grocers*, op. cit., vol. II, pp. 289–91).
50. *Calendar of Patent Rolls, 1452–61*, pp. 227, 334–5 (in 1458 Godfrey was obliged to share his office of garbler with another courtier (ibid., p. 462)).
51. PRO, E404/59/126. Hakedy submitted this bill in January 1443, but had evidently not been paid by the end of October, when he asked for a further sum of almost £21 to be added to the grand total. This was for medicines supplied to the king between January and June 1443 (E404/60/73).
52. *Calendar of Patent Rolls, 1321–24*, p. 2; Matthews, op. cit., p. 29; *idem*, 'King John of France and the English Spicers', *Medical History*, V (1961), p. 68. Other marks of royal favour, ranging from pardons for serious crimes to fur-trimmed robes, are noted by Trease in 'The Spicers and Apothecaries of the Royal Household', op. cit., *passim*.
53. A.R. Myers, *The Household of Edward IV* (Manchester, 1959), p. 118; PRO, E404/64/199; *Privy Purse Expenses of Elizabeth of York*, ed. N.H. Nicolas (London, 1830), p. 49.
54. Beck, op. cit., p. 32; Trease, 'The Spicers and Apothecaries of the Royal Household', op. cit., p. 36; Matthews, *The Royal Apothecaries*, op. cit., pp. 36–7. In 1359 the Black Prince's apothecary, who ranked as a sergeant of his household, received a 'gift' of 20 marks 'to provide himself for the coming expedition' to France (*The Register of Edward the Black Prince*, ed. M.C.B. Dawes (4 vols, London, 1930–3), vol. IV, p. 303).
55. PRO, E101/402/18; 20, f. 40; British Library, Dept of Mss, Add. Ms. 35115, f. 35. Wandsworth (or Waddesworth as he is often known) played a prominent part in City politics, being a representative of Cheap Ward on the Common Council and a warden of London Bridge (*Calendar of the Letter Books of the City of London, H*, pp. 38, 42, 210, 281, 333, 411).
56. *Calendar of Close Rolls, 1341–43*, pp. 574, 590–1, 603. Bartholomew, who came originally from Lucca, belonged to the influential network of Italian spicer-apothecaries resident in Cheapside at this time. His son, Nicholas, followed him in business, and provided drugs for Queen Isabella during her last illness (E.A. Bond, 'Notices of the Last Days of Isabella, Queen of Edward II', *Archaeologia*, XXXV (1853), pp. 462–3), as well as serving overseas with the Black Prince (Matthews, *The Royal Apothecaries*, op. cit., p. 33).
57. PRO, C1/113/52.
58. Harvey, op. cit., pp. 84, 232; *Calendar of Wills Proved and Enrolled in the Court of Hustings*, ed. R.R. Sharpe (2 vols, London, 1889–90), vol. II, pp. 4, 39–40. For details about Adam see Matthews, *The Royal Apothecaries*, op. cit., pp. 27–8.
59. Maryns was quite probably the son or next heir of Thomas Maryns (d.1349), who rose to become master of the Mystery of Apothecaries and Chamberlain of London. His own career was greatly helped by marriage in 1372 to the widow of Adam Carlisle, a wealthy spicer with whom he had served as surveyor of the Grocers' Company. Such was his position in the civic hierarchy that he eventually became alderman of Cripplegate Ward (*Calendar of the Letter Books of the City of London, E*, pp. 232, 291; *F*, p. 191; *G*, pp. 204, 303; *H*, pp. 9, 118, 148, 291. For his will, see *Calendar of Wills in the Court of Hustings*, op. cit., vol. II, p. 248).
60. *Calendar of Wills in the Court of Hustings*, op. cit., vol. II, pp. 299–300.
61. Trease, *Pharmacy in History*, op. cit., Chapter VIII; *Calendar of Patent Rolls, 1292–1301*, p. 224; Borthwick Institute, York, York Registry Wills, vol. V, f. 257v; PRO, C1/111/11–12.
62. *Inventaires Mobiliers et Extraits des Comptes des Ducs de Bourgogne, 1363–1471*, ed. B. and H. Prost (2 vols, Paris, 1902–13), vol. I, no. 2029. The two men stayed together at the *Lion d'Or* in Ghent for ten days, at a cost to the duke of 30 *livres tournois*.
63. *The Complete Works of John Gower*, ed. G.C. Macaulay (4 vols, Oxford, 1899–1902), vol. I, pp. 283–4.
64. PRO, C1/230/53. The two apothecaries were John Clark and John Berell, both discussed below, p. 164. Executors often had to meet quite heavy medical expenses: those of the London draper, Robert Tattersall, for example, paid 14s.6d. to the deceased's apothecary and a mark to his physician (Eton College Records, vol. XLVII, no. 130).

65. *Les Statuts et Règlements des Apothicaires*, op. cit., vol. V, pp. 1215–17; Reutter de Rosemont, op. cit., pp. 186, 194; *Documentazioni Cronologiche per la Storia della Medicina in Venezia*, op. cit., pp. 37–8. In Breslau, in 1370, it was likewise decreed that although apothecaries should be controlled by physicians they should not share the same premises nor make financial arrangements together (Rosemont, vol. I, p. 211).
66. H.R. Lemay, 'Anthonius Guainerius and Medieval Gynecology', in *Women of the Medieval World*, ed. J. Kirshner and S.F. Wemple (Oxford, 1985), p. 324.
67. K. Park, *Doctors and Medicine in Early Renaissance Florence* (Princeton, 1985), pp. 29–31.
68. Myers, *The Household of Edward IV*, op. cit., p. 125.
69. Matthews, *The Royal Apothecaries*, op. cit., p. 52. For the money owed to Clark see PRO, E404/72/2/27, 72/4/5, 76/1/21. Despite these mounting debts, he supplied the Duke of Gloucester with medicines for his campaign in the north in 1482 (E405/70, m. 3), being perhaps mollified by the award of 8d. per day and a robe every Christmas made to him at the beginning of Edward's reign (*Calendar of Patent Rolls, 1461–67*, p. 122).
70. *The Household Books of John Howard, Duke of Norfolk, 1462–1471, 1481–1483* (1 vol. in 2 parts, Stroud, 1992), part I, pp. 304. 504–5.
71. *Calendar of Patent Rolls, 1446–52*, p. 29.
72. *Stonor Letters and Papers*, ed. C.L. Kingsford (Camden Soc., third series, XXIX and XXX, 1919), vol. XXX, no. 271; PRO, Probate Court of Canterbury, 5 Logge; *Calendar of Patent Rolls, 1485–95*, p. 362. There were two John Berells, senior and junior, active as apothecaries at this date (*Calendar of the Letter Books of the City of London, L*, pp. 103, 113, 244).
73. Reutter de Rosemont, op. cit., vol. I, pp. 297–300, 305–8. Lady Pertelote's efforts as a barnyard apothecary, as described in *The Nun's Priest's Tale* (Chaucer, op. cit., p. 200), and below, p. 218, make it clear that people went to their local pharmacist for advice and treatment, probably because a physician was not available.
74. Matthews, *The Royal Apothecaries*, op. cit., p. 55.
75. PRO, E135/8/48, ff. 3–3v. At a salary of £10 p.a., the apothecary was to be paid exactly half what the physician earned and £3 6s.8d. less than the surgeon: a scale which reflects their relative seniority. He was also to receive £20 p.a. for 'drugges gumes, aromates and other necessaries'. In 1532 the Savoy Hospital spent £22 on medicaments (*Valor Ecclesiasticus*, ed. J. Caley and J. Hunter (6 vols, London, 1810–34), vol. I, p. 359), a mere fraction of the 1,500 to 2,000 gold florins set aside annually by its prototype, the Hospital of Santa Maria Nuova, Florence (K. Park and J. Henderson, '"The First Hospital among Christians": The Ospedale di Santa Maria Nuova in Early Sixteenth-Century Florence', *Medical History*, XXXV (1991), p. 182). Not until the Tudor period did English hospitals engage the services of apothecaries on a formal basis, since it was only then that they assumed overtly medical functions. However, some connexion, as found at St Leonard's, York, in 1287 and 1420, probably existed before then (P. Cullum, *Cremetts and Corrodies: Care of the Poor and Sick at St. Leonard's Hospital, York, in the Middle Ages* (University of York, Borthwick Paper LXXIX, 1991), p. 14).
76. *Les Statuts et Règlements des Apothicaires*, op. cit., vol. I, pp. 21–2; Borthwick Institute, York, York Registry Wills, vol. III, ff. 4v–5v (Damme was affluent enough to leave £8 to the friars of York, £10 for the poor, sick and leprous, £2 and a piece of silver plate to the hospital recently founded by John de Roucliffe in Fossgate, York, to which he may have been professionally connected, and over £25 in bequests to friends and family. He owned a large quantity of plate and some fine jewellery as well); IV, ff. 204–204v, 410v–11.
77. PRO, C1/252/13–16, 309/43–44. The period of apprenticeship seems to have grown longer with the passage of time: at Norwich, in 1291, it was six years (L.G. Matthews, 'The Spicers and Apothecaries of Norwich', *Pharmaceutical Journal*, CXCVIII (1967), pp. 5–9); and at London, in 1312, seven (*Calendar of the Letter Books of the City of London, D*, p. 176).
78. W.P. Baildon, 'Notes on the Religious and Secular Houses of Yorkshire', *Yorkshire Archaeological Soc.* (Record Series, XVII, 1894), p. 78. For Bolton's will of 1452 see Borthwick Institute, York, York Registry Wills, vol. II, ff. 315v–16.
79. Siraisi, op. cit., pp. 22–3; *Documentazioni Cronologiche per la Storia della Medicina in Venezia*, op. cit., pp. 37–8; *Les Statuts et Règlements des Apothicaires*, op. cit., vol. I, pp. 6, 21–2. In 1352, for example, at the request of the faculty of medicine of Paris the King of France ordered that no laxatives, syrups, electuaries, pills, clysters, opiates or such like were to be prepared without the supervision and direction of a physician, and that *no medical advice whatsoever* was to be given by apothecaries (ibid., pp. 25–6).
80. *Memorials of London and London Life in the Thirteenth, Fourteenth and Fifteenth Centuries*, ed. H.T. Riley (London, 1868), pp. 273–4; Clark, op. cit., vol. I, p. 80.
81. *The Records of the City of Norwich*, ed. W. Hudson and J.C. Tingey (2 vols, Norwich, 1906–19), vol. II, p. 168.
82. Matthews, *The Royal Apothecaries*, op. cit., p. 46. For a discussion of 'the golden age' see G. Holmes, *Augustan England, Professions, State and Society 1680–1730* (London, 1982), pp. 184–92.

CHAPTER EIGHT

WOMEN AND MEDICINE: CONFLICTING ATTITUDES

But of all this thronge
One came them amonge,
She semed halfe a leche,
And began to preche
Of the Tewsday in weke
Whan the mare doth keke;
Of the vertue of an unset leke;
And her husbandes breke.
With the feders of a quale
She could to Burdeou [Bordeaux] sayle;
And with good ale barme
She could make a charme
To helpe withall a stytch;
She semed to be a wych.

John Skelton, The Tunnyng of Elynour Rummyng

Yea, but now ych am a she,
And a good mydwyfe per De,
Yonge chyldren can I charme,
With whysperynges and whysshynges,
With crossynges and with kyssynges,
With blasynges and with blessynges,
That spretes do them no harme.

For the cowgh take Judas eare,
With the parynge of a peare,
And drynke them without feare
If ye wyll have remedy.
Thre syppes are for the hycock,
And six more for the chycock;
Thus may my praty pycock
Recover by and by.

If ye can not slepe but slumber,
Geve otes unto saynt Uncumber,
And beanes in a serten number
Unto saynt Blase and saynt Blythe;
Geve onyons to saynt Cutlake,
And garlyke to saynt Cyrylake,
If ye wyll shurne the head ake,
Ye shall have them at Quene hythe.

John Bale, A Comedy Concernynge Thre Lawes

Like the lepers and lunatics with whom they were sometimes categorized, women occupied an ambivalent position in the eyes of the medieval Church and the medical profession alike. On the positive side, female saints, headed by the Virgin herself, were venerated for their miraculous healing powers; housewives were expected, as a matter of course, to supervise everything touching the health and welfare of their families; and all the larger hospitals and almshouses (which were almost always religious or quasi-religious institutions) employed women to care for the sick, albeit often in menial positions. Yet, although contemporary literature abounds with examples of fictional heroines noted for their medical skills, the authorities were in practice increasingly hostile towards those women who overstepped the bounds of their amateur or domestic role by setting themselves up as empirics of various kinds. Claims that these freelance practitioners, who ranged from village wise-women and faith-healers to female surgeons carrying on their husbands' or fathers' practices, were involved in the black arts cannot necessarily be taken at face value; but a significant number of them were mistrusted by the ecclesiastical establishment, whose fears found expression in a series of legal measures designed to curb, if not completely suppress, their activities.

In dismissing women as frail creatures at best, susceptible to every temptation and thus forced to accept the yoke of male supremacy, the early Fathers could find all the ammunition they needed in the book of Genesis. God's admonition to Eve ('I will greatly multiply thy sorrow and thy conception, in sorrow thou shalt bring forth children; and thy desire shall be to thy husband, and he shall rule over thee': Genesis 3: 16) held good for all her female descendants, who had inherited this burden of shame. As Tertullian (d.*c.* 235) warned his 'sisters in Christ', even the most pious among them bore 'the sentence of God on your sex': each remained 'the devil's gateway', 'a temple built over a sewer', bringing sin and retribution to man. Because of their carnal appetites and intimate association, through parturition, with the most degrading aspects of human nature, women posed a constant threat to higher spiritual values. They were, in the words of St John Chrysostom (d.407), nothing more than 'phlegm, blood, bile, rheum and the fluid of digested food . . . behind . . . a whitened sepulchre'.[1]

Among the many painful consequences of the Fall were the nausea and discomfort of pregnancy, miscarriage, the agony of childbirth itself, the death, illness or deformity of infants and the attendant risks of medical treatment at the hands of ill-informed doctors. St Augustine of Hippo (d.430) wrote movingly about the suffering endured by women, whose fertility he saw, along with death, famine and disease, as a direct result of Eve's fatal transgression. Even so, his revulsion from the obscenity of conception and birth contributed not a little towards the growing distaste felt by the Church towards womankind. While conceding, for example, that a female could not technically be denied admittance to heaven because of her gender, he stressed that her reproductive organs would first be 'freed from corruption' and transformed to avoid the risk of pollution in paradise. Pollution on earth was, meanwhile, averted by the simple precaution, taken by some parish clergy, of denying burial in consecrated ground to women who were pregnant or had died in labour. As Simone de Beauvoir perceptively remarked, half a century ago, 'the aversion of Christianity in the matter of the feminine body is such that while it is willing to doom its God to an ignominious death, it spares him the defilement of being born . . . the body of the Virgin remained closed'.[2]

These prejudices were reinforced to a considerable extent by current medical theories. The Greek physician Galen (who expressed a degree of admiration for the sexual restraint, if not the actual dogma, of the early Christians) advanced an explanation of female physiology which held good for the next millennium and beyond, and exercised a profound influence outside the ranks of the medical profession. His argument, based on the Hippocratic concept that women were colder and more phlegmatic in their humoral make-up than men, gave added support to stereotypes of female inferiority derived from the biblical account of the Creation and the Fall.

> Now just as mankind is the most perfect of all animals, so within mankind the man is more perfect than the woman, and the reason for his perfection is his excess of heat, for heat is Nature's primary instrument. Hence in those animals that have less of it, her workmanship is necessarily more imperfect, and so it is no wonder that the female is less perfect than the male by as much as she is colder than he.[3]

Humoral theory taught that the phlegmatic complexion was not only cold but also wet, and thus subject to fluidity and change. Mutability, fickleness and lack of purpose therefore seemed quintessentially feminine characteristics; and it is no coincidence that the moon, the planet most closely associated with water, movement and, of course, madness, appeared to be female. The damp, disease-bearing south wind, against which medieval physicians issued so many warnings, was described in the same way. So great were its malign powers that children conceived while it was blowing would almost certainly be girls.[4]

Nor was this all. Besides the fact that Greek philosophers drew a close connexion between heat and the soul (with obvious implications so far as women were concerned), the female of the species was held to be additionally disadvantaged by specific spiritual and physical defects, themselves caused by the privations which she had to endure while still in the womb. Since the right side of the body was considered to be far warmer than the left, it followed logically that sperm from the father's right testicle reaching the right wall of the mother's uterus would produce a boy. As the outcome of what was, quite literally, a *sinister* ('left-hand') conjugation, girls, on the other hand, were vulnerable from the very start to a colder, more hostile environment. In accordance with the teaching of Aristotle, who had maintained that the foetus did not acquire a human soul until some time after conception, medical authorities generally allowed a period of forty days in the case of males, but twice as long for females, who were doomed to moral and intellectual inferiority even before birth.[5]

Furthermore, whereas the genital organs of a male foetus developed *outside* the body, in a female these very same organs became impacted or 'turned inside out', thus making her a botched and bungled version of the ideal, with ovaries instead of testicles and a cervix in lieu of a penis. Or, as the late medieval English reader learned, in more homely speech, 'in the woman for sothe in the stede of the yarde [penis] ys the necke of the moder [womb] . . . and it hath wyth

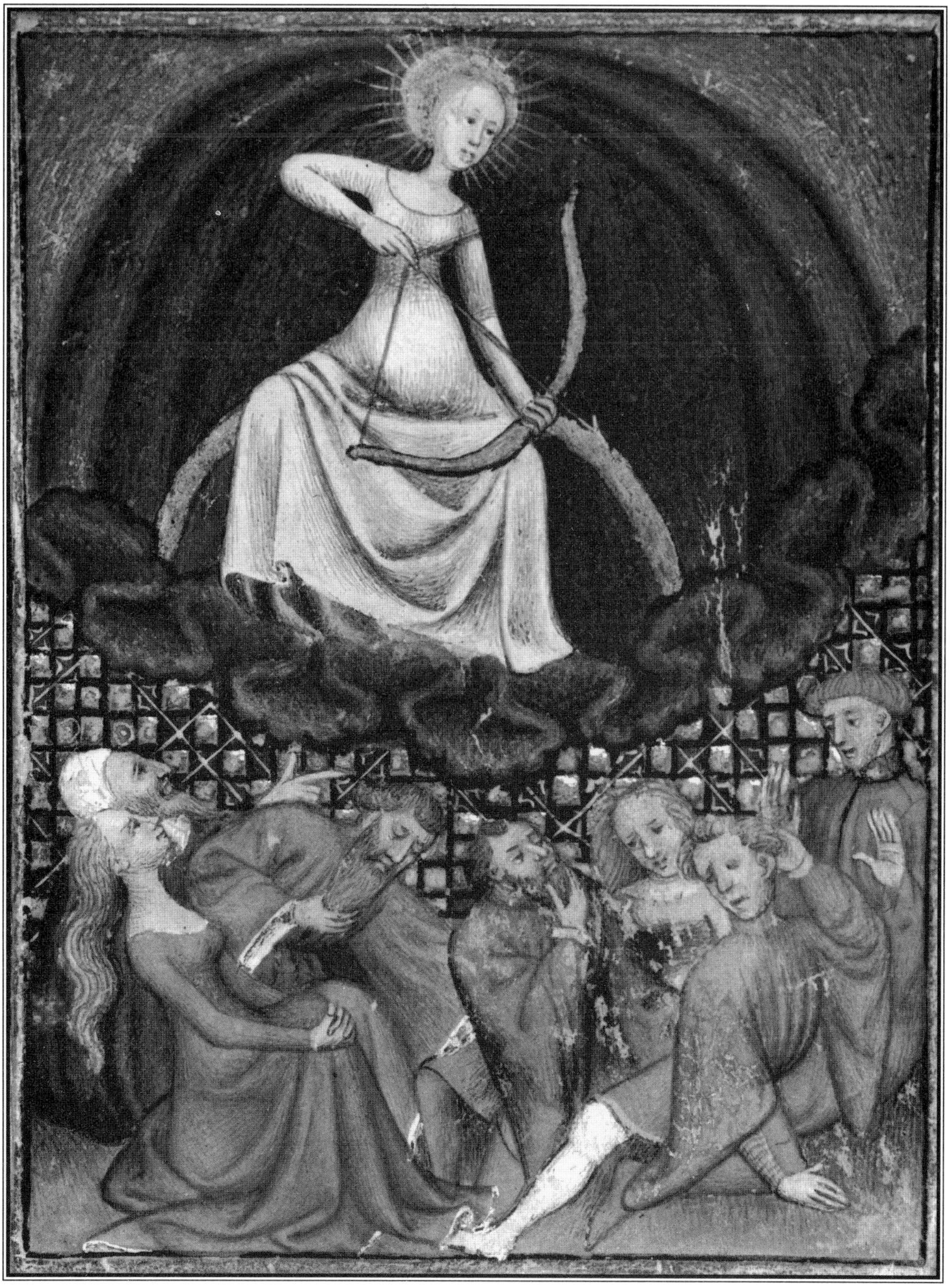

Diana, the huntress and goddess of the moon, strikes down men and women on earth with the arrows of madness. The connection between the moon, traditionally a watery and 'feminine' planet, and insanity served to reinforce ideas about the female sex's inherent instability.

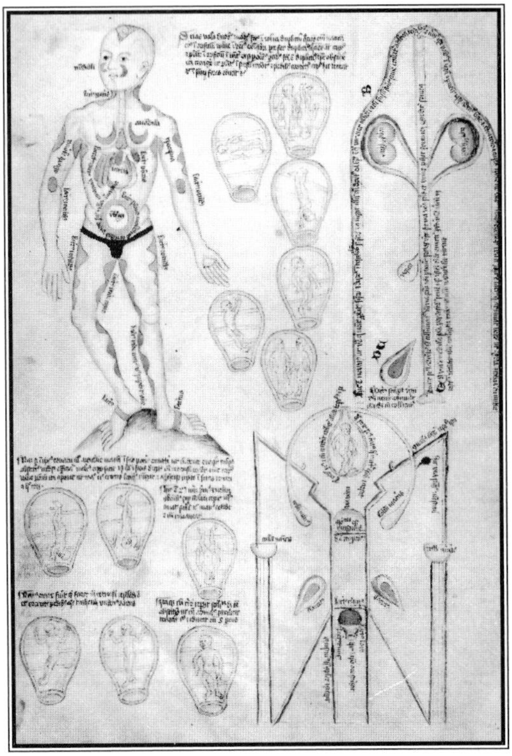

Drawings of the different positions of the foetus in the womb depict the uterus as an open vessel, or sack. But the diagram of the female reproductive tract in the top right-hand quarter of the page, complete with bipartite uterus, emphasizes the perceived similarity between male and female generative organs, and could be used to represent either.

that ij echyng, and yt hath smalle balokkys, netheles brode, and the neke of yt in comparycon to the ballokkys ys in maner of a yerd or a pyntyl y-turned inwarde'. Luckily, this deformity had its compensations, as Galen was quick to point out, since it made possible the propagation of the species. 'You ought not to think that the creator would purposely make half the whole race imperfect, as it were mutilated', he wrote, 'unless there was to be some great advantage in such a mutilation'.[6]

Because their reproductive function assumed such overwhelming importance, women were inevitably defined in terms of the uterus, which male writers had little trouble in describing, without any apparent sense of contradiction, as both a passive, empty vessel *and* a voracious animal. From the former point of view, the female of the species seemed, just like her womb, to be a vacant object awaiting the active male principle to provide her with energy, purpose and fulfilment. 'Everything imperfect naturally desires to be perfected,' observed Albertus Magnus (d.1280), to whom it was self evident that women would regard the sexual act as a temporary means of shedding their defective natures and 'putting on' masculinity. Albertus, a Dominican friar, was prepared to concede that lack of reason rather than inherent evil made women so libidinous, but he did not question other unflattering assumptions about their carnal appetites. Since it was widely understood that conception required the emission of female as well as male semen, and that the former could only be produced in response to pleasure, theologians drew the obvious conclusions: if a woman became pregnant, even when raped, her baser, animal nature must have overwhelmed her moral sense.[7]

The curse of menstruation, first inflicted upon Eve as a result of her fall from grace, came to be seen as another badge of infamy, borne conspicuously by all womankind. Although it was generally accepted that menstrual blood served to nourish the embryo after conception, turned to milk during lactation, and therefore played an essential part in sustaining life, the belief that it was otherwise designed to rid the body of unwanted or harmful humours generated through 'defaute of hete' provided clerical propagandists with yet more powerful weapons in their armoury against the female sex. In helping to make a woman 'clene and hole from syknesse', menstruation turned her, temporarily at least, into the vile creature so despised by the patriarchs. It might constitute a 'stain' rather than a sin, and 'cast a shadow' rather than leaving her 'in total darkness', but monthly purgation still marked yet another falling-away from perfection. The heroic austerities performed by some female visionaries resulted in amenorrhoea (cessation of menses), which was seen not as a consequence of starvation but a proof of sanctity. Colette of Corbie (d.1433) seemed unusually holy because she never menstruated, 'a special grace not heard of in others'. One version of the *Secrets of Women*, a popular work on human reproduction which derived at several removes from the writings of Albertus Magnus and circulated widely in the later Middle Ages, expressed the extreme view that 'women are venomous during the time of their flowers [periods] and so very dangerous that they poison beasts with their glance and little children in their cots, sully and stain mirrors, and on some occasions those men who lie with them in carnal intercourse are made leprous'.[8] Others argued that only diseased and degenerate offspring could result from conception in 'tainted blood'. Children might be stillborn, 'possessed of the devil, or leprous, or epileptic, or hunchbacked, or blind, or malformed, or feeble-minded, or club-headed', but all would bear some badge of ignominy, if only red hair.[9]

Having described how menstrual blood flowed into the uterus 'as filthe into a goter', Bartholomew Anglicus (*fl.*1230) added the further warning that, at its touch, 'fruyt growth noght, but drieth and beth ibrent, and dyeth herbes, and treen leseth here fruyt, irne is frete with roust, bras and metal wexith blake; if houndes etith therof he waxith wood [mad]'. Sick males (and their physicians) were cautioned as a matter of routine against sexual activity during treatment, particular emphasis being placed on the need to prevent 'a womman in tyme of menstrue' from even glancing at the patient, whom she might easily kill. This idea of menstruation as a pathological condition, at odds with nature and harmful to men, retained a powerful hold over the medical establishment for centuries to come: in its identification of menstrual blood as the cause of gonorrhoea in the male *The American Journal of Obstetrics* of 1875 may, for example, be regarded as the direct heir to a long and pervasive tradition.[10]

How far day-to-day relations between ordinary men and women were affected by these and similar ideas remains open to debate: after all, most of the early Fathers relied heavily upon their female acolytes, and their misogyny was often exacerbated by recourse to rhetoric and the desire to strike a polemical note. Even so, the apparent reluctance shown by medical practitioners to treat women's 'intimate' problems may, in some cases, have sprung from distaste as much as from a bashful desire to respect the modesty of their female patients, which was the reason usually given. And it is easy to see how underlying assumptions about female malignity could later be used to justify wholesale persecutions during the witch-hunts of sixteenth- and seventeenth-century Europe, especially as older women, past the menopause, were viewed with even greater alarm than those of child-bearing age.

In keeping with contemporary medical theory, the elderly of both sexes were believed to lack 'natural warmth', but in women this phenomenon seemed particularly dangerous in so far that it rendered them incapable of eliminating the 'many evil humours' which henceforward accumulated unchecked within their bodies. In short, once a woman ceased to menstruate she grew into a repository of poison, and the more impoverished her diet (that is wanting in heat) the worse the malignancy became. Clearly, a penurious old crone surviving by the skin of her few remaining teeth presented a prime target for abuse and denunciation. Others, who were better-off, also had to contend with a degree of prejudice: homilies on 'the governing of the body', for instance, frequently warned men to avoid 'flessheley' dealings with 'wymmen aged', since they could prove both morally and physiologically harmful.[11] Although many an ambitious apprentice or youngster on the make seems happily to have ignored this advice when the prospect of marriage to a rich dowager presented itself, some remained cautious. The animosity often shown by men in a position of authority

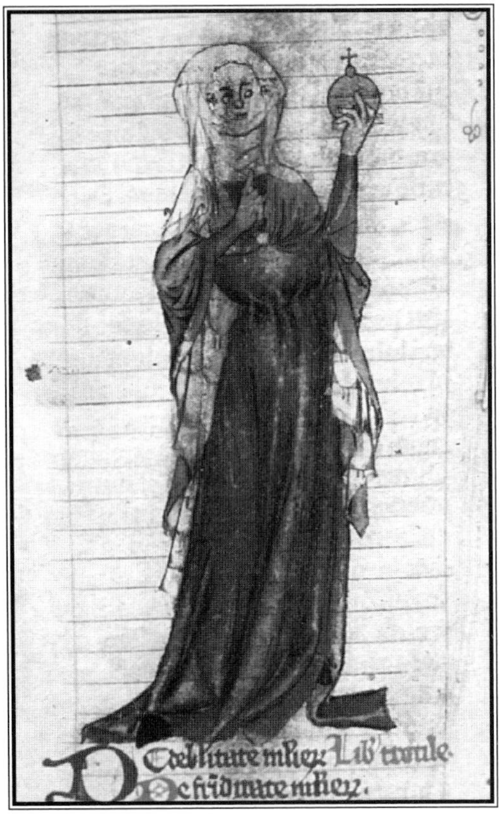

Trotula, portrayed in a flattering light as the queen or empress of midwives, in a twelfth-century Italian manuscript. Ironically, however, the work on gynaecology attributed to her was produced by a male physician, and represents an academic tradition very different from that which she herself followed.

towards female healers, who tended to be of mature years, probably had as much to do with fear and deep-seated mistrust as it did with the more immediately obvious question of professional competence.

The ambivalent status of women who made a living as empirics and midwives is illustrated by the posthumous fate of Dame Trotula of Salerno, the reputed author of a famous work on gynaecology and of a handbook which, significantly under the circumstances, dealt with the enhancement of female beauty (*De Ornatu Mulierum*). Recent research has shown that the real, historical Trotula did in fact produce a substantial guide to medicine, as practised on a day-to-day basis by her female contemporaries, at some point during the twelfth century, but that almost all her writing has been lost. The corpus of more academically orientated texts later attributed to her was in fact written by a man for the use of male physicians, and had little, if anything, to do with her at all.[12] Yet partly because of her assumed familiarity with the questionable subject of cosmetics, and no doubt also on account of her sex, the legendary Trotula soon developed a split personality: one half of her remained in the medical pantheon, while the other was thrown out on to the streets to peddle her wares as a flamboyant charlatan and procuress. By the mid-thirteenth century this wayward alter-ego had effectively become the patron saint of quacks and mountebanks, at least as portrayed by the French satirist, Rutebeuf:

> Good people, I'm not one of these impoverished preachers or poor traders in simples who pitch up in front of churches with their tattered old cloaks, carrying boxes and bags, and who spread out a carpet: why, they have more bags than dealers in pepper and cumin! Oh no, I'm not one of *that* crowd, but I'm in the service of a lady who is called Madam Trotula of Salerno: she wears a kerchief round her head and brows, hung about with gold chains down to her shoulders. You may be sure she's the wisest woman in the four corners of the earth. My mistress sends us all over the place to different countries . . . to kill wild animals, to extract unguents, to give remedies to those whose bodies have fallen prey to diseases. My mistress has given me clear orders to deliver, wherever I go, a few words of advice to those folk who gather around me . . . so off with your hoods, lend an ear, and just look at these herbs, which my mistress has sent along![13]

Medieval readers would certainly have detected more than a passing reference to 'Dame Trot' in the character of the lubricious old bawd who gives Fair Welcoming a distinctly unsentimental education about women in *The Romance of the Rose*. A cynical sensualist, bent on revenging herself against the men who betrayed her in her youth, she personifies the two predominantly female vices of concupiscence and deceit. The various tricks and embellishments, including hair-dye and face cream, which she recommends to every latter-day Eve, were, allegedly, part of the stock in trade of the village wise-woman, along with an even less acceptable store of knowledge (real or imaginary) about contraception, abortion and 'the arts of love'. Not content, then, with simply ameliorating the painful consequences of human sexuality, such creatures actually went so far as to encourage it. And, what seemed even worse in the eyes of the clergy, they often did so with the help of spells, incantations and other illicit devices. In denouncing the 'old courtesans and go-betweens and others of that ilk . . . who beguile patients with holy water, prayers to God and other tricks', Henri de Mondeville (d.*c.* 1320) spoke not merely on behalf of the medical establishment to which he belonged, but of the Church as well.[14]

Magic was, as we have seen, an integral component of medieval medicine, and although most practitioners, from the highest court physician to the humblest leech, had recourse to the occult, women tended to invite the greatest suspicion. Other considerations apart, their limited formal training and scant resources made them dependent upon herbal remedies and charms, both of which alarmed the ecclesiastical courts because of their potential connexion with sorcery and the black arts. And through this association with a dark, pagan world of ritual and superstition the wise-woman sometimes seemed to pit herself against Christ himself. As Haukyn, the Active Man, explains in *The Vision of Piers Plowman*:

> And whan I may noght have the maistrie, swich malencolie I take
> That I cacche the crampe, the cardiacle [chest pains] som tyme,
> Or an ague in swich an angre, and som tyme a fevere
> That taketh me al a twelvemonthe, til that I despise
> Lechecraft of Oure Lord and leve on [believe in] a wicche,
> And seye that no clerc ne kan – ne Crist, as I leve –
> To the Soutere [cobbler] of Southwerk, or of Shordych Dame Emme.
> And seye that [God ne] Goddes word gaf me nevere boote,
> But thorugh a charme hadde I chaunce and my chief heele.[15]

The 'old wytche' who specializes in a bizarre mixture of black and white magic, maleficent to some, beneficent to others, is a recurrent feature of contemporary literature, emphasizing, yet again, the mixed feelings she, and other members of her sex, aroused. John Bales's comic, but still sinister, crone, Idolatria, some of whose remedies are quoted at the start of this chapter, can do untold damage to her enemies, while curing those she favours by reciting the *Ave Maria* and 'other charmes of sorcerye'. The author may, perhaps, have had in mind a real London witch of the period, who confessed, in 1528, to employing a combination of simples and prayers to treat the sick. Margaret Hunt's testimony is of considerable interest, since it appears that her knowledge of plant lore and the efficacy of charms was acquired from another wise-woman in Wales, named Mother Elmet. Although some of these herbal remedies were intended to combat spells and ward off evil, and thus had an occult rather than a directly medicinal purpose, she seems otherwise to have been a devout, if naïve, Christian, and prayed earnestly to the Trinity for each of her patients. She was, even so, bound over to abjure her heresy and abandon her practice.[16]

Concern that women misused prayers out of ignorance, or else deliberately and heretically employed them to call up demons or familiars, had led earlier, in 1438, to the trial of another faith-healer, Agnes Hancock, before the Bishop of Somerset's commissary. Agnes, who stood charged of invoking the help of an aerial spirit ('*quos vulgus* "feyry" *appellant*') to cure sick children, denied any involvement in sorcery, but, when she was allowed the opportunity to recite the conventional prayers she claimed to use, her defence collapsed.[17] Given that in England witchcraft did not become a statutory offence bearing the death penalty until 1542, that previously all but the most politically motivated cases of necromancy were heard before the ecclesiastical rather than the secular courts, and that exponents of 'white' or even 'grey' magic were generally required to do no more than renounce their methods of treatment, on pain of a more severe penalty, she and all the other individuals, men as well as women, who faced prosecution under similar circumstances may be said with hindsight to have escaped quite lightly.[18] But they still stood to lose their principal means of earning a living if they obeyed the orders of the court; and, if they did not, the threat of degrading physical punishment, loss of goods or even excommunication from the ranks of the faithful hung over them. However skilful they may have been, however successful in healing or comforting the sick, however little real harm they may have done, their activities raised a number of moral and theological questions. From the female point of view, at least, the answers were rarely encouraging.

Yet if mankind had been burdened with original sin because of Eve's folly, it was now offered the prospect of eternal salvation through the Virgin Mary, whose growing theological importance during the later Middle Ages not only helped to improve the lot of women, but also promoted the development of a cult intimately involved with healing (colour plate 2). Hailed as the 'modir of lyf, cause of al our welthe, fyndere of grace and of our medecyne', she was commonly held to possess unlimited intercessionary powers, even over the dead.[19] Henry, Duke of Lancaster, described her as a devoted nurse, whose calm and soothing presence made bearable the painful treatment administered by her son, Christ the Physician:

> Since I have been given such a good nurse, who cares for me so tenderly in my sickness, and binds up my wounds so carefully and so well, it would be quite outrageous if I were not patient; nor could it be beyond her skill to cure me however ill I might be. This kind nurse is the gentle Virgin Mary, our Blessed Lady and your gentle mother, dear Lord. And it is a wonderful custom that, when anyone is suffering terribly, a woman is found to be with him; for she is able to minister to him far more solicitously and do everything for him in a much more agreeable fashion than a man. And therefore, gentle Lord, I am greatly bound to thank you with all my heart, since it pleased you to entrust me to such capable hands.[20]

Shrines dedicated to the Virgin thus often became pilgrimage centres for the sick. That of Our Lady of Walsingham in Norfolk attracted the faithful from all ranks of society and all parts of the country, in search of either a cure for their own maladies or help for incapacitated loved ones. On learning of her husband's illness, in September 1443, Margaret Paston promptly dispatched an expensive 'ymmage of wax' to the shrine and made arrangements to go there herself and pray for his recovery, although as a local landowner she faced a less arduous journey than most. A decade later, Henry VI's queen, Margaret of Anjou, travelled up from London, in

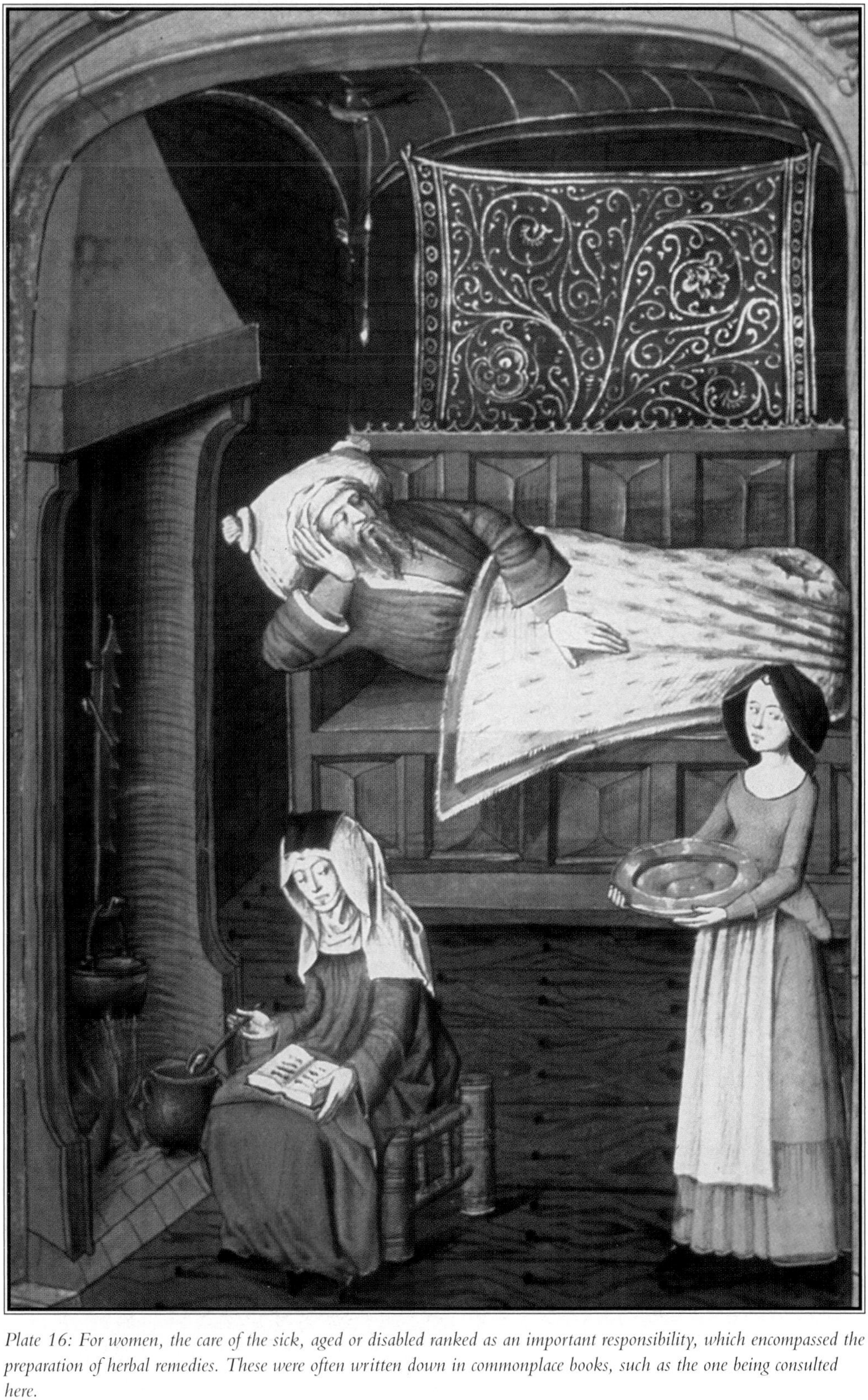

Plate 16: For women, the care of the sick, aged or disabled ranked as an important responsibility, which encompassed the preparation of herbal remedies. These were often written down in commonplace books, such as the one being consulted here.

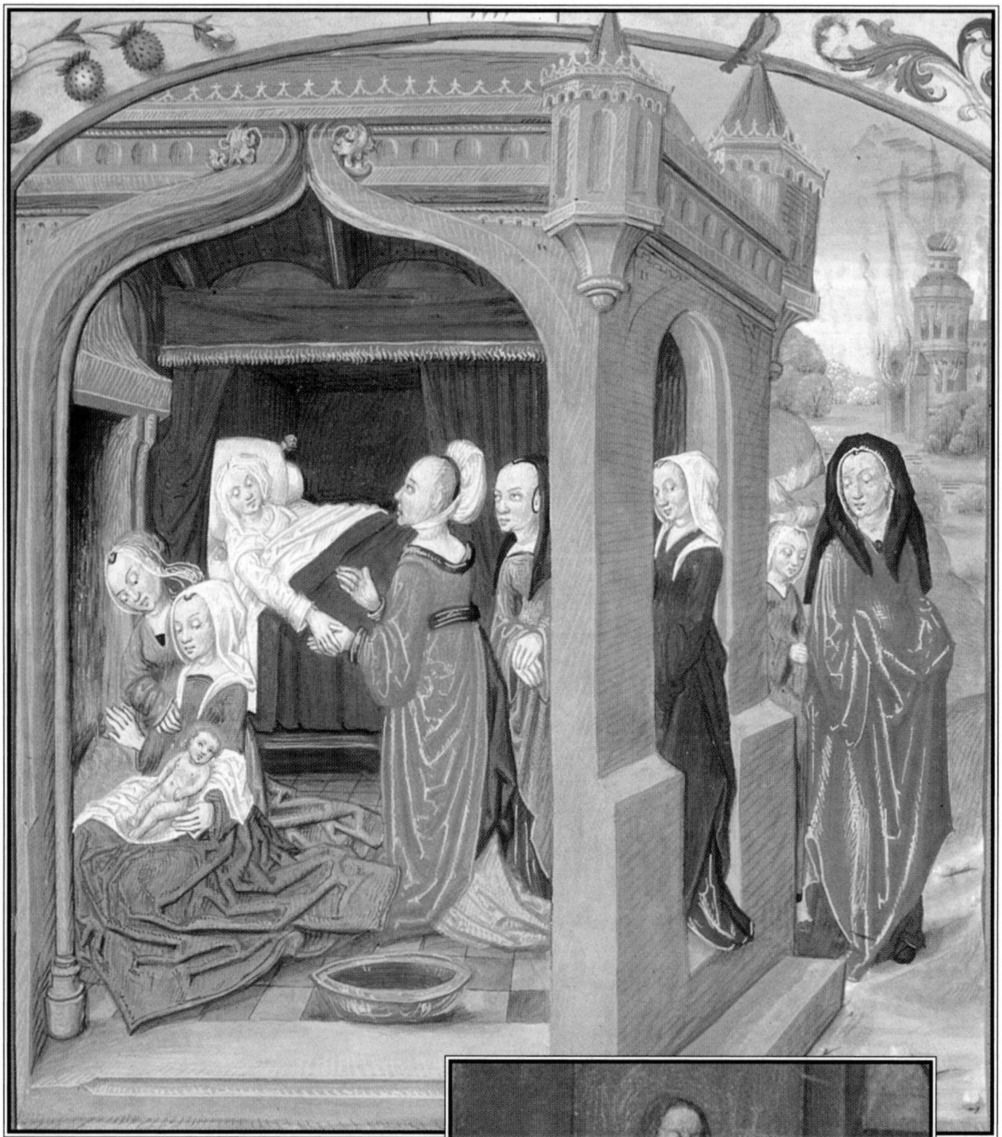

Plate 17: At all levels of society female friends and relatives offered support and encouragement to women in labour. Seen through medieval eyes, the birth of Alexander the Great brings many visitors to the bed of Olympias, who is able to benefit from their collective experience.

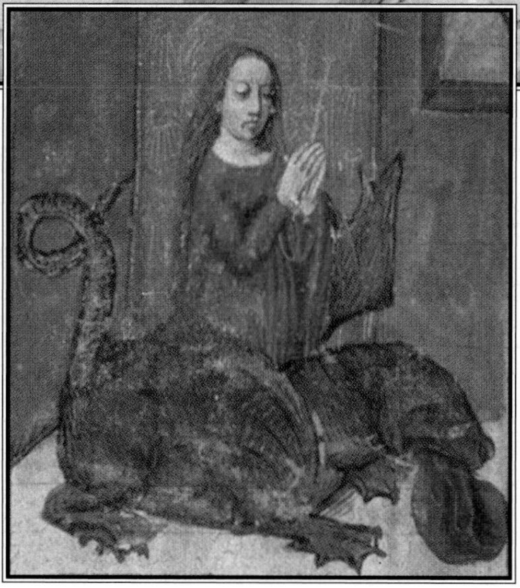

Plate 18: During her protracted martyrdom, St Margaret of Antioch was swallowed by a dragon, from whose belly she burst unscathed. For this reason, along with her readiness to protect women in labour, she became a patron saint of childbirth.

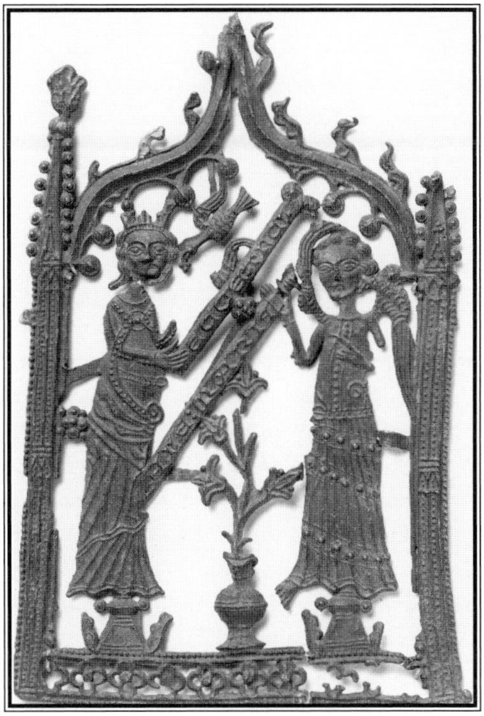

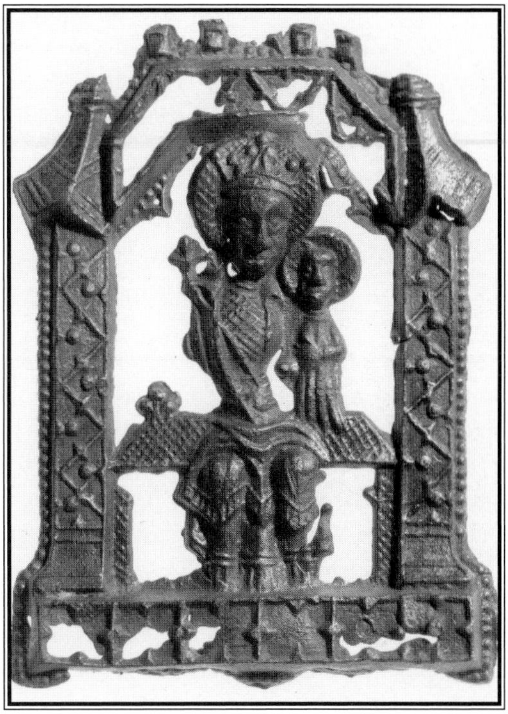

Two fourteenth-century pewter pilgrim badges from the shrine of Our Lady of Walsingham, Norfolk. One depicts the Annunciation, the other the Virgin and Child.

the hope that an appeal to the Virgin would enable her to produce an heir. Her offering of 'a tablet of gold garnished in the borders . . . with ten troches of pearl, five sapphires and five spinel rubies of rose-red, with an angel in the middle having at the head a cameo . . . and holding between its hands a cross garnished with a ruby and nine oriental pearls' was valued at £29, and ranked as one of her most expensive purchases. Clearly, she regarded it as a worthwhile investment. Another visitor to Walsingham at this time was Cecily, Duchess of York, who awaited with trepidation the next in a series of difficult confinements.[21]

Pregnant women naturally enlisted the protection of the mother of Christ, making use of 'birth girdles' and similar devices, inscribed with charms and prayers invoking her name (as discussed in Chapter IV). Towards the close of the Middle Ages other female members of the Holy Kindred, whose popularity reflects a more measured acceptance of the realities of family life, childbirth and fertility, also became the focus of cults supported by the laity. How much easier it must have been for harassed parents to identify with a matriarch, such as St Anne, who had reputedly been married three times and was the grandmother of Christ and six of his disciples[22] (colour plate 3). Although she had gone to the stake in defence of her virginity, St Margaret of Antioch was likewise believed to intercede on behalf of women in labour, for whom she had prayed to God at the time of her martyrdom:

> And specyally to the I beseche
> To alle wymmen whiche of childe trauayle,

For my sake, oo lorde, be thou her leche,
Lat my prayere un-to hem availe,
Suffre no myschief tho wymmen, lorde, assaile,
That calle to me for helpe in theire greuaunce,
But for my sake save hem fro myschaunce.
Lat hem, lorde, not perisshe in theire chyldynge,
Be thou her comforte and consolacyoun,
To be delivered thurgh grace of thym helpynge,
Socoure hem, lorde, in theire tribulacyoun[23] (colour plate 18).

Even though the Church looked askance at some of these practices, individual clerics continued to condone them, not least because of the additional income which they helped to generate. The monk who delivered 'Our Lady Gyrdelle' to Henry VII's pregnant queen in 1502 was, for example, paid 6s.8d. for his pains, and many religious houses were happy to oblige their patrons in similar ways. After the Reformation, however, strenuous efforts were made to prevent midwives from deploying the 'girdles, purses and such superstitious things' to which they had previously had recourse.[24] The struggle proved long and difficult, being compounded by devotion to the numerous lesser female saints associated with miracles of healing throughout Britain. St Dwyn's shrine at Llandwyn, for example, drew large numbers of pilgrims, whose offerings (given on behalf of their animals as well as themselves) made the prebend the most affluent in Wales. St Edburga of Minster and St Ethelburga of Barking were also noted for their miraculous cures, as was St Ethelfleda, although her predilection for taking cold baths at dead of night sprang from a desire to subdue rather than cleanse the flesh. Lepers as well as the blind were reputedly made whole at St Milburga's tomb at Wenlock, where several dramatic incidents took place.[25]

Wells, such as those connected with St Mindred at Exning and St Sidwell at Exeter, were sought out by men and women who hoped to wash away their diseases with purifying holy water. Most notable in this respect was St Winefrede's shrine at Holywell, near the estuary of the River Dee, which was favoured as a place of resort by the sick throughout the Middle Ages, even after the saint's remains had been solemnly transferred to Shrewsbury Abbey in the twelfth century. According to Adam of Usk, Henry V himself travelled between the two places *on foot* in 1416; and since one of his leading captains, Richard, Earl of Warwick, subsequently left a handsome bequest to the saint's altar at Shrewsbury, it looks as if they both held her in particular regard. The cult of St Frideswide of Oxford, on the other hand, exercised a more local and specific attraction, for approximately two-thirds of her recorded miracles were performed on females, such as the blind girl who awoke one morning after sleeping on the steps of Frideswide's tomb to find that she could see. Since they were recorded by clerics, these accounts often contain jibes at the expense of medical practitioners, largely because of incompetence or venality, and the list of Frideswide's miracles is no exception. Indeed, the tale of a young boy left for dead on his parents' table by an Oxford surgeon who had bungled an operation, only to be revived by the saint herself (and later to become mayor), presents a damning indictment of the profession.[26]

A second, very different area in which women were extolled, if not actually venerated, for their healing skills is to be found in the pages of the chivalrous romance. Here convention demanded that the hero should engage in single combat with at least one supernaturally powerful opponent and, more often than not, be put to rights afterwards by a female healer of gentle birth.

Since the enemy might well take the form of a dragon or hideous giant, the neighbouring chatelaine could face quite a challenge, but her medical expertise rarely proved wanting. Gottfried von Strassburg's (*fl.* 1210) version of the legend of *Tristan* provides a particularly good description of one of these gifted ladies in the person of Queen Isolde, who is 'versed in herbs of many kinds, in the virtues of plants, and in the art of medicine', and who alone is able to cure the maimed knight.

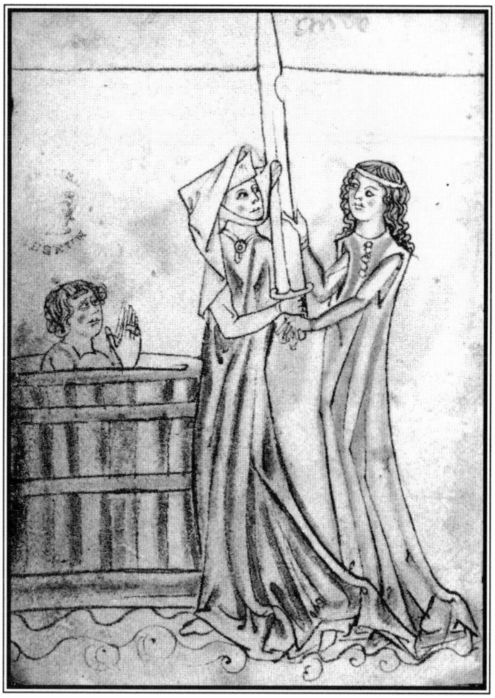

At a later stage in the Tristan legend, the wounded hero recuperates in a medicinal bath. Unfortunately, an embedded fragment of Morold's sword reveals his true identity, and Isolde realizes that she has saved the life of her sworn enemy.

During the course of a long and terrible fight, Tristan has been wounded by the poisoned sword of his enemy, Morold. Despite the latter's warning that only his sister, Queen Isolde, can save him, Tristan cuts off his head, and is thus left to die slowly without any apparent hope of relief. At last, goaded by pain, he resorts to the desperate step of disguising himself as a minstrel and seeking her out across the Irish Sea in Dublin. Once there, he lodges with a leech, who is himself powerless to help, but at least manages to arrange a meeting with Isolde, the finest doctor in the land. 'Now, if I were to speak at length and deliver you a long discourse on my lady's skill as a physician', writes the narrator, 'on the marvellous efficacy of her medicines and how she treated her patient what good would it do and what would be the point of it? A seemly word sounds better in noble ears than one from a druggists box.' Sure enough, Tristan is fully healed, only to fall in love with the queen's beautiful daughter and bring tragedy on them both.[27]

When retelling this story for the benefit of English readers over two hundred years later, Sir Thomas Malory chose to depict the princess rather than her mother as the 'noble surgeon' to whom Tristan owes his life. Of greater interest, however, is his account of the young man's suffering before he sails for Ireland: at this stage 'all manner of leeches and surgeons, both . . . men and women' are called in to examine him, and 'a right wise lady', famous for her knowledge of poisons, suggests the only possible cure.[28] It has usually been assumed that figures such as Isolde, who ministered to the heroes of courtly romance, represent a flight of fancy on the part of their creators, as far removed from reality as the exploits of the dragon-slayers themselves. Certainly, Malory's Dame Lynet and her benign sisterhood, accustomed to replacing lost intestines, limbs and occasional heads at astonishing speed, may safely be dismissed as sheer fantasy on the part of one who was all too familiar with the bloody toll of medieval battles; but there is plenty of evidence to suggest that others were modelled, albeit at several removes, on real women renowned for their understanding of physic.[29]

Although, unlike Queen Isolde, she failed to save her patient, Elizabeth Ryman, the wife of one of the senior retainers of Thomas, Earl of Arundel, was clearly a person of no mean accomplishments. Having been invalided back from the siege of Harfleur while in the last stages of terminal illness, the earl made his will at Arundel Castle in October 1415, leaving her the impressive sum of 50 marks (equivalent to the annual income of a wealthy landowner) specifically for the care she had shown him both before and during his last illness, as well as instructing his trustees to pay her an additional £10 p.a. for life, also out of gratitude. Elizabeth must have enjoyed an enviable reputation as a nurse, because in June 1421 she was commanded by Henry V himself to travel to Paris with his new queen, who was then pregnant, as one of her private entourage. Nor was his confidence misplaced: after the birth she was ordered to 'watch and attend' the baby prince at Windsor, being made responsible for his welfare after Queen Katherine returned to France in May 1422. She herself was struck down by 'infirmity, old age and weakness' two years later, when she received an honourable discharge, along with a further pension of £20, albeit only after appealing to the government for financial assistance.[30] Her successor, Joan Astley, drew twice this amount, which indicates clearly enough the value placed upon senior nursing staff in the royal household. So too does the fact that Joan's three assistants were later admitted to the prestigious confraternity of St Albans Abbey, a mark of favour customarily reserved for persons of far superior status. It is worth stressing that although birth (or the right connexions by marriage) mattered to a certain extent, skill in the art of 'nurture' ranked as the primary qualification for a post which rarely, if ever, assumed the aspect of a sinecure. Anyone considered suitable to undertake the care of high-born infants was obviously guaranteed an appropriate standard of living while their charges remained in the nursery, and some, who inspired great affection, continued to enjoy the benefits of patronage for years afterwards. Edward IV's old nurse, Elizabeth of Caux, was still collecting an annuity of £20 in 1482, just before he died; and James II of Scotland, whose family was noted for its kindness and generosity in this respect, gave a dowry of £40 to the daughter of Janet Liddale, who had looked after him, at a fee of £10 p.a., throughout his early life.[31]

For every Elizabeth Ryman or Joan Astley there were, however, thousands of obscure women who devoted their lives to the young, the sick or the aged, usually without leaving much, if any, evidence behind them in the records. The 'wedoo in Busshe Lane', London, who cared for John Russell while he was suffering from the 'gret pokkes', at a fee of 3s.4d. a week, is unusual only because a passing reference to her ministrations has survived. Sometimes a grateful invalid, such as the New Romney MP, James Lowys (d.1454), would remember in his will the nurses who had tended him, but more often than not their services were simply taken for granted. This was no doubt because women were expected to look after relatives and other dependants as a matter of course[32] (colour plate 16).We may note, for instance, one of many vituperative attacks made upon the mystic, Margery Kempe (b.1373), whose pursuit of the celibate life led her to live apart from an ageing husband. On finding him 'half alive, all streaked with blood' after a fall, the neighbours vilified her as little short of a murderess, since she had so flagrantly disregarded her obligation to cherish him in his dotage. How different from the tale of the young wife, recommended by the knight of la Tour-Landry as a model to his own daughters because of her devotion to an incontinent 'right auncien' husband, whom she nursed until the end.[33] Margery had probably neglected other important duties in her search for spiritual health: given the cost and relative inaccessibility of professional medical treatment and the corresponding popularity of folk remedies, culled from the herb garden and the kitchen, most women had little choice but to accept major roles as healers, whether in the confines of their own homes or more publicly in nunneries, hospitals or the communities in which they lived.

A manual of instruction written in the early 1390s by an elderly Parisian for the guidance of his young bride provides an interesting, if idealized, picture of the medieval *bourgeoise*, busy about her daily tasks. These centered upon the care of her husband, with particular emphasis on the need for cleanliness and proper food, but she was also supposed to assume responsibility for the health and well-being of their domestic staff. 'If one of your servants fall ill', the *Menagier* instructed, 'do you lay all common concerns aside, and do you yourself take thought for him full lovingly and kindly . . . seeking to bring about his cure.'[34] A large section of the tract is devoted to gardening, partly because the lady of the house had to supply fruit and vegetables for the kitchen and see that her employees were adequately fed. Of equal importance, however, was the need to cultivate a fully stocked herber so that all the necessary ingredients for routine medicaments and prophylactics lay immediately to hand. In this instance, the author does no more than list the most useful plants and provide hints about the best way of growing them, but there was no shortage of simple vernacular guides (often in verse so they could easily be memorized) explaining how to prepare and administer herbal remedies in the home.

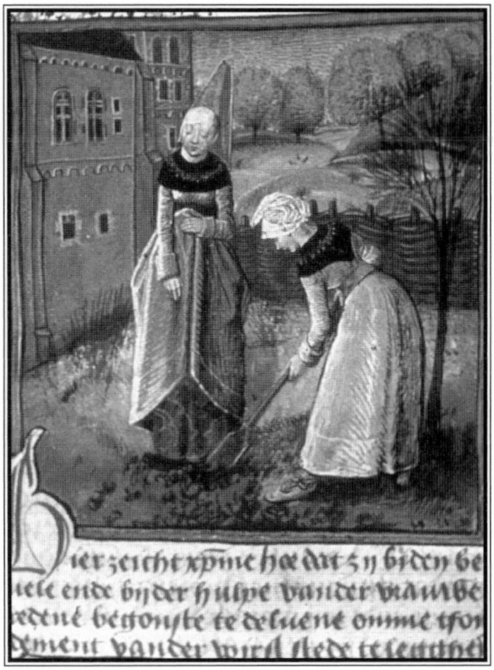

Working under the direction of her mistress, a female servant prepares a herber for planting just below the windows of their residence. The cultivation of medicinal plants was an important female activity at all levels of society, from cottage garden to castle.

Contrary to certain preconceived ideas about the limitations of medieval horticulture, even a fairly modest garden could produce a profusion of medicinal plants. The Dominican friar Hugh Daniel, who has been described as the father of English botany, grew over 250 herbs ('my xij score and xij erbis') in his physic garden at Stepney during the later fourteenth century. His knowledge of wild and domestic flora was probably unrivalled at the time, but many of his contemporaries, especially women, must have shared this interest, acquiring a sound practical understanding of the subject. We can, indeed, infer as much from the many surviving collections of vernacular remedies, which take for granted the ability not only to recognize a wide variety of plants but also to find substitutes when necessary. A brew widely recommended to ease the pain of wounds and bruises contained a mixture of comfrey, marigold, knapweed, yarrow, wood avens, root of wallwort, 'baynwort', clover, herb Robert, wild sage, black harehound, mouse-ear hawkweed, dock, common polipody, greater celandine and madder, all of which it was assumed the housewife would either grow herself or gather from the fields and hedgerows.[35]

Perhaps Chaucer had this very drink in mind when describing the 'fermacies of herbes and eek save' prepared for the wounded combatants in *The Knight's Tale*: given the high level of violence and injury in medieval society, women must have devised quite a number of soothing potions for their battered kinsmen. Problems of identification and nomenclature, as well as regional variations, likewise encouraged the domestic herbalist to experiment, thus increasing her familiarity with different species and types of plants. Daniel himself records how Elizabeth, Lady Zouche (d.1380/1), 'the best godys leche of Bryzthlond [Britain] in women', used to substitute one kind of wild sage for another when the need arose, evidently scouring the countryside for it, since it was to be found 'only in wodish places as under busschys'.[36]

To protect and preserve her family and servants, the medieval chatelaine had to cultivate the skills of an apothecary as well as a herbalist. The making of pills, electuaries, ointments and other compound medicines was a complicated matter which called for binding agents, such as flour, wax, honey and animal fat from the larder. The pounding, mixing, stirring, sieving and blending required came easily enough to women used to running their own kitchens; and it is by no means unusual to find instructions for cooking 'a good sawce for a rosted capon', mending 'broken stone pottes' or even for producing home-made soap interspersed in contemporary notebooks alongside remedies for the stone, nosebleeds or swollen feet. A clerk employed by John Howard, the future Duke of Norfolk, actually set aside a few lines when compiling household accounts for 1464 to note down two such remedies for eye strain, evidently in the hope that they could be made up by one of his master's female servants. The demand for salves and washes to ease tired eyes was enormous, bringing to mind Thomas Hoccleve's complaint about the bad backs, stomach pains and blurred vision endured by professional scribes, who must have relied heavily on such palliatives. Even elementary receipts might require additional ingredients which had to be bought from a specialist and prepared at home: white ginger for cramp; myrrh and frankincense for haemorrhoids and a wide range of skin diseases; mastic and turpentine for wounds; olive oil and mercury for removing dead flesh and concealing anything that looked like leprosy; powdered almonds, alum and white lead for erysipelas; nutmeg for tremor of the head and limbs; and, of course, 'treacle' for those who felt 'rygth evyll att ese' or under the weather, especially during epidemics.[37]

The surgeon, John of Arderne, expressed some contempt for 'the medycinez of ladiz', citing two cases where he had been called in to make good the damage caused by amateur leechcraft.[38] Cauterization and other drastic surgical techniques, which were often the only means of arresting the spread of infection in an age before antibiotics, clearly lay beyond the scope of most women. Yet a respectable number of their cures, based on tried and tested folk remedies passed on from one generation to the next, may well have proved quite effective. A mid-fourteenth-century account by the Icelandic chronicler Abbot Arngrimr Brandsson of emergency measures employed to repair a fractured skull shows the female healer involved (whose gentle birth and spiritual qualities are, significantly, established at the start) in the best possible light. Even Arderne would have commended her restraint in allowing Nature a free hand in the case of a man injured in a fall from the top of a cliff:

> He is taken home to the dwelling of a certain lady who was pious and had a fine understanding of how to aid those in need of help. She cuts around the fracture in the skull and removes the splinters that had been crushed into small particles, then cleans the wound and purifies it, as much as she dared to do, right down to the outer membrane. . . . The opening in the head was now as big as three finger widths in each direction. But what is there to say about an application or salve for healing, but that the lady takes water moss . . . and fills the wound with it, then binds it up, and does not unbandage it until three nights have passed. . . . Within a few days, he was a completely well man.[39]

At least such a comparatively benign form of treatment (the water moss was probably held to possess supernatural properties, since it came from a holy well) did less positive harm than some of the aggressive measures advocated by proponents of academic medicine. Their knowledge often derived from texts marred by scribal errors and misinterpretations, rather than practical instruction of the kind Margaret Hunt had received from Mother Elmet; and they were disposed to favour rare, expensive *materia medica* instead of utilizing whatever plants might be available. We should, however, be wary of dismissing women as heirs to a folk tradition and nothing more, for there can be little doubt that many of good family, like Lady Zouche, made a serious study of medicine. It was, indeed, expected of them as part of their duty to society: Sir Thomas More, for example, wanted his daughter to devote herself to physic as well as the Scriptures; and others held regular consultations with 'learned men' to improve their grasp of theory.[40]

The Paston women, who are unusually well documented, thanks to the survival of their correspondence, regarded the medical profession with a degree of scepticism which confirms that not all doubts about competence were one-sided. Having turned, first and foremost, to the Virgin Mary, Margaret Paston's next move in dealing with a husband lying sick in London was to beg him to return home as soon as possible since she could look after him far better than anyone else. Later on, in 1464, she was even less inclined to mince words: 'for Goddys sake', she warned him, 'be ware what medesynys ye take of any fysissyanys of London. I schal never trust to hem be-cause of yowre fadre and myn onkyl, whoys sowlys God assoyle.'[41] Perhaps mindful of this advice, her son, Sir John (d.1504), put all his faith in his wife's ability, begging her

> in all hast possybyll to send me by the next swer [reliable] messenger that ye can gete a large playster of your *flose ungwentorum* for the Kynges Attorney James Hobart; for all his dysease is but in hys knee. He is the man that brought yow and me togedyrs, and I had lever then a xl li. [£40] ye kond with your playster depart hym and hys peyne . . . ye must send me wryghtyng hough it shold abyd on hys kne vnremevyd, and houghe longe the playster wyll laste good, and whethyr he must lape eny more clothys a-bowte the playster to kepe it warme or nought.[42]

The ointment in question appears to have been Lady Margery's version of 'a goode entrete for ach and brusid blode', made by melting bacon fat with grease from a neutered boar, adding wax and powdered incense, blending in ground wheat and rye and then pounding the mixture with a mortar until it looked like honey and could be stored in a box. When needed, the paste was spread on cloth or a piece of leather and applied twice daily. The indiscriminate use of what one surgeon scornfully dismissed as 'potage in maner maad of eerbis and swynes greece and water and whete flour' was criticized in vain by medical writers, which suggests that, if not actually effective, such concoctions caused less pain than the radical methods sometimes favoured by experts.[43] We do not know how quickly Hobart recovered, if at all, but he at least survived for thirteen more years.

Honor, Lady Lisle, also established a reputation for skill in the preparation of medicines, and was regularly approached by her husband's friends and retainers for help. She even appears to have achieved some success in treating the bladder stone, although her famous powder had undesirable side-effects, as this letter of 1535, from Lord Edmund Howard, reveals:

> Madame, so it is I have this night after midnight taken your medicine, for the which I heartily thank you, for it hath done me much good, and hath caused the stone to break, so

> that now I void much gravel. But for all that, your said medicine hath done me little honesty, for it made me piss my bed this night, for the which my wife hath sore beaten me, and saying it is children's parts to bepiss their bed. Ye have made me such a pisser that I dare not this day go abroad . . . and though my body be simple yet my tongue shall be ever good and especially when it speaketh of women.[44]

It was, none the less, one thing for women to treat members of their immediate circle and quite another for them to offer their services on the open market in direct competition with experienced professionals. Here, a far more negative attitude prevailed, as the authorities became less tolerant of individuals (of both sexes) who did not conform to their requirements. Although female empirics were hardly rare in medieval England, the introduction of regulations in the fifteenth and early sixteenth centuries designed to restrict the practice of physic and surgery to a narrowly defined group of university graduates and guildsmen made life increasingly difficult for those of them who hoped to continue working within the confines of the law. As control over the licensing of practitioners fell into the hands of the Church, so women found themselves increasingly open to attack, and not just as potential witches. At the beginning of the fifteenth century, for example, Joanna Lee, the widow of one of Henry IV's soldiers, petitioned the king for help, claiming that her husband's death on active service had left her destitute, 'with no means of supporting herself except by the physic which she has learned'. Suspicion of itinerant female practitioners seems to have been rife: she begged in vain for letters patent under the Great Seal, which would have enabled her 'to travel safely about the countryside without let or hindrance on the part of those who revile her because of her art'.[45]

Hostility also came, needless to say, from the upper reaches of the medical establishment: surgeons derided women for their superstition and incompetence, while physicians insisted upon the importance of an academic education. Some, such as the Italian Professor of Medicine, Anthonius Guainerius, whose *Treatise on the Womb* appeared while Joanna Lee was attempting to set up in practice, might privately recommend recourse to a wise-woman when all scientific methods had failed (or, significantly, in cases demanding a knowledge of gynaecology), but in public they continued to mock.[46] The stereotype of the female empiric who kills her patients through a combination of vanity and ignorance had a long history and a secure future. When he came to examine the subject in his medical encyclopaedia, the priest John Mirfield (d.1407) had simply to transcribe a passage from Bruno of Calabria's *Magna Chirurgica*, written a century and a half earlier:

> at the present time, not only ignorant men – but what is much worse and must be judged yet more horrible – vile and presumptuous women usurp that office to themselves and abuse it, since they have neither learning nor skill. Whence, because of their stupidity, the worst kind of mistakes are made, oftentimes involving the death of the patient; since they operate neither wisely nor with proper diagnosis, but casually, and are wholly ignorant of the causes and names of the diseases which they declare that they know how to heal and can heal.[47]

As this quotation makes clear, the question of gender was theoretically subordinate to that of formal training. Yet in practice the conviction that 'an illiterate person is hardly capable of completely performing the function of a physician' effectively ruled out women altogether, since literacy was judged by the ability to read and write Latin, which females of low or middling status would have been unable to do. Needless to say, women could, and did, protest that familiarity at first hand with the writings of Aristotle did not necessarily make one a better physician, but generally to no avail. In Paris efforts were made as early as 1271 to restrict the activities of herbalists, apothecaries and empirics of both sexes; and a rigid code of practice, approved by the French king in 1352, deprived them even of the freedom to prescribe pills or let blood.[48]

From the outset the Parisian faculty of medicine showed great zeal in defending its monopoly against women. Several were brought under threat of excommunication before the ecclesiastical courts, the most notable being Jacqueline Felicie, who was accused in 1322 of practising as a physician without the necessary medical knowledge. She claimed, with supporting witnesses, to have cured several people where licensed graduates had failed, and maintained that her female patients much preferred to be treated by one of their own sex. 'It was better and more fitting', she argued, 'that a wise and sagacious woman, experienced in the art of medicine, should visit another woman to examine her and to inquire into the hidden secrets of her being, than that a man should do this.' Furthermore, because of their modesty and shame, 'many women have died in their illnesses since they were unwilling to have a physician who might learn their innermost secrets'. Although, as we shall see, this line of reasoning was successfully deployed in England to justify the translation of works on gynaecology and obstetrics, it carried no weight with the University of Paris, and Jacqueline was found guilty.[49]

The struggle against freelance practitioners continued in France throughout the Middle Ages, with 'literacy' or the possession of recognized academic or craft qualifications as the principal test of professional competence. Appeals of 1325 and 1330 made by the faculty of medicine of the University of Paris to Pope John XXII for help in suppressing the 'old women and soothsayers' who persistently ignored the regulations suggest that other, darker prejudices were also at work; but in court, at least, women were judged by their ability to read and comment upon the standard medical texts, or, in the case of female surgeons, to produce a valid permit. Perretta Petonne, who failed on both these counts in 1411, alleged that several other women were then working openly in the city as unlicensed surgeons, so it looks as if the authorities still had far to go.[50]

Female leeches and wise-women catered to a widespread demand for relatively cheap and painless treatment, and on these grounds alone were perceived as a threat by the emergent medical profession. Their apparent lack of formal training seemed an embarrassing handicap to the small but growing body of physicians, apothecaries and surgeons who were anxious to establish the academic and technical credentials of their calling. That many of the moving spirits were clergymen, predisposed to view the opposite sex with fear and suspicion, may further help to explain some of the mounting pressure to exclude women from practice, which inevitably followed the expansion of university faculties and the growth of restrictive craft guilds. It is, however, important to remember that in most parts of Europe women were not specifically singled out from the general run of charlatans, quacks and itinerant herbalists against whom sporadic warfare was waged until comparatively recent times.

Whereas in Valencia regulations of 1329 stipulated that 'no woman may practise medicine or give potions, under penalty of being whipped through the town; but they may care for little children and women, to whom, however, they may give no potion', discrimination elsewhere assumed a rather more subtle guise. The evident inability of scatter-brained females to memorize or use a wide range of *materia medica* without killing the customer served as a pretext for their prohibition as apothecaries in certain late medieval cities; and in others, such as Nuremberg, where they were allowed to make only 'juices and elixirs' for public consumption, further restrictions were introduced in the early sixteenth century because of alleged amateurism and sharp practice. Yet accusations of ignorance, however ill-founded, were not always enough to drive them from the field, for although the authorized practice of physic was clearly out of bounds to women, surgery, in theory, at least, remained just within their grasp.[51]

By insisting simply upon the possession of an appropriate diploma or evidence that a full apprenticeship had otherwise been served, most of the craft guilds which monitored the work of barbers and surgeons did not specifically exclude women; and a small number of them were in fact admitted, usually by virtue of pre-existing family connexions. In Naples and Frankfurt, for example, a handful of licensed females remained active throughout most of the late Middle Ages, the Frankfurt practitioners being noted for their specialization in eye surgery, which required a delicate hand rather than physical strength. For about fifty years, from the Black Death until 1408, the medical guild of Florence also opened its doors to women (who tended to fare rather better in Italy than elsewhere in Europe), but although empirics continued to play an important part in its affairs, henceforth they seem to have been exclusively male.[52]

In England, too, enough evidence has survived of guild membership by women surgeons and barbers to suggest that initially, at least, they encountered little active resistance. Most, even so, were closely related to male members of the craft, from whom they learned their skills: 'Katherine *la surgiene* of London, daughter of Thomas the surgeon and sister of William the surgeon', who appears in *c.* 1286, was probably destined from birth to follow in the family business. Her female descendants may well have done likewise, for the oath of admission taken by the wardens of the Surgeons' Mystery of London in the late fourteenth century refers unambiguously to their authority over men *and* women 'undertaking cures and practising the art of surgery'. It is interesting to note that at this time the monks of Westminster Abbey harboured few reservations about the employment of female surgeons or even *medicae*, occasionally retaining both, albeit at a lower rate of pay than their male counterparts. And customers patronizing the barbers' shops of London were also served by women: the complaint made in 1413 by the Archbishop of Canterbury about the City barbers' sacrilegious disregard of the Sabbath (see above, p. 137) describes how not only they, but also their wives, sons, daughters, apprentices and servants had persistently broken the law with regard to Sunday trading. Perhaps they were busy offering cut-price treatment to the patients of their rivals, the surgeons: at all events, practitioners of both crafts clearly relied heavily upon female dependants. The London surgeon Nicholas Bradmore held his apprentice, Agnes Woodcock, in such high regard that he left her a red belt with a silver buckle and 6s.8d. in his will of 1417, although she may, ironically, have been one of the last of her sex to receive formal training in the City.[53]

From the date of its foundation in 1379, the Guild of Barbers of Lincoln admitted sisters as well as brothers, who marched together in procession on feast days. A similar arrangement obtained in both Norwich and Dublin; and in York male and female barbers were bound by identical regulations, drawn up at some point before 1413. From the provision that 'no man or woman whatsoever shall engage in the art of surgery, nor in the extraction of teeth nor in anything else pertaining to the barbers' craft in this city, unless they are under the direction of a master barber of this city or another who has been authorized to practise his craft' we may reasonably assume that both sexes could expect the same basic level of tuition. Although women were allowed to take apprentices for the standard term of five years in York, these must usually have been girls, unless the circumstances of marriage or widowhood placed a female surgeon temporarily in charge of her husband's practice.[54]

Yet, however much liberty they may have enjoyed at first, women had disappeared from the ranks of the London surgeons by the 1430s; and, although their sisters in York fared rather better, they, too, eventually came under pressure from male colleagues. Fortunately for them, the civic authorities were far from unsympathetic: a general by-law of 1529 permitted the widows of freemen, without exception, to 'occupy theyr husbands crafts, occupatons and misterys and tayke bothe journay men and apprentices'; and the ordinances of the Barbers still contained references to women at the end of the century. The council was obliged to intervene directly, in 1572, on behalf of one Isabell Warwick, confirming that she 'hath skill in the scyence of surgery and hath done good therin' and insisting that she should be allowed to continue her work 'without lett' of any of the local guildsmen.[55] If accredited female practitioners were now experiencing the full force of prejudice and professional rivalry, the situation for other women, who operated outside the privileged confines of an urban élite, grew correspondingly worse.

Being far smaller in size and less well organized than its French counterpart, the English medical profession made no real attempt to assert itself until the fifteenth century; and even then another ninety years were to elapse before effective, protectionist legislation on the continental model could be set in place. A parliamentary petition of 1421 protested about the practice of physic by 'many unconnyng and unapproved in the forsayd science', while demanding that a draconian penalty of 'long emprisonement', accompanied by an entirely unrealistic fine of £40, should be imposed on all offenders, male or female; but although it commanded the support of both Houses and the Crown, the bill remained a dead letter. Matters were not helped by the failure of the proposed joint college of physicians and surgeons, which aimed, just two years later, to drive these same 'unconnyng and unapproved' empirics off the streets of London by providing reasonably priced treatment for all. How far prospective members of the college would, in practice, have been able to keep their solemn oath, abjuring all forms of 'bigilyng, evyle, sophisticacion or untrouthe' is a moot point; but it was clearly intended to distance them even further in the public eye from the old cobbler-women of Southwark and their kind.[56]

Battle was resumed in the parliament of 1512–14, with the passage of an act 'Concerning Phesicins and Surgeons'. This painted the alarming picture of

> a grete multitude of ignorant persones of whom the grete partie have no maner of insight in [medicine] nor in any other kynde of lernyng. Some also can [know] no lettres on the boke, so far furth that common Artificers as Smythes, Wevers and Women boldely and custumably take upon theim grete curis and thyngis of great difficultie. In the which they partely use socery and which crafte, partely applie such medicyne unto the disease as be verey noyous and nothyng metely therfore, to the high displeasoure of God, great infamye to the faculties and the grevous hurte, damage and distruccion of many of the Kynge's liege people. . . .[57]

Henceforward, all practitioners of medicine in London or within seven miles of the capital were to submit themselves for examination and formal certification to their bishop and a board of professionals, comprising either four physicians or a group of master surgeons, while elsewhere bishops were to enlist expert help with the licensing process as they saw fit. The act, which imposed a more viable fine of £5 on those who failed to comply, provided the authorities with an effective weapon along the lines of the French model, and before long the city's empirics were being 'sued, troubled and vexed' accordingly. The establishment, by royal charter in 1518, of the College of Physicians of London was further intended to clear such 'malicious persons' off the streets, not least through the introduction of an even more stringent system of supervision and the punishment of offenders. Significantly, however, the Church retained sufficient power to ensure that the religious orthodoxy and reputation of applicants for licences would, in practice, assume paramount importance. Such was the Church's fear of witchcraft and other occult practices (most notably on the part of midwives) that the question of skill was often ignored altogether.[58]

The empirics fought back. Although strictly well outside the period covered in this book, their petition to the 1542–44 parliament describes a traditional type of medicine practised throughout the Middle Ages by

> divers honest persones as well men as women, whome God hath endued with the knowledge of the nature, kinde and operacion of certeyne herbes, rotes and waters, and the using and ministering of them to suche as been pained with custumable diseases, as womens brestes being sore, a Pyn and the Web [ulcers and conjunctivitis] in the eye, uncoomes [abcesses] of handes, scaldinges, burninges, sore mouthes, the stone, strangurye [painful urination] saucelin [swollen face] and morfew [scurvy], and suche other lyke diseases, and yet the saide persones have not takin any thing for theyre peynes and cooning, but have mynistred the same to the poore people oonelie for neighbourhode and goddes sake and of pitie and charytie. . . .[59]

And, despite its preoccupation with repressive measures against witchcraft, the House of Commons did in fact prove receptive to the idea that quackery was a relative concept.

This chapter has presented some contrasting views of the female healer, which reflect a wider range of contemporary attitudes towards her sex as a whole: the solicitous chatelaine or obedient nurse stood as far from Dame Trot as the Virgin Mary did from Eve. Women inspired confusion and fear in the medieval male, but so too did the prospect of illness and suffering, against which a wife, mother, herbalist or empiric might possibly offer relief. And, more to the point, a woman was, in many cases, quite capable of providing the same, or even better, care than a practitioner of physic with his degrees or a surgeon with his diplomas. The unreliability, discomfort and cost of professional treatment, as well as an obvious preference on the part of ordinary people for traditional remedies, ensured that women of all types, from housewives to witches, would continue for generations to provide basic medical care in the community. There were, indeed, two particular areas in which their expertise had always been recognized, and in which they were allowed, if not actually encouraged, to develop specialist skills. These deserve to be examined in more detail, and are considered next.

NOTES

1. M. Warner, *Alone of All Her Sex: The Myth and Cult of the Virgin Mary* (pbk, London, 1976), p. 58. For further examples of medieval misogyny see *Woman Defamed and Woman Defended*, ed. A. Blamires (Oxford, 1992), Sections 1–6.
2. G. McMurray Gibson, 'Saint Anne and the Religion of Childbed: Some East Anglian Texts and Talismans', in *Interpreting Cultural Symbols: Saint Anne in Late Medieval Society*, ed. K. Ashley and P. Sheingorn (Athens, Georgia, 1990), p. 98; S. de Beauvoir, *The Second Sex*, trans. H.M. Parshley (pbk, London, 1988), pp. 199–200; E. Pagels, *Adam, Eve, and the Serpent* (pbk, London, 1990), pp. 63, 133–4. The Gnostics interpreted the Genesis myth quite differently, as Professor

Pagels points out, hailing Eve as 'the Physician, and the Woman, and She Who Has Given Birth' (ibid., p. 66). Augustine's ideas about original sin and disease are discussed above, pp. 7–8.

3. *Galen on the Usefulness of the Parts of the Body*, ed. M.T. May (2 vols, Cornell, 1968), vol. II, p. 630. For more about the impact of these views see V.L. Bullough, 'Medieval Medical and Scientific Views of Woman', *Viator*, IV (1973), pp. 485–501; and for Galen on Christianity, R.L. Wilken, *The Christians as the Romans Saw Them* (Yale, 1984), pp. 68–93.

4. See above, pp. 41–2.

5. U. Ranke-Heinemann, *Eunuchs for Heaven: The Catholic Church and Sexuality*, trans. J. Brownjohn (London, 1990), p. 61.

6. Wellcome Library, Western Ms. 290, ff. 31–31v; *Galen on the Usefulness of the Parts of the Body*, op. cit., vol. II, pp. 628, 630. See T.W. Laqueur, *Making Sex: Body and Gender from the Greeks to Freud* (Harvard, 1990), Chapters I–III, *passim*, for a fuller discussion of this theory.

7. J. Cadden, *Meanings of Sex Difference in the Middle Ages* (Cambridge, 1993), pp. 94–5, 143.

8. *Medieval Woman's Guide to Health*, ed. B. Rowland (Kent, Ohio, 1981), pp. 58–9; D. Jacquart and C. Thomasset, *Sexuality and Medicine in the Middle Ages* (Cambridge, 1988), p. 129; Cadden, op. cit., pp. 174–5; C.W. Bynum, *Holy Feast and Holy Fast: the Religious Significance of Food to Medieval Women* (University of California Press, 1987), p. 138.

9. Ranke-Heinemann, op. cit., p. 13. The author also discusses the commonly held belief that similar afflictions were visited upon children conceived at times when the Church demanded abstinence, pp. 120–3.

10. *On the Properties of Things: John Trevisa's Translation of Bartholomaeus Anglicus De Proprietatibus Rerum*, ed. M.C. Seymour and others (3 vols, Oxford, 1975–88), vol. I, p. 154; *Lanfrank's 'Science of Cirurgie'*, ed. R. von Fleischhacker (Early English Text Soc., CII, 1894), p. 55; V.L. Bullough and M. Voght, 'Women, Menstruation and Nineteenth-Century Medicine', *Bulletin of the History of Medicine*, XLVII (1973), p. 67.

11. Jacquart and Thomasset, op. cit., p. 75; British Library, Dept of Mss, Sloane 775, f. 54.

12. J.F. Benton, 'Trotula, Women's Problems, and the Professionalization of Medicine in the Middle Ages', *Bulletin of the History of Medicine*, LIX (1985), pp. 30–53.

13. Rutebeuf, *Oeuvres Complètes*, ed. M. Zink (2 vols, Paris, 1989–90), vol. II, p. 247. Another version of this passage is quoted in C.H. Talbot, *Medicine in Medieval England* (London, 1967), p. 142.

14. Guillaume de Loris and Jean de Meun, *The Romance of the Rose*, ed. and trans. C. Dahlberg (New England, 1983), pp. 216–52; Jacquart and Thomasset, op. cit., pp. 110–15; M.C. Pouchelle, *The Body and Surgery in the Middle Ages*, trans. R. Morris (Oxford, 1990), p. 52.

15. William Langland, *The Vision of Piers Plowman*, ed. A.V.C. Schmidt (Oxford, 1978), p. 158 (B passus XIII, vv. 333–41). Southwark remained a popular refuge for exponents of the black arts: some years later one Alice Huntley of Kent Street reputedly left 'dyverses mamettes for wychecraft and sorsery' buried in a cellar (C.T. Martin, 'Clerical Life in the Fifteenth Century', *Archaeologia*, LX (1907), pp. 373–4).

16. *The Complete Plays of John Bale*, ed. P. Happe (2 vols, Woodbridge, 1985–6), vol. II; G.L. Kittredge, *Witchcraft in Old and New England* (Cambridge, Mass., 1928), pp. 34–5.

17. *The Register of John Stafford*, ed. T.S. Holmes (Somerset Record Soc., XXXI–XXXII, 1915/16), vol. I, pp. 325–7. For the theological background, see *Fasciculus Morum: A Fourteenth-Century Preacher's Handbook* ed. S. Wenzel (Pennsylvania, 1989), pp. 576–87. It is worth noting that just seven years before Agnes stood trial Joan of Arc was accused, among other things, of using rings and conjurations to cure illness. This she denied: *Procès de Condamnation de Jeanne d'Arc*, ed. P. Tisset (3 vols, Paris, 1960–71), vol. I, pp. 85, 101, 194, 217–18.

18. K. Thomas, *Religion and the Decline of Magic* (pbk, London, 1984), pp. 525–6, 541, 554–8.

19. Thomas Hoccleve, *Hoccleve's Works: The Minor Poems*, ed. F.J. Furnivall and I. Gollancz (Early English Text Soc., extra series, LXI, 1892, LXXIII, 1925, reprinted in one vol. 1970), p. 43.

20. Henry of Lancaster, *Le Livre de Seyntz Medicines*, ed. E.J. Arnould (Oxford, 1940), p. 233.

21. *Paston Letters and Papers of the Fifteenth Century*, ed. N. Davis (2 vols, Oxford, 1971–6), vol. I, p. 218; C. Rawcliffe, 'Richard, Duke of York, the King's "Obeisant Liegeman", a New Source for the Protectorates of 1454 and 1455', *Historical Research*, LX (1987), p. 257; A.R. Myers, 'The Jewels of Queen Margaret of Anjou', *Bulletin of the John Rylands Library*, XLII (1959–60), pp. 115, 124. For the use of wax images, see above, pp. 22–4.

22. E. Duffy, *The Stripping of the Altars: Traditional Religion in England* c. *1400*–c. *1580* (Yale, 1992), pp. 181–2; McMurray, op. cit., pp. 95–110.

23. John Lydgate, *The Minor Poems: Religious Poems*, ed. H.N. MacCracken, (Early English Text Soc., CVII, 1911, reprinted 1961), p. 190.

24. *Privy Purse Expenses of Elizabeth of York*, ed. N.H. Nicolas (London, 1830), pp. 78, 197; *Visitation Articles and Injunctions*, ed. W.H. Frere (Alcuin Club Collections, XIV–XVI, 1910), vol. II, pp. 58–9. For the magical aspect of birth-girdles, see above, pp. 96–7.

25. *The Oxford Dictionary of Saints*, ed. D.H. Farmer (Oxford, 1978), pp. 114, 118, 137, 139, 279.

26. Ibid., pp. 280, 356–7; D.J. Hall, *English Medieval Pilgrimage* (London, 1965), pp. 18–34; R.C. Finucane, *Miracles and Pilgrims: Popular Beliefs in Medieval England* (London, 1977), pp. 66, 92, 127–9. For examples from Italy relating to the

miracles of St Chiara of Montefalco (d.1308) see N.G. Siraisi, *Medieval and Early Renaissance Medicine* (pbk, Chicago, 1990), pp. 40–2, 171; and for pilgrimages generally, above, pp. 21–4.

27. Gottfried von Strassburg, *Tristan*, ed. A.T. Hatto (pbk, London, 1967), pp. 138–68.

28. Thomas Malory, *Le Morte d'Arthur*, ed. J. Cowen (pbk, 2 vols, London, 1986), vol. I, p. 316.

29. Ibid., pp. 265, 274–5, 281–2, 296–7. An interesting account of female healers in the fiction of the period appears in M.J. Hughes, *Women Healers in Medieval Literature* (New York, 1943, reprinted 1968). Her work has been extensively used, but not always acknowledged, by subsequent writers on the subject.

30. *The Register of Henry Chichele*, ed. E.F. Jacob (Canterbury and York Soc., XLII, 1937), pp. 75–6; *Calendar of Patent Rolls, 1416–22*, p. 368; *1422–29*, p. 254; *Calendar of Fine Rolls*, vol. XV, p. 306; I am grateful to Dr L.S. Clark for providing these references.

31. R.A. Griffiths, *The Reign of King Henry VI* (London, 1981), pp. 51–2; C.D. Ross, *Edward IV* (London, 1975), p. 7; PRO, E405/70, Easter 22 Edward IV, m. 1; *The Exchequer Rolls of Scotland, 1406–36*, pp. 436, 471, 575; *1437–54*, pp. 386, 436, 498.

32. F.M. Getz, 'To Prolong Life and Promote Health: Baconian Alchemy and Pharmacy in the English Learned Tradition', in *Health, Disease and Healing in Medieval Culture*, ed. S. Campbell, B. Hall and D. Klausner (Toronto, 1992), p. 148; Canterbury Cathedral, City and Diocesan RO, Consistory Court Wills, Register VII, ff. 67–8.

33. *The Book of Margery Kempe*, ed. W. Butler-Bowdon (Oxford, 1954), pp. 235–7; *The Book of the Knight of la Tour-Landry*, ed. T. Wright (Early English Text Soc., XXXIII, 1868), p. 155.

34. For an early edition in English see *The Goodman of Paris*, ed. G.G. Coulton and E. Power (London, 1928), p. 220; and for a more recent French one, *Le Menagier de Paris*, ed. G.E. Brereton and J.M. Ferrier (Oxford, 1981), p. 136.

35. J. Harvey, 'Henry Daniel: A Scientific Gardener of the Fourteenth Century', *Garden History*, XV (1987), pp. 81–93; *The Thornton Manuscript* (Scolar Press, 1975), f. 310.

36. Geoffrey Chaucer, *Works*, ed. F.N. Robinson (Oxford, 1970), p. 43; British Library, Dept of Mss, Arundel 42, f. 22 (quoted in full in J. Harvey, *Medieval Gardens* (pbk, London, 1990), p. 130).

37. British Library, Dept of Mss, Sloane 4, ff. 50, 87, 90–1, 96; Sloane 983, ff. 12, 50, 50v, 55, 73v, 82v, 90, 90v; *The Household Book of John Howard, Duke of Norfolk, 1462–1471, 1481–1483* (1 vol. in 2 parts, Stroud, 1992), part I, p. 280; *Paston Letters*, op. cit., vol. I, p. 243.

38. John of Arderne, *Treatises of Fistula in Ano*, ed. D. Power (Early English Text Soc., CXXXIX, 1910), pp. 44–6, 49.

39. I. McDougall, 'The Third Instrument of Medicine: Some Accounts of Surgery in Medieval Iceland', in *Health, Disease and Healing in Medieval Culture*, op. cit., pp. 69–74.

40. C. Opsomer-Halleux, 'The Medieval Garden and Its Role in Medicine', in *Medieval Gardens*, ed. E.B. MacDougall (Dunbarton Oaks, 1986), pp. 95–113; A.L. Wyman, 'The Surgeoness: The Female Practitioner of Surgery 1400–1800', *Medical History*, XXVIII (1984), p. 31.

41. Paston Letters, op. cit., vol. I, pp. 218, 291.

42. Ibid., p. 628.

43. *A Leechbook or Collection of Medical Recipes of the Fifteenth Century*, ed. W.R. Dawson (London, 1934), pp. 107–9; *Lanfrank's 'Science of Cirurgie'*, op. cit., p. 42.

44. *The Lisle Letters*, ed. M. St Clare Byrne (5 vols, Chicago, 1981), vol. II, no. 399. See also vol. V, nos. 1280, 1541–2.

45. PRO, SC8/231/11510. This petition is discussed in E. Power, 'Some Women Practitioners of Medicine in the Middle Ages', *Proceedings of the Royal Soc. of Medicine*, XV (1922), pp. 20–3. C.H. Talbot and E.A. Hammond (*The Medical Practitioners in Medieval England* (London, 1965), p. 100) argue that Joanna, the leech who provided medicine shortly afterwards for certain monks at Westminster, may have been the petitioner, but this seems most unlikely.

46. H.R. Lemay, 'Anthonius Guainerius and Medieval Gynecology', in *Women of the Medieval World*, ed. J. Kirshner and S.F. Wemple (Oxford, 1989), pp. 317–36.

47. G.R. Owst, *Literature and the Pulpit in Medieval England* (Oxford, 1961), pp. 349–50; *Johannes de Mirfeld: His Life and Work*, ed. P. Horton-Smith-Hartley and H.R. Aldridge (Cambridge, 1936), p. 123.

48. *Chartularium Universitatis Parisiensis*, ed. H. Denifle and A. Chatelain (4 vols, Paris, 1897–9), vol. I, pp. 488–90; vol. II, pp. 16–17.

49. P. Kibre, *Studies in Medieval Science: Alchemy, Astrology, Mathematics and Medicine* (London, 1984), article no. XIII, pp. 7–12.

50. Ibid., pp. 12–14, 17–18; M. Wade Labarge, *Women in Medieval Life* (London, 1986), pp. 177–8. The French universities continued to invoke the full force of the law against female practitioners: in the 1440s, for example, Jeannette Camus was first imprisoned and then expelled from Dijon for practising medicine; and in 1462 the barbers of Reims forbade Isabelle Estevent from taking over her husband's premises, even though he wished her to do so (E. Wickersheimer, *Dictionnaire Biographique des Médecins en France au Moyen Age* (Paris, 1936), pp. 397, 506).

51. M. Green, 'Women's Medical Practice and Health Care in Medieval Europe', *Signs*, XIV (1989), p. 448. As J.M. Riddle notes, 'scholastic or theoretical medicine was so voluminous, so vigorous to learn, so intricate to implement that it required the best minds, not the neighbourhood midwife, the old woodsman who could repair a broken bone of dog

or man alike, or the leech who knew the herbs' ('Theory and Practice in Medieval Medicine', *Viator*, V (1974), p. 183).

52. M.E. Wiesner, *Working Women in Renaissance Germany* (Rutgers, 1986), p. 50; Green, op. cit., pp. 442–4; K. Park, *Doctors and Medicine in Early Renaissance Florence* (Princeton, 1985), pp. 71–5. In 1247 the Confraternity of the Barbers of Arras welcomed sisters as well as brothers, but it is not known if they practised the craft (J. Le Goff, *The Birth of Purgatory*, trans. A. Goldhammer (London, 1984), pp. 327–8).

53. Talbot and Hammond, op. cit., p. 200; B. Harvey, *Living and Dying in England 1100–1540: The Monastic Experience* (Oxford, 1993), pp. 83, 85–6; *Memorials of London and London Life in the Thirteenth, Fourteenth and Fifteenth Centuries*, ed. H.T. Riley (London, 1868), pp. 352, 593–4; T. Beck, *The Cutting Edge: Early History of the Surgeons of London* (London, 1974), pp. 56, 75.

54. *English Gilds*, ed. T. Smith, L.T. Smith and L. Brentano (Early English Text Soc., XL, 1890), p. 27; *Annals of the Barber Surgeons of London*, ed. S. Young (London, 1890), p. 576; *York Memorandum Book 1376–1419* (Surtees Soc., CXX, 1911), pp. 207–10; Wyman, op. cit., p. 27.

55. *York Memorandum Book*, op. cit., pp. l–li; D. South and J.F. Power, *Memorials of the Craft of Surgery* (London, 1886), pp. 59–70; *The Victoria County History of the County of York*, ed. W. Page (3 vols, 1907–13, reprinted 1974), vol. III, p. 453. It is interesting to compare the conduct of the barber-surgeons of York with those of Nuremberg, who described one of their female competitors as '*Winckelartztin*' ('a person who works in dark corners') (Wiesner, op. cit., p. 51).

56. *Rotuli Parliamentorum*, vol. IV, p. 158 (quoted above, p. 120); Beck, op. cit., p. 66.

57. *Statutes of the Realm*, vol. III, 3 Hen. VIII, c. 11. This act has been consistently misdated by historians, who cite the date of summons (28 Nov. 1511) rather than the actual date of assembly (4 Feb. 1512) of the parliament.

58. G. Clark, *A History of the Royal College of Physicians of London* (2 vols, Oxford, 1964), vol. I, pp. 54–66; J.R. Guy, 'The Episcopal Licensing of Physicians, Surgeons and Midwives', *Bulletin of the History of Medicine*, LVI (1982), pp. 528–42.

59. *Statutes of the Realm*, vol. III, 34 and 35 Hen. VIII, c. 8.

CHAPTER NINE

WOMEN AND MEDICINE: THE MIDWIFE AND THE NURSE

For as moche as ther ben manye women that hauen many diuers maladies and sekenesses nygh to the deth and thei also ben shamefull to schewen and to tellen her greuaunces unto eny wyght, therefore I schal sumdele wright to herre maladies remedye, praying to God ful of grace to sende me grace truly to write to the plesaunce of God and to all womannes helpyng. And thowgh women haue diuers evelles and many great greuaunces mo than all men knowen of, as I seyd, hem schamen for drede of repreving in tymes comyng and of discuryng off uncurteys men that loue women but for her lustes and for her foule lykyng. And yf women be in dissese, suche men haue hem in despyte and thenke nought how moche dysese women haue or than they haue brought hem into this world. And therefore, in helping of women I wyl wright of women prevy sekenes the helpyng, and that oon woman may helpe another in her syknesse and nought diskuren her previtees to suche uncurteys men.

Medieval Woman's Guide to Health

However jealously they may have defended their professional monopoly in other areas, medieval medical practitioners were prepared to concede that certain basic aspects of obstetrics and gynaecology, as well as the general care of the sick in hospitals and nunneries, were essentially female preserves. If only because of the dynastic and economic aspirations of their wealthier patients, physicians and surgeons retained a vested interest in the efficient working of the female reproductive system, although their concern tended to manifest itself at a theoretical rather than a practical level. By and large, the routine business of examination and treatment, as well as delivery in childbirth, was left, out of decency, ignorance and perhaps even – as suggested in the previous chapter – distaste, to midwives and other knowledgeable women. The conventional reluctance of physicians to affront the modesty of their female patients, and the latter's evident fear of revealing intimate parts of their anatomy to men, which was the argument usually advanced for employing an obstetrix, has led some historians to assume that the world of academic medicine showed little interest in women's health; but this is to ignore the pervasive influence of classical ideas about their bodies.[1]

So long as the wives and daughters of landowners and merchants (who most frequently had resort to medical experts) were valued as breeding stock, problems about fertility and procreation continued to exercise the profession. Provided they kept their place and accepted direction, midwives and nurses posed no direct threat, and were therefore tolerated, even encouraged: they consulted manuals written for their guidance by men, worked as men's assistants and assiduously administered the interventionist and sometimes aggressive types of therapy recommended by male physicians. They were, moreover, expected to enlist 'qualified' help in emergencies – at least when the affluent and well-connected seemed at risk. The apparent readiness of certain contemporary medical authorities, such as Guy de Chauliac, to dismiss obstetrics as a field 'haunted by wommen', upon which 'it byhoueth not to dwelle moche', may possibly reflect a degree of contempt for the female body, but it also serves as a reminder that some of these 'wommen' had, by dint of long experience, acquired practical skills which men, whatever their qualifications, could never expect to attain and had thus, albeit grudgingly, to recognize.[2] Every now and then they clung tenaciously to this knowledge, refusing to share it with their superiors. The midwives of Heilbronn were clearly reluctant to divulge professional secrets when required to do so in the late fifteenth century, and were reprimanded accordingly. 'If you should be called before the local . . . physicians . . . to be asked and examined about your trade', ran the ordinance, 'you should not resist, but be respectful, and give the correct information to the best of your experience.'[3]

Other male medical writers appreciated the value of collaboration, or at least association, with such women. While seeking to distance himself as a '*vir scientificus*' from the unlearned lay healer, the Italian physician Anthonius Guainerius constantly stressed the important role of the female assistant or midwife in dealing with gynaecological cases. To her fell the task of physically examining the patient and reporting her symptoms, administering any medicines which required contact with the breasts, abdomen or genitals, and, in certain cases, of giving advice on intimate personal matters. Unlike some of his colleagues, Guainerius was also prepared to admit that women might possibly succeed in diagnosing and curing 'female problems' on their own, a view which he shared with his distinguished predecessor, Soranus of Ephesus (d.*c.* 129).[4]

From the time of its composition, in the second century AD, Soranus' great work on gynaecology had proved extremely influential, and his teachings, transmitted through a variety of medical compendia, continued to command respect throughout the medieval period. His insistence that the midwife should be 'literate, with her wits about her, possessed of a good memory, loving work, respectable and generally not unduly handicapped as regards her senses, sound of limb, robust and . . . endowed with long, slim fingers and short nails' is in itself worth noting. But he goes on to recommend other, quasi-academic qualifications, which suggest a high standard of professional competence and a close working relationship with the physician:

> We call a midwife faultless if she merely carries out her medical task; whereas we call her the best midwife if she goes further and in addition to her management of cases is well versed in theory. And . . . if she is trained in all branches of therapy (for some cases must be treated by diet, others by surgery, while still others must be cured by drugs); if she is moreover able to prescribe hygienic regulations for her patients, to observe the general and the individual features of the case, and from this to find out what is expedient. . . . She will be unperturbed, unafraid in danger, able to state clearly the reasons for her measures, she will bring reassurance to her patients, and be sympathetic. . . . She must be robust on account of her duties but not necessarily young as some people maintain. . . . She will be well disciplined and always sober, since it is uncertain when she will be summoned to those in danger. She will have a quiet disposition, for she will have to share many secrets of life.[5]

The notion that women should have access to literature about health, written clearly in the vernacular for ease of comprehension, resurfaced during the fifteenth century, when numerous

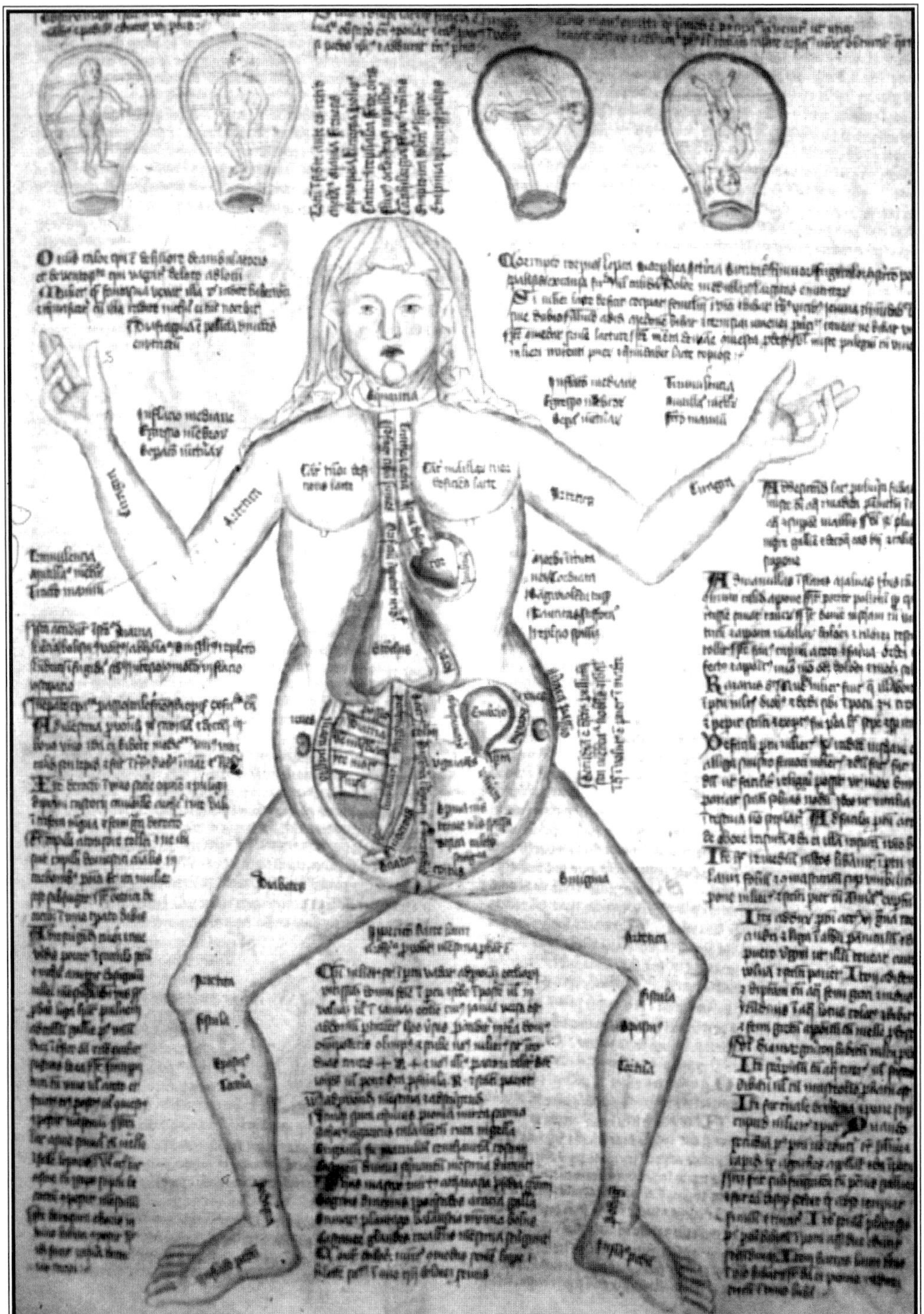

The traditional series of squatting anatomical figures often included a representation of the female internal organs. The artist has drawn an embryo on the left-hand side of the body and placed the kidneys far apart at the level of the navel. Above the head are four sketches of presentations in the uterus.

scientific works were being translated and simplified for the use of ordinary layfolk. 'Because whomen of oure tonge donne bettyr rede and undyrstande thys langage than eny other', it seemed obvious that those who were literate should instruct the rest, 'and help hem and conceyle hem in her maledyes, withowtyn shewyng here dysese to man . . .'.[6] But these manuals contained exactly the same advice and remedies as other medical handbooks: firmly based on humoral theory and a conventional view of female pathology, they prescribed a harsh regime of purging, vomiting, fumigation, pessaries and phlebotomy to keep the reproductive organs in working order.

Although dismissed by Soranus as arrant nonsense, the idea of the migratory uterus, prowling about the body 'like a wild animal', was accepted by most physicians as a means of explaining certain maladies of the heart and lungs (*suffocacio matricis*), as well as other specifically gynaecological conditions. Once lodged painfully in the chest, the uterus was believed to emit noxious fumes which initially rose to the brain and then descended to the heart, causing loss of consciousness and respiratory difficulties. In order to drive it back to its proper place, the patient had to inhale the fumes of 'exceptionally odious' things, such as burning horsehair, smoking coals, old shoes and pitch, while at the same time her genitals were anointed with 'fragrant oils' and fumigated with sweet-smelling herbs in a manner likely to attract the recalcitrant beast. In the case of a prolapsed uterus the process was reversed, being made marginally less disagreeable by the added provision of herbal baths.[7]

Besides prescribing a range of treatments for gynaecological disorders in general, some of these English texts, which derived from a variety of sources, including Soranus and the ubiquitous 'Trotula', were designed to help the midwife by providing information (both written and diagrammatic) about difficult presentation and other obstetrical problems. It is, even so, unlikely that more than a handful of these women could lay claim to anything like the impressive level of formal training advocated in classical times. In his foreword to the 1545 edition of *The Byrth of Mankynde*, a manual on obstetrics recently translated from German for the popular market, the physician Thomas Reynalde spoke of the need for proper guidance, if only at second hand. Since the book's first appearance, he noted with approval, 'many ryght honourable ladyes, and other worshypfull gentlewomen' had taken it along to confinements so that they could read appropriate passages to the midwife, who was presumably illiterate.[8]

Knowledge of contemporary medical

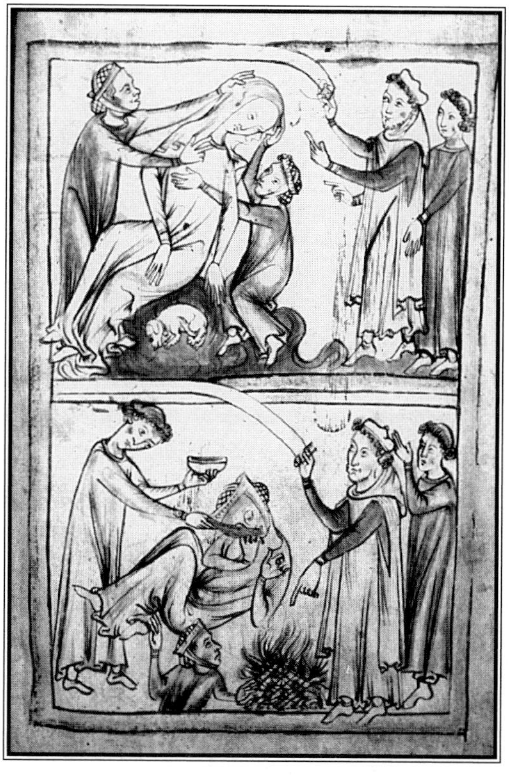

An attempt to revive a swooning patient with the smell of burnt feathers. Quite possibly the physician suspects a migratory uterus is to blame, as the inhalation of unpleasant odours was believed to drive the beast home. At the same time, the genital area was massaged with sweet-smelling ointments to lure it downwards.

theory is, on the face of things, unlikely to have made midwives any more adept, and may, indeed, have proved something of a mixed blessing; but it is significant that no steps were taken in late medieval or Tudor England to ensure, either by a process of apprenticeship or examination, that they possessed any *practical* qualifications, or that supply kept pace with demand. In this instance, the authorities, who were normally so vociferous in their defence of professional standards, seem to have been either indifferent to the need for proper tuition, or else afraid that it might give the obstetrix ideas above her station. Perhaps the presence at confinements of experienced female friends, relatives and social superiors was considered enough to keep the midwife alert (colour plate 17). The obligation to attend 'wymmen in theyr childbedde' ranked high among the charitable works customarily expected of high-born ladies, who were called upon to offer advice as well as financial and moral support on such occasions.[9]

Here, as in so many other areas of medical activity, the English lagged far behind their continental neighbours. Fourteenth- and fifteenth-century French midwives might be licensed by either the clergy or the municipal authorities where they worked, but it was generally understood that they would first be examined by a physician, and would always have served an apprenticeship. Sometimes, as at Lille, their competence was actually assessed by the women who employed them, while elsewhere they remained in the pay of local authorities, and had to make themselves available as required.[10] The great majority of German cities likewise soon came to appreciate the benefits of careful regulation. In Nuremberg an annual oath was demanded of the city's sixteen or so midwives from 1417 onwards; a group of matriarchs from the ruling élite subsequently assumed supervisory and disciplinary powers over them; and, at the beginning of the next century, rules were laid down about their use of drugs, the recruitment and training of apprentices and, most important of all, the provision of care for rich and poor alike. The Nuremberg council also established a precise rate of fees, designed to ensure that any expectant mother, however humble, would receive help during labour, if necessary at the taxpayer's expense.[11]

Although midwives had ranked as sworn civic officials in Constance as early as 1379, the introduction of formal codes of practice was very much a late fifteenth-century phenomenon: Regensburg came first in 1452, then Munich in 1488, Freiburg six years later and Strasburg at the turn of the century. By this point regulatory measures were growing increasingly complex, as one city copied another and the criteria of skill and personal suitability began to assume paramount importance. The Munich ordinances, which read very much like the quotation from Soranus given above, accentuated the need to treat the poor with compassion, a common, if no doubt optimistic, aspiration. In urging midwives, who earned far less than barbers or surgeons, to content themselves with a heavenly reward for philanthropic works, the Frankfurt city fathers can have been expressing little more than a pious hope; and they were, indeed, otherwise chiefly concerned about practical rather than spiritual matters.

Due stress was naturally placed upon the need to employ women of good character, who would report illegitimate births and suspected cases of infanticide, as well as performing their religious duties (including emergency baptisms) properly at all times, but the emphasis throughout these various decrees fell upon the immediate comfort and safety of mother and child. Midwives were, for instance, ordered to attend anyone who might call upon them, irrespective of wealth or social position, never to try to boost their earnings by taking on more than one delivery at once, and, similarly, to avoid hastening the birth or agitating the mother so they could move on to the next confinement. In Nuremberg the term of apprenticeship lasted for four years, during which time it was evidently assumed that the trainee would have mastered certain basic texts, such as Rosslin's *Rosegarden for Midwives*, the precursor of a spate of sixteenth-century handbooks of variable quality, such as the one mentioned above.[12]

Despite the fact that the *Malleus Maleficarum*, a witch-finders' manual compiled by two German inquisitors in 1485, had identified midwives as potentially the most vulnerable of all women to the snares of diabolism, and, once entrapped, the most evil and dangerous, these municipal codes seem to have been far more exercised about the question of technical proficiency than possible involvement in the black arts.[13] In England, however, such evidence as does survive about the place of the midwife in society suggests a very different set of priorities. Her lowly status, her lack of professional recognition and her association (in the eyes of the Church at least) with a variety of disreputable activities compounded the problem, as did the poor rate of pay, which led many women to take up midwifery as a part-time occupation when times were hard, combining it with the kind of freelance practice which already caused so much alarm to the medical establishment.

A few well-connected midwives found favour at Court or in baronial households and prospered accordingly: the one who delivered Thomas, future Duke of Clarence, in 1387 received a gift of 40s.; and by the end of the next century a standard fee of £10 p.a. was considered appropriate for women such as Margery Cobbe and Agnes Massy, who supervised royal confinements.[14] But rewards on this scale were few and far between, and not all midwives brought credit on their calling. Agnes Marshall, of Emswell in the diocese of York, was presented before the Church courts in 1481 both for employing dubious incantations and for her lack of experience ('*non habet usum neque scienciam obstritricandi*').[15] Clearly, sporadic attempts were being made to remove the worst offenders, although the criteria were essentially moral or religious rather than practical: so far as the Church was concerned Agnes's superstition posed a far greater threat than her ignorance.

The ecclesiastical authorities were particularly anxious that, in the event of a child being born dead or dying, the midwife should be able to discharge her primary responsibility and save its soul through baptism. Parish priests were required to teach the appropriate procedure, which, in desperate circumstances following the mother's death, might require surgery in order to rescue (i.e. christen) the infant:

> And thaghe the chylde bote half be bore
> Hed and necke and no more,
> Bydde hyre spare, never the later,
> To crystene hyt and caste on water;
> And but scho mowe se the hed,
> Loke scho folowe hyt for no red;
> And yef the wommon thenne dye,
> Teche the mydwyf that scho hye
> For to undo hyre wyth a knyf,
> And for to save the chyldes lyf,
> And hye that hyt crystened be,
> For that ys a dede of charyte.[16]

Concern lest the child's soul might be lost through the midwife's negligence was aggravated by the greater and more terrible fear that she might use, or make available to others, the flesh of an

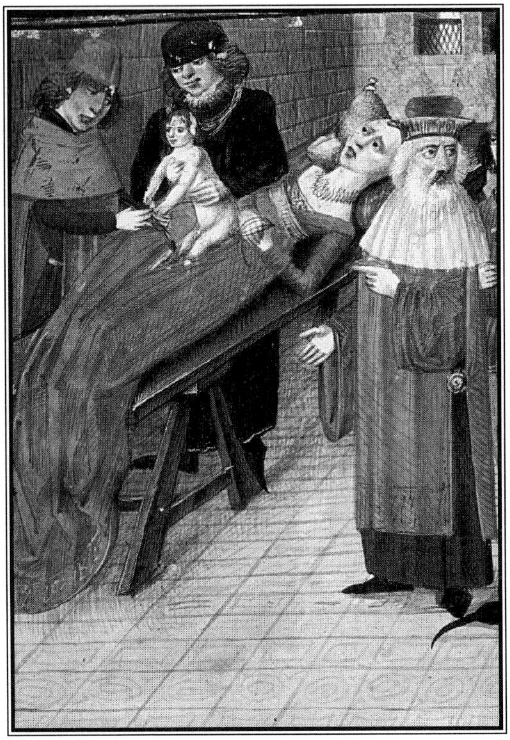

The delivery of Julius Caesar (which gave its name to the surgical procedure involved) imagined by a medieval artist. Far removed from the traditionally female preserve of the childbed, Aurelia lies on what looks uncomfortably like a dissecting table, as the surgeon removes her child and the priest baptizes him.

unbaptized infant for satanic purposes.[17] So long as the belief in witchcraft persisted, midwives remained open to accusations of complicity with the devil, and for this reason alone (although clerical prejudices about women in general and parturition in particular clearly played their part) they had to tread carefully.

Long before the Reformation resort to charms and other occult devices during labour could provoke a hostile reaction, as Agnes Marshall found to her cost; and from the 1530s onwards the list of forbidden activities widened to include anything which smacked of popish or Marian superstition. Prayers which might previously have been recited over a woman in the throes of a difficult labour by the local priest himself now seemed at best unorthodox and at worst charged with sinister implications:

> In the name of the Father + and the Son + and the Holy Ghost +, Amen. Mary gave birth to Christ, Anne gave birth to Mary, Elizabeth gave birth to John the Baptist. Mary gave birth to Our Lord Jesus Christ without shame and without sorrow. In his name and through the merits of St Mary the Virgin, his mother, and of St John the Baptist we order you to come out, child, whether you are male or female, from your mother's womb, without dying or causing her death. + In the name of the Father + the Son + and the Holy Ghost + Amen.[18]

Many hitherto acceptable practices, followed as a matter of course during confinements, now carried with them the risk of interrogation before the Church courts: in 1538, for example, the midwives of the diocese of Salisbury were warned 'to beware that they cause not the woman, being in travail, to make any foolish vow to go in pilgrimage to this image or that image after her deliverance, but only to call on God for help'; and a few years later those of Gloucester and Worcester faced questioning to see if they used 'any prayers or invocations unto any saint, saving to God in Christ, for the deliverance of the woman, [or] any salt, herbs, water, wax, cloths, girdles or relics, or any such like thing'. Although, from time to time, the diocesan courts took steps to investigate 'disorder or evil behaviour concerning the said midwives', and thus, to a limited extent, to enforce general standards of conduct, the campaign against 'witchcraft, charms, sorcery, invocations or prayers' took priority over other considerations. The medical writer Andrew Borde, who argued in the mid-sixteenth century that any woman seeking to practise should first be presented to the bishop 'by honest women of great gravity' and then instructed, examined and approved by a physician, seems largely to have been ignored. His claim that such measures would not only reduce infant mortality but would also help women to avoid miscarriages certainly fell on deaf ears. The first English oath for midwives, introduced in the diocese of Canterbury in 1567, placed godliness above training or practical experience, of which no mention was made at all.[19]

Although it evidently mattered little to the ecclesiastical authorities of the time, the question of competence has proved a controversial subject for twentieth-century historians, who are anxious for reasons of their own either to extol the merits of wise-women and female empirics as proponents of 'natural' childbirth, or else to compare them unfavourably with the male midwives and doctors who came after them. This is, for the medieval and Tudor period, at least, a largely futile exercise, since we have so little evidence of actual practice, and no meaningful statistics whatsoever to rely on. The encyclopaedist Bartholomaeus Anglicus (*fl.* 1230), who wrote about motherhood and childcare with unusual insight, provides a matter-of-fact definition of the midwife as:

> a womman that hath craft to helpe a womman that travaileth of childe, that sche bere and bringe forthe here childe with the lasse woo and sorwe. And for the childe schulde be i-bore with the lasse travaile and woo sche annoyntith and bawmeth the modir wombe, and helpith and comfortith here in that wise. Also sche fongith [delivers] the child out of the wombe, and kettith his navel foure ynche long. With water sche wasschith awey the blood of the childe, and bawmeth hym with salt and hony to drye up the humours and to comforte his lymes and membres, and swathith hym in clothis and cloutis.[20]

The practice of swaddling, or wrapping up a newborn baby in cloth bands was not, as might be supposed, a traditional folk custom, but yet another example of the ubiquitous influence of humoral theory. Since human life appeared to be a continuous, ineluctable process of dessication from the fluidity of the womb to the dust of the grave, it was necessary to prevent premature loss of moisture after birth by protecting all or part of the recently exposed body. Unformed, malleable limbs also needed support, lest they became misshapen, although the midwife had to be very careful in case she herself caused deformity by binding the child too tightly. Warnings about the need for regular exercise must often have gone unheeded, while the risk of skin infections was high.[21]

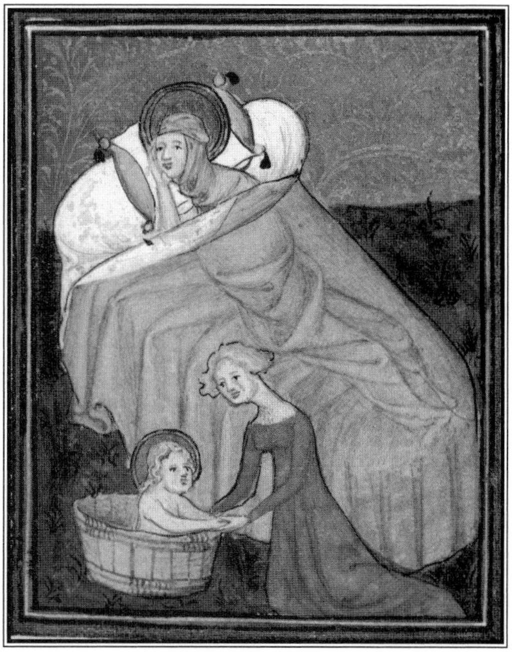

The newly born Virgin Mary is washed by a midwife as her mother, St Anne, rests in bed. Although the Immaculate Conception became a dogma of faith in 1438, artists continued to emphasize St Anne's humanity as a parent and her empathy with ordinary mothers.

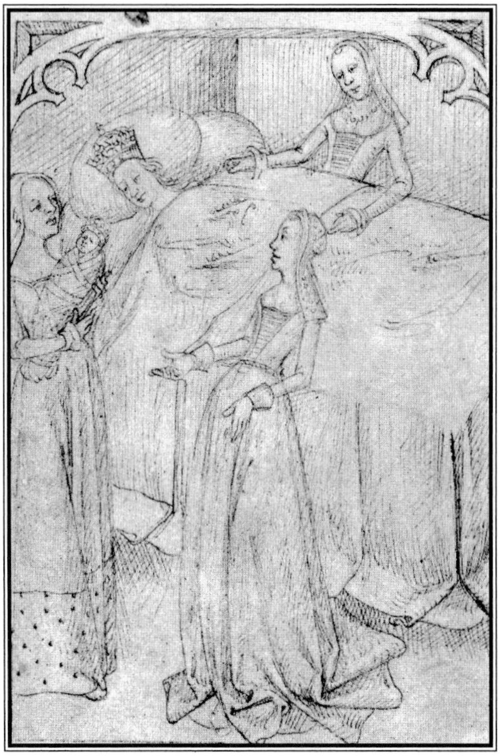

The birth of Henry VI at Windsor in 1420. Unlike most members of their calling, the midwives and nurses who cared for the future king enjoyed a high level of remuneration. Already wrapped in swaddling bands to retain his moist humours and straighten his limbs, Henry is presented to his mother, Queen Katherine.

Sickly infants and weak, undernourished mothers enfeebled by earlier pregnancies were generally at risk; and difficult presentations or post-natal complications all too easily proved fatal. Bartholomaeus' reflection that 'the more woo and sorwe a womman hath in travaile of childe, the more heo loveth that childe whenne he is i-bore' underlines the fact that childbirth was a daunting experience for the healthiest of women. Could an obstetrix actually make matters worse? There is some reason to believe that, even for those who survived labour relatively unscathed, unnecessary discomfort may have been caused by the midwife's compulsion to intervene. From Soranus onwards, physicians had recommended stretching the vagina (a potential source of infection from dirty nails and unwashed hands) and bearing down heavily on the abdomen to hasten delivery, both of which procedures could cause serious problems.

According to some, the midwife's chief function was actually 'to massage the stomach of the woman in labour with ointments to make the child appear as quickly as possible'. Preoccupation with speed sometimes led to harmful tugging and wrenching at whatever parts of the child's anatomy might appear first, as well as to potentially fatal injuries occasioned by the overhasty or forcible removal of the placenta (a malpractice which, in Nuremberg, carried with it the threat of corporal punishment). Even though they may have been better qualified to deal with emergencies, professional midwives were tempted to rush the birth, as the above-mentioned ordinances testify. Instructions that they should not 'use any gruesome or clumsy tools to damage or pull out the child, like long hooks and similar things', or attempt surgery without the approval of an expert, were by no means uncommon, although extreme measures could not always be avoided. Wise-women and part-time midwives employed by rural communities and the urban poor were no doubt able to deal with routine confinements, where the risk lay in their lack of personal hygiene rather than any want of experience. An examining hand which had previously tended the sick, bandaged wounds or even cared for a diseased animal posed a serious threat to the welfare of mother and baby. Not until 1560 was specific mention made (in the first set of regulations for Parisian midwives) of the advisability of washing one's hands and removing any rings before attempting a delivery.[22]

Contemporaries had quite different reasons for mistrusting the female empirics who operated on the fringes of respectability. One of the many undesirable attributes of 'Dame Trot' and other fictional old crones posturing as *medicae* was their command of a lore of unholy knowledge about contraception and abortion, which they used to corrupt the young. Midwives were especially well placed to provide such advice, and must often have done so, drawing not only upon folk custom but also on the thinly disguised 'remedies' available in vernacular medical compilations. Restrictions upon the use of harmful drugs by German midwives, who had to swear that they would eschew anything to do with abortion, were intended to prevent them from falling into temptation. For, however great the demand for this service may have been, it still constituted an act of open defiance against the Church. From the eleventh century onwards the papacy had adopted an uncompromising line with regard to all forms of contraception: 'fleischly deedes' between husband and wife were permissible only if the latter wanted children, wished to avoid illnesses caused by the retention of evil humours or feared that they might otherwise be driven to commit the far worse sin of adultery.[23]

Under no circumstances was interference with the natural process of 'childbigetyng' theologically acceptable, and couples were solemnly warned against any attempts to prevent conception or terminate pregnancy, which would, if successful, lay them open to the charge of homicide. Yet some clerics, and especially those with scientific backgrounds, were not so inflexible, preferring the more measured approach adopted by the medical profession, which allowed a period of up to eighty days before the foetus acquired a human soul. Nor did ordinary men and women experience much difficulty in adjusting their consciences: that many tried to limit the size of their families seems likely from the evidence of recent studies of late medieval urban population, not to mention the Church's growing anxiety about the use of illegal methods, from *coitus interruptus* (which, as one fourteenth-century English vicar philosophically observed, had long ceased to be regarded as sinful by his flock) to abortion.[24] Popular homiletic literature contained direct attacks on such practices, evidently with little hope of success:

> Zyf men or womman be so wylde
> To fordo a getyng of a chylde
> Wyth wurde or dede, syn hyt ys gete,
> With mete or drynk that they do yete,
> Or other strenkthe, that hyt dye,
> Than they doun ful grete folye;
> With sl[au]ghter hast thou there hyd,
> That thy lecherye ys nat kyd.[25]

The Lollards, never slow to miss an opportunity for maligning the established religious orders, blamed nuns for the illicit trade in abortifacients (presumably because they often cared for unmarried mothers), but midwives and wise-women were understandably regarded as the chief culprits by the Church. Like Adelheit von Stutgarten, an abortionist sent into exile from Selestat for three years in 1409, they were said to supply their clients with 'concoctions or roots' designed to induce miscarriage. Adelheit's customers included 'many respectable women', who presumably knew enough about conventional medicine to have access, through books of household remedies, to prescriptions for pessaries, fumigations and potions adaptable for the same purpose. The popularity of 'emmenagogues' or drugs to stimulate the menses, the frequent recommendation of herbal drinks or douches for removing a dead foetus, and the ubiquity of quasi-magical devices, '*ut mulier non concipat*', confirm the impression that information, however unreliable, was widely disseminated and thus, by inference, actively sought.[26] The following 'cure', ostensibly intended to encourage menstrual bleeding, could well have been one of Adelheit's own, and although recorded by a man for use in a gynaecological handbook, hardly differs in tone or content from traditional folk medicine:

> Take the rote of marche [smallage], of the quantite of thy fynger all grene and larde it with the rote of pelettre of spayne [pellitory], and syth put that rote in erthe a yene a xiiij nyght or iij wokes, then take it up and wype it clene and put it in here privey membre, a day and a nyght, afture ward take it oute and a noynte yt with oyle of lorer [laurel] or with mete oyle and put it yn efte sonys and let it lye tyl sche hafe hyre purgacioun: *for though ther were a ded childe in here wombe it wold bringe it oute*. . . . But or sche underefonge [inserts] this supposytore thou shalt sethe savyn and myntes and puliall [pennyroyal] and bay levys yn watre and let the woman setten over that watre a gode whyle.[27]

The relaxed attitude towards illegitimacy characteristic of the upper and middle classes of late medieval England did not necessarily extend to the poor, whose offspring would have been a burden on the community. Priests, too, were keen to destroy the evidence of their misdemeanours, sometimes with fatal consequences. Early in the sixteenth century the chaplain of Alne in Yorkshire accidentally killed his servant and their unborn child ('*destruit puerum in utero suo et eciam mulierem*') with a potion which he had reputedly given to other women in similar circumstances. Perhaps the lethal brew contained savin, the 'rough herbe' and popular abortifacient purchased on a special trip to London by the rector of Leaden Rothing, whose pregnant mistress miscarried immediately after consuming it. Plants such as tansy, parsley, mint and cress were also employed for this purpose, along with willow leaves and seeds, ivy and the bark of white poplar; but, although they may have been quite effective when picked at the right time, properly prepared by a skilled herbalist and administered in appropriate quantities, the termination of pregnancy could rarely be guaranteed. Some concoctions were too revolting to drink in adequate doses, others could prove fatal and the vast majority were simply useless. It is therefore no wonder that many girls chose instead to perform vigorous exercises with a rolling pin or similar instrument on their spreading waistlines or else seek refuge in the hospitals and almshouses set up to help women 'that had done a mysse, in truste of good mendement'.[28]

At the Hôtel Dieu in Paris a special room was set aside for pregnant women, who could call upon the services of a *ventrière*, or professional midwife, her assistant and at least one of the nursing sisters. An average of eighty or so orphaned or abandoned children (some of whom had been delivered there) gained admittance every year, constituting a sizeable proportion of the four or five hundred inmates to be found at any given time.[29] Although St Leonard's, York, one of the largest hospitals in England, accommodated barely half this number (just over two hundred), and most institutions catered for a mere handful of patients, limited provision was still made for expectant mothers without homes or apparent means of support. Whatever moral judgements may have been passed against those who were unmarried, the fate of '*poveres femmes enseintez*' in general aroused a good deal of sympathy, not least among the Members of the 1414 parliament, who urged that they and other unfortunates should receive better treatment. Some hospitals, including St Thomas's, Canterbury, and Holy Trinity, Salisbury, recognized a particular responsibility in this quarter, the latter having been founded to help orphans, widows and 'lying-in women' above all others.[30]

The need for maternity services for the destitute single woman was particularly acute in London: St Mary's, Bishopsgate, opened its doors to them, as did St Bartholomew's (which lay conveniently near the stews in Cock Lane, Smithfield). Both houses undertook to support and educate any infants whose mothers died there in childbirth, which, partly because of malnutrition, seems to have been a frequent event. Across the river, in Southwark, Richard Whittington (d.1424) had donated eight beds to St Thomas's Hospital for the use of girls desperate for anonymity ('he commaundyd that alle the thyngys that ben doon in that chambyr shulde be kepte secrete . . . for he wolde not shame no yonge women in noo wyse for hyt myght be cause of hyr lettyng of hyr maryage'); but not all his fellow-citizens showed such compassion. On drawing up his will in 1479, John Don the elder, another wealthy London mercer, deliberately excluded 'common beggars' and 'women in childbed' from his generous bequests to local hospitals.[31]

Unlike its modern counterpart, the medieval English hospital served only the poor – the rich expected to be nursed in the comfort of their own homes – and performed a variety of functions besides tending the sick. In fact, some institutions categorically refused to admit anyone with a serious illness or embarrassing disability, lest they upset the peaceful round of prayer and ritual necessary for spiritual as well as physical regeneration. They catered instead for people with particular, not necessarily medical, needs, such as pilgrims, the blind, cripples, elderly priests or impoverished widows, children and honest tradesmen who had fallen on hard times. St John's Hospital, Bridgwater, for example, refused to countenance lunatics, epileptics, lepers or victims of contagious diseases, pregnant women, infants and 'intolerable persons', opening its doors only to 'the poor, infirm (i.e. chronically disabled) and needy'. Nor would it accept the well-to-do and sometimes disruptive boarders who often lodged in hospitals on a temporary basis or elected to retire there as pensioners in search of sheltered accommodation. But, in common with almost all other foundations, whatever their purpose, it employed women to look after the inmates. They were to be 'of good conversation and report', prepared to work hard at all times (a qualification felt in this instance to exclude persons of gentle birth) and dedicated to a life of service and prayer.[32]

In theory, if not in practice, nursing the sick poor was seen as a laudable vocation, earning respect and admiration on earth and a lasting reward in heaven. *The Golden Legend*, a popular compilation of saints' lives and exemplars of Christian conduct for the laity, provided, in the story of St Elizabeth of Hungary (d.1231), a model for female readers:

> In order to give shelter to pilgrims and to the homeless, she had a large house built at the foot of her lofty castle. In this house she cared for a great multitude of the sick, visiting them each day, maugre the steepness of the way, ministering to their needs and exhorting them to patience. And although she was sorely distressed by the least taint of the air, she shrank not from the sores of the sick, even in the summer weather, for the love of God. She applied their remedies, cleansed their wounds with the veil of her head, and handled them with her own hands, paying no heed to the protestations of her handmaidens. . . . And once, in caring for a one-eyed child whose body was covered with scabs, she bore him to the privy in her own arms seven times in one night, and gladly washed his soiled bed-clothing. She cared for a woman with dreadful leprosy in the same manner, bathing her, putting her in bed, cleansing and bandaging her sores, applying her salves, cutting her fingernails, and kneeling at the sick woman's feet to loosen the laces of her shoes. She urged the sick to confess their sins and to receive the Holy Communion; and once when an old woman refused to do this, Elizabeth had her chastised with a whip.[33]

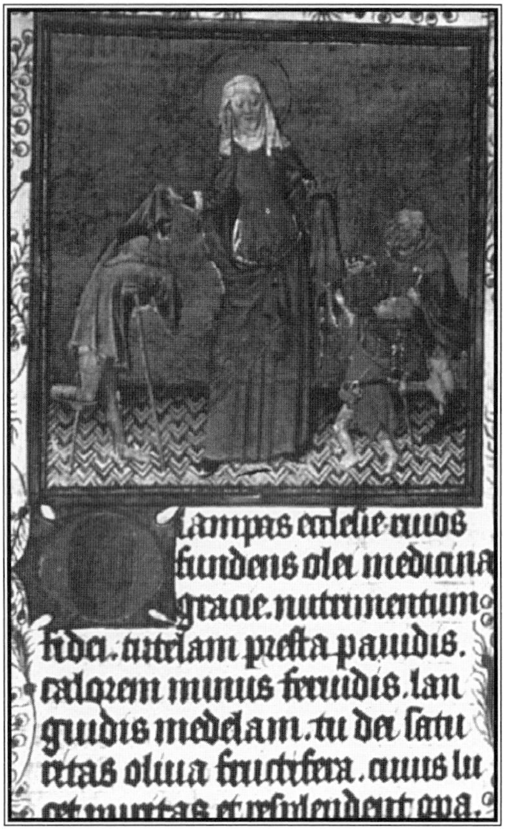

St Elizabeth of Hungary was extolled as the personification of charity and a model to other women. Here she clothes a crippled beggar while (metaphorically) offering her crown to two other supplicants.

Among the extremes of self-abasement practised by holy women of the stamp of St Catherine of Siena and Angela of Foligno was a desire not merely to nurse the diseased and dying, but actually to drink the water used to wash their sores or even the pus itself. Perhaps, as one historian has suggested, these bodies became a substitute for Christ's, which was regularly consumed at mass, and the task of ministering to them a mortification of the flesh. Advice literature for women, such as Christine de Pisan's *Treasure of the City of Ladies*, struck a more temperate note, encouraging charitable work, especially among the sick and destitute, but never once suggesting that it was necessary to become personally involved in their care. On the contrary, recognizing the value of a well-publicized royal visit, Christine urged 'the good princess' to tour hospitals 'in all her grandeur, accompanied magnificently', since this would raise the spirits of the poor as she passed among them.[34]

During the high Middle Ages a few great ladies, including Henry I's queen, Matilda, and many female religious had devoted themselves to the care of lepers as a mark of Christian piety, but nursing in hospices and almshouses seems invariably to have been the preserve of poor women, who were often themselves dependent on public assistance.[35] Their wealthy sisters were, however, expected to provide funding and medical services: those who did not accept this responsibility were condemned as 'mannishe and not womanly, whiche is a vice in womanhode', harsh and lacking compassion (colour plate 20). Laurette de Saint-Valèry might look like a man because of her facial hair ('*barbata faciei seipsa exhibit virum*'), but her generosity to the poor and her decision to learn physic so that she could treat them offered more reliable proof of her femininity.[36] The legendary kindness (which did not, significantly, extend to single mothers) of Emma, Duchess of Aquitaine, was likewise held up as an example to all her sex:

> she enquered thorugh every parishhe for pore men and women that were wedded and had children, and had not wherewith to susteyne hem, and for suche and for diverse sikenesses or other adversitees might not laboure ne travaile, and upon poure women in gesynge [childbirth], alle suche pepille, and mani other, she releved and comforted with almesse of her charitable devocion. And also she hadde her medicines and surgens forto hele and medicine alle suche as were needfulle, wher thorugh that for her bounte and goodnesse, God hath shewed mani miracles for her.[37]

With the exception of segregated houses for lepers and of hostels for the accommodation of pilgrims, medieval English hospitals fell into two basic categories: the older and larger monastic institutions, such as St Leonard's, York, and St Bartholomew's, Smithfield, which often followed the Augustinian rule; and almshouses or *maisons dieu* run in accordance with the patrons' wishes either by the Church or a designated secular authority. A survey of English and Welsh religious houses in the Middle Ages has estimated that almost 70 per cent of the 1,100 or so hospitals identified belonged to the latter group, although several endowments never really got past the planning stage, while others, dependent on the goodwill of trustees and executors, collapsed after the death of their founders.[38]

In the hospital priories, most routine nursing work was undertaken by professed sisters, novices and maidservants, while the brothers saw to the spiritual welfare of their charges. If the latter sometimes helped to prepare medicine or supervise difficult cases, no such change of role was permitted to the sisters. Indeed, in 1414, the nurses at St James's Hospital, Thanington, were ordered not to 'stand or sit in any way round or near the altars or . . . presume to serve the priests celebrating the divine offices'. Strict obedience was expected, if not always forthcoming: at St Katherine's Hospital, by the Tower of London, sisters swore to live chastely 'with a pure heart and clean body', submitting to the master in all things and surrendering any private possessions. Perhaps a few had grown tired of the obligatory 'habit of religion', since ordinances of 1351 specifically banned the wearing of 'green, red or striped stuff, which might tend to dissolution'.[39]

Women in the larger hospitals shouldered a heavy burden of duties, not the least of which was the washing of quantities of bedlinen and clothing in all weathers. The Hôtel Dieu in Paris boasted an impressive complement of forty sisters, thirty novices and sixteen domestics, but there was still no respite from back-breaking physical labour:

> The work in this house is extremely taxing, as quite often here day must become night, and night day, so the sick poor can be tended . . . cleaned up, washed, put to bed, bathed, dried, fed, given drinks, carried from one bed to another and lifted; so beds can be made and remade, personal linen washed out every day in clean water and cloths warmed to wrap around the patients' feet; so every week between eight and nine hundred sheets can be laundered, rinsed out in clean water and put in the wash tub; so ashes can be kindled and wood thrown into the furnace; so the sheets can be washed in the River Seine, whether it is freezing, windy or raining, then hung out on walk-ways in summer or dried by a great fire in winter and then folded up; so the dead can be buried, and other innumerable, laborious and exhausting services can be performed. . . . Some patients, hard to look after and impossible to please, abuse [the nurse] with hostile and defamatory language, while others, in a frenzy brought on by sickness, strike and wound her, and others pull at her clothing.[40]

At the Hôtel Dieu a prioress who had worked her way up through the ranks, starting as a novice in the laundry, was responsible for all the nursing staff, as well as managing a budget well in excess of £500 a year, most of which went on linen. It is unlikely that the principal sister at St Leonard's, York (known in 1383 as Matilda '*la* huswyf' and in 1416 as 'Alice '*materfamilias*'), enjoyed more than a fraction of this authority, although her duties were demanding enough, and her establishment of seven or so professed sisters, various lay brothers and other servants, including cooks and a laundress, was not always amenable to discipline.[41] Nurses found it dispiriting to do such heavy manual work, year in, year out, without much in the way of encouragement or support, or even adequate food and clothing.

In England, where many monastic hospitals faced serious financial difficulties, exacerbated by upheavals in the property market following the Black Death, morale inevitably suffered. As early as 1303, for instance, the seven sisters at St Mary's, Bishopsgate, were being deprived of their rightful share of food, and had to raid the endowment fund to pay for new habits. The overall picture of maladministration and managerial incompetence at St Mary's was, indeed, depressing, and had grown worse by the following century. An episcopal visitation of 1431 found that the sisters remained ill-fed, badly housed and poorly clothed, and had, to the bishop's dismay, begun consorting with the brethren in the kitchens as they collected the patients' even less appetizing fare. His insistence upon a proper procedure for the admission and training of novices suggests that the prior had been trying to raise money by selling off accommodation to women who had no intention of helping with the sick and destitute. Although the foundation statutes of hospitals made it abundantly clear that entry to the sisterhood should be a matter of vocation and merit rather than a commercial transaction, many houses began to demand fees from their new probationers. At Norman's Hospital, Norwich, for example, the master required a flat payment of ten marks, and then compounded his offence, in the late fifteenth century, by allowing the sisters' stipends to fall over two months into arrears. The size of the fee, which came to more than the annual salary of a master mason, makes it unlikely that these particular women would have been prepared to undertake menial duties in return for the promise of a secure old age, but others were not in a position to refuse.[42]

During an inspection of St Bartholomew's Hospital, Smithfield, in 1316, Bishop Segrave of London had actually been obliged to spell out the minimum recommended diet (in terms of both quantity and quality) necessary for the sisters, who may have been too undernourished to perform their tasks properly. At all events, Segrave gave them a pointed reminder that their primary responsibility lay towards the sick. Things did not improve: in 1375 the master, Richard Sutton, faced public accusations of immorality with one of the sisters, although he clung to office despite this and other alleged offences.[43] Standards do not seem to have been very much higher at St Thomas's, Southwark, where brothers and sisters were warned for the second time to avoid '*confabulaciones*' and other exchanges likely to arouse suspicion, and regular checks were deemed essential to monitor the quality of the nursing. Not until just before the Reformation, however, did the house acquire its unsavoury reputation as a 'bawdy hospital' because of the master's flagrant immorality.[44]

The founders of the almshouses and other non-monastic hospitals which sprang up in increasing numbers during the later Middle Ages were keenly aware of the problems caused by inadequate and badly managed resources, lack of vocation and poor discipline. As merchants, landowners or high-ranking members of the secular clergy they themselves possessed considerable financial and administrative experience; and they sought, from the very outset, to impose strict regulations upon their endowments. But the founding and upkeep of even the most unpretentious *maison dieu* was an expensive, time-consuming business: many small ones were never intended to last for more than a few years, representing instead short-term acts of philanthropy on the part of pious men and women who had welcomed the sick poor into their homes. The rest relied for their day-to-day survival upon women, sometimes inmates but more often specially recruited housekeepers, whose contribution to the smooth running of the medieval equivalent of the 'old folk's home' was little short of heroic. The female attendant at Ford's Hospital, Coventry, had to look after five elderly married couples, 'see them clean kept in their persons and houses, and for dressing of their meats, washing of them and ministering all things necessary to them'. In addition to these duties, her counterpart at the Higham Ferrers almshouse was expected to visit all the sick at night, 'please every poor man to her power' *and* refrain from 'brawling or chiding' if her charges proved cantankerous. To sisters at God's House, Southampton, fell the subsidiary task of winnowing corn, sometimes (at least in lean years) without any hired help.[45]

Although most of their time was spent laundering, cleaning and cooking, these women and others like them throughout the country had to undertake a variety of quasi-medical duties, and must have grown quite experienced in the specific requirements of geriatric care. Yet their status remained comparatively low, often little higher than that of a domestic servant, and the small size of English charitable institutions gave them little scope for either advancement or independence. Not until the early sixteenth century could London boast anything like Nuremberg's Heilig Geist Spital, founded by a wealthy merchant in 1339 and run with great efficiency by the city council. Three women in particular occupied positions of authority there: the *custorin*, who, like the prioress at the Hôtel Dieu in Paris, had general care of the sick; her assistant, the *meisterin*, who ran the kitchens and recommended suitable diets for the patients; and the *schauerin*, or 'gate-keeper', whose main responsibility was to inspect all potential inmates for contagious diseases and distribute food to the poor. We shall return to the question of medical expertise and treatment in hospitals later, but it is worth noting that each of these officials evidently possessed a reasonable level of diagnostic ability, as well as some training in general principles relating to the *regimen* of health[46] (colour plate 19).

Henry VII never lived to see the opening of his hospital at the Savoy, which was still at the planning stage when he died in 1509, and took many years to complete. It was far smaller than its prototype, the Ospedale di Santa Maria Nuova, which catered for the sick poor of Florence. Described by one historian as 'arguably the first Western European hospital in the modern sense of the word', the Ospedale offered medical and surgical treatment of the highest order to the occupants of its 230 or more beds, as well as serving the city with a public dispensary and clinics for outpatients. The duties of the hundred or so nurses were explained to King Henry as he embarked on his new foundation:

> First, they receive sick women in the hospital and care for them. . . . The rector of the hospital appoints a female infirmarer and nurses, with exactly the same responsibilities as in the men's hospital. The women include several skilled in surgery, for experience is the mistress of all things. These have many remarkable cures to their credit and are even more trusted than the men. About ten women are responsible for making the bread for the sick and the well of both sexes. . . . The women change duties each week, replacing each other in a fixed order. Ten take care of the cooking and prepare the food. Fifteen do the laundry, scalding, cleaning, washing, drying and folding it each day. Eight look after the chickens, hens, geese and ducks, of which there are incidentally 1,000. . . . The rector of the hospital appoints one woman to keep the linen clothes, another the woollens, and another the bedlinens, the napkins and the cloths. Another looks after the room containing the sacred objects.[47]

Given 'the nature and weakness of the female sex', the hospital authorities felt it was particularly important to keep their nurses 'busy and diligent, cultivating and observing charity, piety and patience'. This point was not lost on the king's trustees, who drew heavily upon the Italian model when compiling their own ordinances. Although conceived on a far more modest scale, by contemporary English standards the Savoy Hospital offered unusually opulent facilities for a hundred poor and preferably sick men. The nursing staff comprised a matron, whose salary of £4.6s.8d. had to cover living expenses and clothing, and twelve unmarried women over the age of thirty-six. (Even if it protected the patients from the risks posed by a menstruating woman, Walter Suffield's requirement that the four sisters who worked at St Giles's Hospital, Norwich, should be at least fifty was clearly unrealistic in view of the heavy tasks required of them.) At 10d. a week, each nurse's allowance comprised just half of the assignment made to the house's four canons, reflecting her subordinate position in the official hierarchy. But she still had to work hard for her keep. Every evening the matron and one of her assistants would join the master in supervising admissions, another nurse would examine the newcomers, and two more would ensure that they took proper baths, if necessary consigning their clothes to a delousing oven. The matron made her rounds of the sick with a physician and surgeon twice a day, in the morning and again in the afternoon, checking that all was in order and giving out further instructions with regard to diet and medication. Since each inmate had his own bed (a luxury not available at either the Hôtel Dieu or the Ospedale di Santa Maria Nuova) with three pairs of sheets, two blankets, a linen cover and a counterpane embellished with a Tudor rose, the most important room in the hospital, and certainly the busiest, must once again have been the laundry.[48]

The cruciform, Italianate structure of the Savoy Hospital, with individual cubicles for the sick in the north and south transepts of the church, was a radical departure from the conventional layout of the English medieval hospital, which usually placed the patients in the nave only. At St Mary's, Bishopsgate, for example, the church served as an open ward of 180 beds in two rows, facing each other across the nave. The principle that everyone should be able to see the altar, take part in services and more devoutly contemplate their own mortality was, however, universal. As noted at the beginning of this book, the hospital or almshouse was primarily a religious institution, where the inmates could immerse themselves in prayer and contemplation, repair the damage done to their immortal souls and, when the time came, be sure of a decent Christian burial.[49]

The reluctance of certain institutions to admit the acutely sick, the insane, or pregnant women sprang, in part, from a desire to concentrate upon these spiritual obligations, which would obviously have been disrupted, and perhaps even devalued, by more demanding patients. While happy to feed, clothe and tend elderly and feeble inmates, or those likely to recover fairly soon from exhaustion, hunger or cold, they were neither prepared nor equipped to provide much in the way of specialist medical care. Larger hospitals, with fewer restrictions on admittance, were thus left to cope with the seriously ill, although it is now impossible to tell exactly what sort of therapy might have been given. Whereas the great French and Italian houses retained physicians and surgeons on a formal basis throughout the fifteenth century and earlier, no attempt was made to follow their example across the Channel until King Henry drew up his plans for the Savoy. Historians have combed the evidence for possible connexions between English hospitals and the medical profession before then, but are generally convinced that little, if any, expert help was available for the average patient.[50]

Such neglect ought to have proved beneficial, for once settled in a clean, quiet environment with regular meals and plenty of rest the sick pauper may well have had a far greater chance of survival

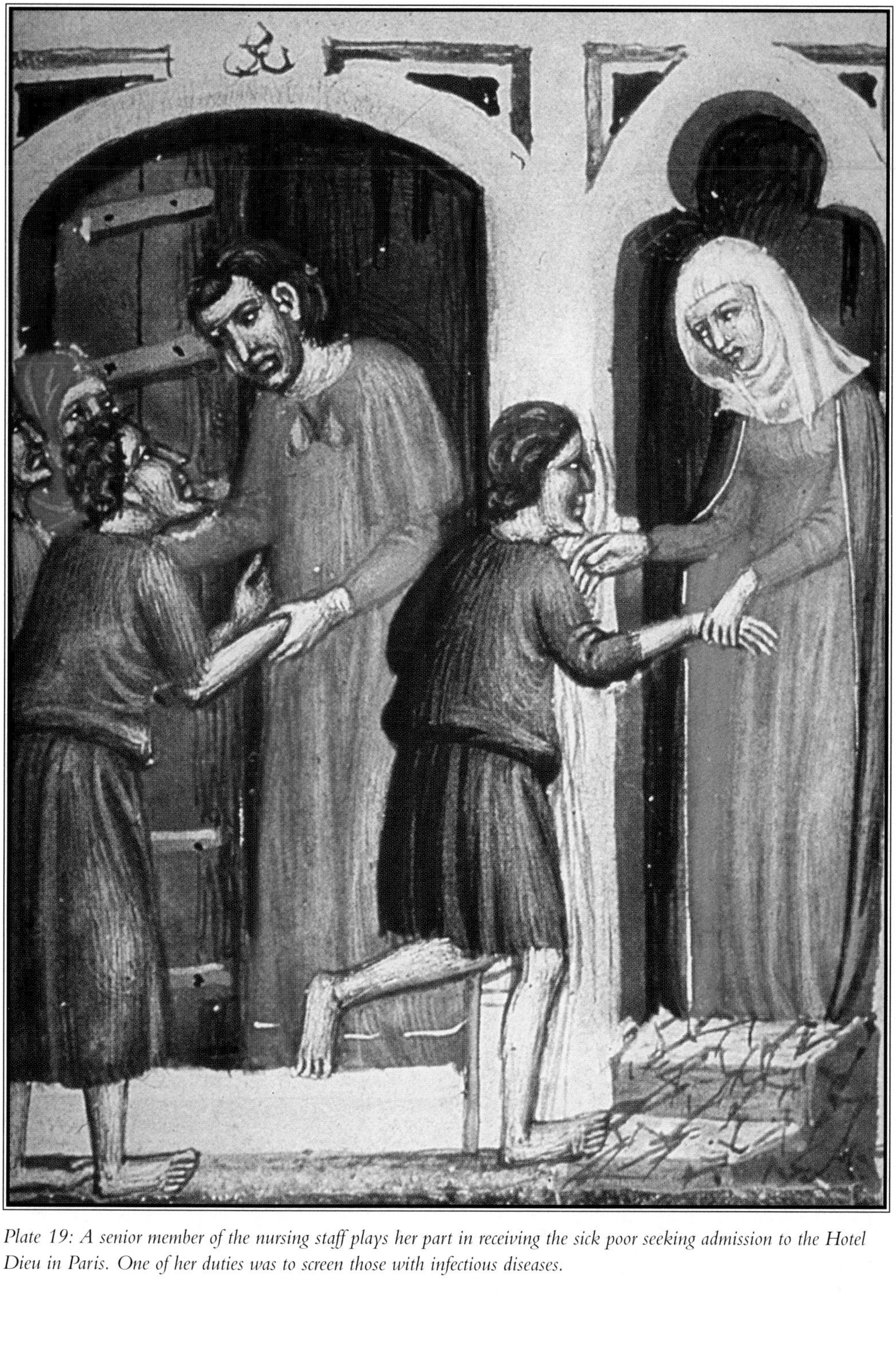

Plate 19: A senior member of the nursing staff plays her part in receiving the sick poor seeking admission to the Hotel Dieu in Paris. One of her duties was to screen those with infectious diseases.

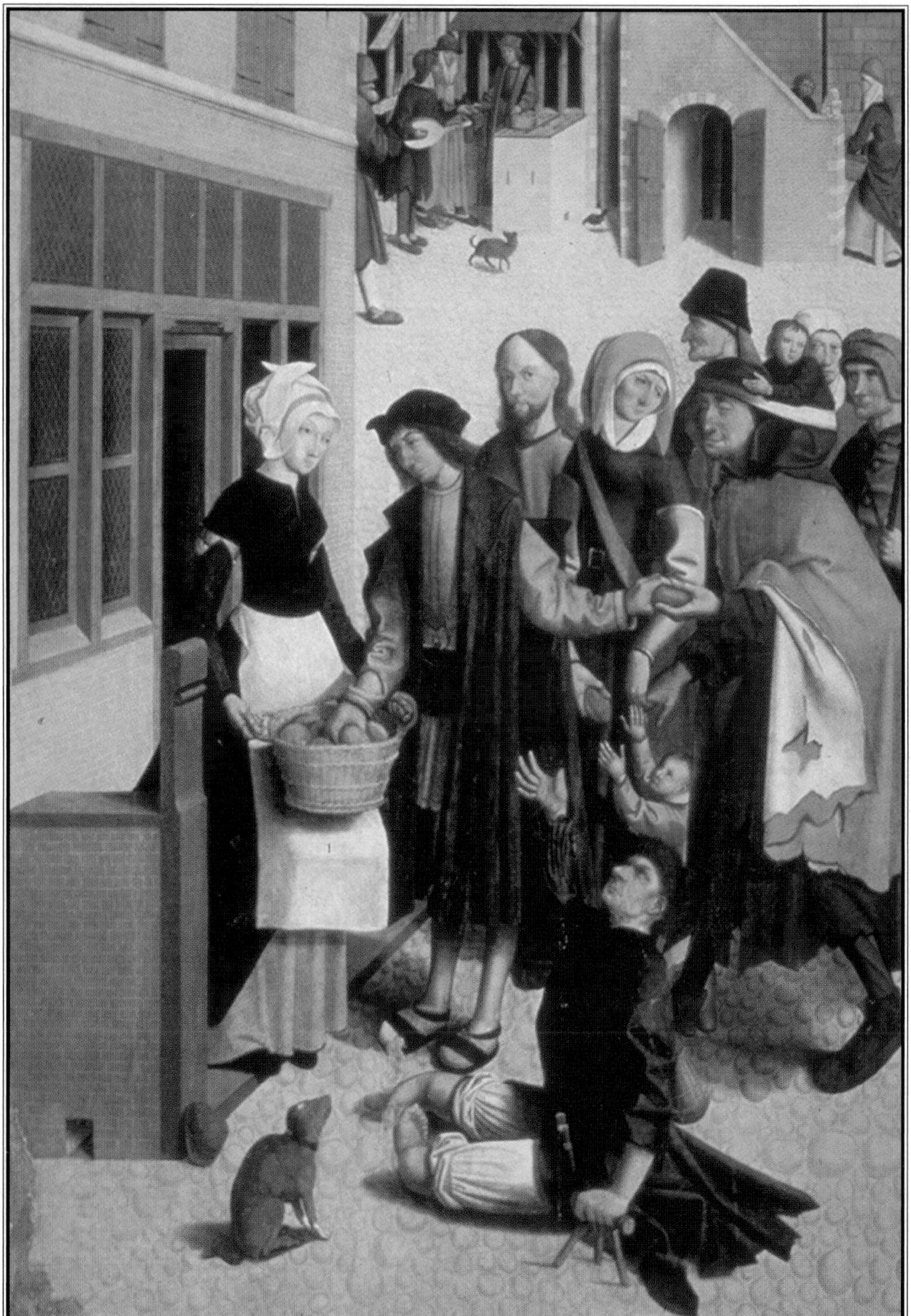

Plate 20: The obligation to help the needy fell especially upon women. In this early sixteenth-century Dutch painting of the seven works of mercy a nursing sister helps to feed sick and crippled paupers. Christ (third from left) looks on approvingly.

than his wealthy contemporaries, weakened by purges, blood-letting and other potentially dangerous remedies as deployed by trained practitioners. Yet he, too, probably suffered to a certain degree, since the rudiments of medical theory were well enough understood in English hospitals. Some nursing sisters were actually designated *medicae*, or female physicians: Abbess Euphemia, who spent forty years at Wherwell Priory, and a nun named Ann at St Leonard's, York, in 1276, both carried this title, as did several women associated with monastic houses but not actually resident in them.[51]

We have seen in Chapter IV how the Church's initial hostility to medical practice as a presumptuous challenge to the will of God softened considerably over the centuries. Bernard of Clairvaux may have castigated monks for seeking other than divine help when they fell ill, but his adversary, Peter Abélard (d.1142), had no such reservations about the benefits of leechcraft. In a letter to his erstwhile mistress, Héloïse, who had by then become Abbess of the Paraclete, he urged that the sick should be given whatever baths, food or luxuries they needed, as well as constant nursing:

> The infirmary must be equipped with everything necessary for their illness . . . medicaments, too, must be provided according to the resources of the convent, and this can be more easily done if the sister in charge has some knowledge of medicine. Those who have a period of bleeding should also be in her care. And there should be someone with experience of blood-letting, or it would be necessary for a man to come in amongst the women for this purpose.[52]

Given that the Paraclete was not a hospital and the number of sick at any one time there must have been comparatively small, Abélard's insistence on the need for proper training is indicative of the importance attached to nursing and therapeutic skills in female monastic communities. Lanfrank of Milan's complaint that phlebotomy, a surgeon's craft, was all too frequently left 'to barbours and to wymmen' may, indeed, have been levelled against some religious, for we know that Augustinian sisters offered blood-letting and other medical services to people from their local communities, very much as outpatients are treated today.[53] The legend of Robin Hood, an implausible figure in any monastic waiting-room, casts an interesting light on this practice. Feeling listless and unable to eat, he decides to visit his cousin, the Prioress of Kirklees, in whose proficiency as a phlebotomist he has every confidence. But she has been suborned by his enemies, and deploys her instruments to deadly effect:

> And downe then came dame prioresse,
> Downe she came in that ilke,
> With a pair off blood-irons in her hands,
> Were wrapped all in silke.
> 'Sett a chaffing-dish to the fyer', said dame prioresse,
> 'And stripp thou vp thy sleeue:'
> I hold him but an vnwise man
> That will noe warning leeve.
> Shee laid the blood-irons to Robin Hoods vaine,
> Alacke, the more pitye!
> And pearct the vaine, and let oute the bloode,
> That full red was to see.

And first it bled, the thicke, thicke bloode.
And afterwards the thinne,
And well then wist good Robin Hoode
Treason there was within.[54]

A more reassuring picture of the medieval nun, solicitously tending her charges, comes from the pen of René of Anjou, the father-in-law of Henry VI. In his allegorical romance, *Le Livre du Cueur d'Amours Espris*, Heart, Desire and Generosity arrive at a hospital for wounded lovers, and are admitted by the elderly infirmarian, who attends the gate day and night to receive the needy. She takes them to meet Dame Pity, the prioress, a gentle figure, busy on her nightly rounds, visiting each patient, comforting him and prescribing the appropriate medicines. Another sympathetic *medica* appears in Jean Cuvelier's biography of the Breton commander, Bertrand Duguesclin (d.1380), whose extreme ugliness as a child led his mother to neglect and abuse him. Her attitude changed, however, when the nun who had been summoned to treat her (and who may, as a converted Jewess, have received specialist medical training) hailed the boy as the future saviour of France, forgetting in her excitement to leave the medicine she had already prescribed and made up.[55]

Unfortunately, neither literary nor archival sources are forthcoming about the remedies which were dispensed on such occasions. The relative paucity of information in English hospital accounts about the purchase of drugs or spices commonly used in pharmacology does not mean that patients lacked for medication (any more than the absence of references to physicians implies a want of proper care), but it appears that most cures were produced, like the housewife's, from the contents of the herb garden and kitchen, without recourse to an apothecary. Women were particularly adept at this kind of traditional herbal medicine, which may, perhaps, have been further developed with the help of standard reference works from the hospital library and consultations with the more learned brethren.[56]

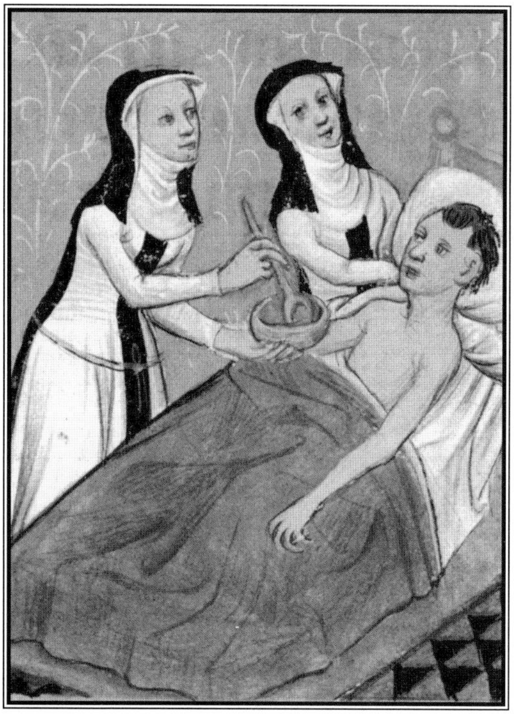

Although primarily concerned with the spiritual health of their patients, medieval hospitals aimed to provide a clean, calm atmosphere, in which rest, regular, if spartan, meals and careful nursing would either hasten recovery or lessen the suffering of the terminally ill.

At its best, the great strength of the medieval English hospital and infirmary lay in the quality of the nursing. Although they rarely obtained much in the way of recognition at the time, and have been woefully neglected by historians ever since, the matrons, sisters, housekeepers and maids considered in this chapter undertook demanding and often unpleasant work under difficult conditions. Some quite possibly lacked any real sense of vocation, and fell far short of the rigorous ideal:

> To kepynge of the seke in the fermery, schal be depute suche a suster by the abbes that dredeth God, hauyng a diligence aboute hem for hys loue, and kan skylle for to do seruyse to them, stronge and myghty to lefte them up, and lede them from place to place whan nede is, to the chirche or fermery chapel, and kan exhorte, styrre and comforte them to be confessed, and receyve the sacramentes of holy chirche. Ofte chaunge ther beddes and clothes, geue them medycynes, ley to ther plastres, and mynyster to them mete and drynke, fyre and water, and al other necessaryes, nyghte and day, as nede requyrethe. . . . Not squaymes to wasche them, and wype them, or auoyde them, nor angry nor hasty, or unpacient thof one haue the vomet, another the fluxe, another the frensy, whiche nowe syngethe, nowe cryethe, nowe lawghethe, nowe wepithe, nowe chydethe, nowe fryghtethe, nowe is wrothe, now wel apayde, ffor ther be some sekenesses vexynge the seke so gretly and prouokynge them to ire, that the mater drawen up to the brayne alyenthe [alienates] the mendes. And therfor they owe to haue moche pacience withe suche, that they may therby gete them an euerlastyng crowne.[57]

Such a combination of spirituality, skill, patience and dedication must have been rare indeed. Dame Margaret Chesham, the sub-cellaress at Gracedieu Priory, who complained at length to Bishop Alnwick of Lincoln, in 1440, because she had been forced to tend the sick in the infirmary, 'sleeping with them, and looking after them by day and night, washing them and doing all else like a laywoman', cannot have been alone in resenting her lot.[58] But the underlying humanity and compassion for suffering, so evident in the foundation charters and ordinances of many late medieval hospitals and almshouses, still found sufficient practical expression to bring comfort and relief to the unfortunate, and offer a promise of salvation to those who cared for them.

NOTES

1. *Medieval Woman's Guide to Health*, ed. B. Rowland (Kent, Ohio, 1981), p. xv. For a reassessment of this view, and evidence of male interest in 'women's problems' see M. Green, 'Women's Medical Practice and Health Care in Medieval Europe', *Signs*, XIV (1989), pp. 442–3.
2. *The Cyrurgie of Guy de Chauliac*, ed. M.S. Ogden (Early English Text Soc., CCLXV, 1971), p. 530.
3. E. Shorter, *A History of Women's Bodies* (London, 1983), p. 38.
4. H.R. Lemay, 'Anthonius Guainerius and Medieval Gynecology', in *Women of the Medieval World*, ed. J. Kirshner and S.F. Wemple (Oxford, 1989), pp. 317–36.
5. *Soranus' Gynaecology*, ed. O. Temkin (Johns Hopkins, 1956), pp. 5–7. For the background to Roman gynaecology see R. Jackson, *Doctors and Diseases in the Roman Empire* (London, 1988), pp. 86–9.
6. *Medieval Woman's Guide to Health*, op. cit., p. 14. See also R.H. Robbins, 'Medical Manuscripts in Middle English', *Speculum*, XLV (1970), p. 406.
7. *The 'Sekenesse of Wymmen'*, ed. M.R. Hallaert (Brussels, 1982), pp. 49–55; Rowland, op. cit., pp. 29, 87–97.
8. R. Barkai, 'A Medieval Hebrew Treatise on Obstetrics', *Medical History*, XXXIII (1989), pp. 96–119; J. Donnison, *Midwives and Medical Men* (London, 1988), p. 21; T.G. Benedek, 'The Changing Relationship between Midwives and Physicians during the Renaissance', *Bulletin of the History of Medicine*, LI (1977), p. 553.
9. Advice literature for women stressed the charitable aspects of giving help in childbirth. See, for example, *The Book of the Knight of la Tour-Landry*, ed. T. Wright (Early English Text Soc., XXXIII, 1868), pp. 136–7, 193.
10. D. Jacquart, *Le Milieu Médical en France du XIIe au XVe Siècle* (Hautes Études Médiévales et Modernes, series 5, XLVI, 1981), pp. 48–9.
11. M.E. Wiesner, 'Early Modern Midwifery', in *Women and Work in Pre-Industrial Europe*, ed. B.A. Hanawalt (Indiana, 1986), pp. 94–9.
12. *Eadem, Working Women in Renaissance Germany* (Rutgers, 1986), pp. 55–61.
13. Donnison, op. cit., p. 18.

14. J.H. Wylie, *History of England under Henry IV* (4 vols, London, 1898), vol. IV, p. 158; *Calendar of Patent Rolls, 1467–77*, pp. 155, 547; *Privy Purse Expenses of Elizabeth of York*, ed. N.H. Nicolas (London, 1830), pp. 102, 208.
15. *Fabric Rolls of York Minster*, ed. J. Raine (Surtees Soc., XXXV, 1858), p. 260.
16. John Myrc, *Instructions for Parish Priests*, ed. E. Peacock (Early English Text Soc., XXXI, 1868, revised 1902), pp. 3–4.
17. This fear was not uniquely English: a midwife named Perrette de Rouen was imprisoned for seven years in Paris and then set in the pillory for procuring a stillborn child so that the flesh could be used to cure leprosy. A royal pardon, issued in 1408, allowed her to resume her calling (D. Jacquart, *Dictionnaire Biographique des Médecins en France au Moyen Age* (Hautes Études Médiévales et Modernes, series 5, XXXV, 1979), p. 222).
18. T. Hunt, *Popular Medicine in Thirteenth Century England* (Cambridge 1990), p. 90. See above, pp. 95–7, for further details about the use of charms in childbirth.
19. *Visitation Articles and Injunctions*, ed. W.H. Frere (Alcuin Club Collections, XIV–XVI, 1910), vol. II, pp. 58–9, 292, 356–7, 372; Donnison, op. cit., p. 21; G.N. Clark, *A History of the Royal College of Physicians of London* (2 vols, Oxford, 1964), vol. I, pp. 66–7. Arrangements for the *medical* supervision and examination of midwives had already been made in Zurich, where, for the first time, in 1544, doctors were called in to give instruction (Shorter, op. cit., p. 41).
20. Bartholomaeus Anglicus, *On the Properties of Things: John Trevisa's Translation of Bartholomaeus Anglicus' De Proprietatis Rerum*, ed. M.C. Seymour and others (3 vols, Oxford, 1975–88), vol. I, p. 305.
21. L. Demaitre, 'The Idea of Childhood and Child Care in Medical Writings of the Middle Ages', *Journal of Psychohistory*, IV (1977), pp. 472–3. For a general discussion of the subject of childbirth see P.P.A. Biller, 'Childbirth in the Middle Ages', *History Today*, XXXVI (1986), pp. 42–9.
22. Bartholomaeus Anglicus, op. cit., vol. I, p. 303; Shorter, op. cit., pp. 49–63; Wiesner, *Working Women*, op. cit., pp. 60–1; E. Coyecque, *L'Hôtel Dieu de Paris au Moyen Age* (2 vols, Paris, 1889–91), vol. I, p. 100; Benedek, op. cit., pp. 555, 557.
23. R. Pecock, *The Reule of Crysten Religioun*, ed. W.C. Greet (Early English Text Soc., CLXXI, 1927), pp. 341–2; Wiesner, 'Early Modern Midwifery', op. cit., p. 98; *eadem, Working Women*, op. cit., pp. 60–1.
24. P.P.A. Biller, 'Birth Control in the West in the Thirteenth and Early Fourteenth Centuries', *Past and Present*, XCIV (1982), pp. 3–26; *idem*, 'Marriage Patterns and Woman's Lives: A Sketch of a Pastoral Geography', in *Woman is a Worthy Wight: Women in English Society* c. *1200–1500*, ed. P.J.P. Goldberg (Stroud, 1992), pp. 70–9.
25. B.D.H. Miller, 'She Who Hath Drunk Any Potion', *Medium Aevum*, XXXI (1962), p. 191; *Robert of Brunne's Handlyng Synne*, ed. F.J. Furnivall (Early English Text Soc., CXIX, 1901), p. 263.
26. D. Jacquart and C. Thomasset, *Sexuality and Medicine in the Middle Ages* (Cambridge, 1988), pp. 88–94; Shorter, op. cit., pp. 183–8; Wellcome Library, Western Ms. 626, ff. 280–2. In 1322 the apothecaries of Paris were expressly forbidden to sell abortifacients without the authorization of a registered practitioner, a ruling subsequently adopted in Basle and other European cities (L. Reutter de Rosemont, *Histoire de la Pharmacie à travers les Ages* (2 vols, Paris, 1931), vol. I, pp. 210, 305–8.
27. *The 'Sekenesse of Wymmen'*, op. cit., p. 37. The italics are mine. For a series of remedies designed to induce menstruation ('*ad provocandum igitur menstruum*') see also T. Hunt, op. cit., pp. 239–40, 258–60.
28. *Fabric Rolls of York Minster*, op. cit., p. 272; A. Macfarlane, 'Illegitimacy and Illegitimates in English History', in *Bastardy and its Comparative History*, ed. P. Laslett and others (London, 1980), pp. 76–7.
29. Coyecque, op. cit., pp. 100–1.
30. *Rotuli Parliamentorum*, vol. IV, pp. 19–20; R.M. Clay, *The Medieval Hospitals of England* (London, 1909), pp. 8–9, 89–90; P.H. Cullum, *Cremetts and Corrodies: Care of the Poor and Sick at St. Leonard's Hospital, York, in the Middle Ages* (University of York, Borthwick Paper LXXIX, 1991), pp. 9–10, 30.
31. *Calendar of Close Rolls, 1343–46*, p. 432; *1349–54*, pp. 414–15; *The Historical Collections of a Citizen of London*, ed. J. Gairdner (Camden Soc., new series, XVII, 1876), p. ix. PRO, Probate Court of Canterbury 2 Logge; C. Rawcliffe, 'The Hospitals of Later Medieval London', *Medical History*, XXVIII (1984), pp. 2, 12.
32. M. Carlin, 'Medieval English Hospitals', in *The Hospital in History*, ed. L. Granshaw and R. Porter (pbk, London, 1990), p. 25. See also M. Rubin, 'Development and Change in English Hospitals, 1100–1500', ibid., p. 49.
33. *The Golden Legend of Jacobus de Voragine*, ed. and trans. G. Ryan and H. Ripperger (New York, 1969), pp. 681, 685.
34. C.W. Bynum, *Holy Feast and Holy Fast: The Religious Significance of Food to Medieval Women* (University of California Press, 1987), pp. 144–5, 166, 171–2, 182; Christine de Pisan, *The Treasure of the City of Ladies*, trans. S. Lawson (pbk, London, 1985), p. 53.
35. Matthew Paris, *Chronica Majora*, ed. H.R. Luard (7 vols, London, 1872–84), vol. II, p. 130. For another example of a high-born nurse caring for lepers see Thomas of Monmouth, *The Life and Miracles of St William of Norwich*, ed. A. Jessopp and M.R. James (Cambridge, 1896), p. 31.
36. E. Wickersheimer, *Dictionnaire Biographique des Médecines en France au Moyen Age* (Paris, 1936), p. 522; *The Book of the Knight of la Tour-Landry*, op. cit., p. 136.
37. *The Book of the Knight of la Tour-Landry*, op. cit., pp. 136–7.

38. D. Knowles and R.N. Hadcock, *Medieval Religious Houses of England and Wales* (London, 1971), pp. 310–410, *passim*. The percentage figures are Professor Martha Carlin's.
39. Clay, op. cit., pp. 154–5; C. Jamison, *The History of the Royal Hospital of St Katherine* (Oxford, 1952), pp. 28–32.
40. Coyecque, op. cit., vol. I, pp. 34–5.
41. *Collection de Documents pour Servir a l'Histoire des Hôpitaux de Paris*, ed. M. Briele and others (4 vols, Paris, 1881–7), vol. III, pp. 4–6, 57–60, 75–91; Clay, op. cit., p. 154.
42. *The Victoria County History of London*, ed. W. Page (London, 1909), pp. 530–4; *Visitations of the Diocese of Norwich, 1492–1532*, ed. A. Jessopp (Camden Soc., new series, XLIII, 1888), p. 14.
43. *The Victoria County History of London*, op. cit., pp. 520–4.
44. Ibid., pp. 538–41; *Letters and Papers of Henry VIII*, vol. XI, no. 168; New College, Oxford, Archives, Ms. 3691, *passim* (I am grateful to Professor Carlin for providing me with a copy of this document).
45. Clay, op. cit., pp. 155–6; P.H. Cullum, 'Poverty and Charity in Early Fourteenth-Century England', in *England in the Fourteenth Century*, ed. N. Rogers (Stamford, 1993), p. 146.
46. Wiesner, *Working Women*, op. cit., pp. 38–9. Although intended to support a hundred blind and paralysed men, William Elsing's London hospital, founded in 1329, initially housed only thirty-two, and was beset by financial and disciplinary problems (*The Victoria County History of London*, op. cit., pp. 535–7).
47. K. Park and J. Henderson, '"The First Hospital Among Christians": the Ospedale di Santa Maria Nuova in Early Sixteenth-Century Florence', *Medical History*, XXXV (1991), p. 186.
48. R. Somerville, *The Savoy* (London, 1960), pp. 29–32. For Santa Maria Nuova see Park and Henderson, op. cit., *passim*, and J. Henderson, 'The Hospitals of Late Medieval and Renaissance Florence', in *The Hospital in History*, op. cit., p. 81; and for Norwich, C.B. Jewson, *History of the Great Hospital Norwich* (Norwich, 1980), pp. 1–11.
49. Rawcliffe, op. cit., p. 12.
50. Carlin, op. cit., pp. 29–31; Henderson, op. cit., pp. 81–2; Coyecque, op. cit., vol. I, p. 97; M. Rubin, *Charity and Community in Medieval Cambridge* (Cambridge, 1987), pp. 148–53. It should, however, be noted that physicians and surgeons were regularly called in to treat the brothers and sisters, if not the sick poor, in English religious houses.
51. Cullum, op. cit., p. 13; E. J. Kealey, 'England's Earliest Women Doctors', *Journal of the History of Medicine*, XL (1985), p. 477.
52. *The Letters of Peter Abélard*, ed. B. Radice (pbk, London, 1974), pp. 215–16. For the attitude of the Church see above, pp. 84–5.
53. *Lanfrank's 'Science of Cirurgie'*, ed. R. von Fleischhacker (Early English Text Soc., CII, 1894), pp. 18–19.
54. *The English and Scottish Popular Ballads*, ed. F.J. Child (5 vols, Folklore Press, New York, 1957), vol. III, pp. 104–5.
55. *Oeuvres Complètes du Roi René*, ed. le Comte de Quatrebarbes (4 vols, Angers, 1845–6), vol. III, 97–9; *Illustrations from the Life of Bertrand Duguesclin by Jean Cuvelier*, ed. H.Y. Thompson (London, 1909), p. 8.
56. Cullum, op. cit., pp. 14–15. The master of the infirmary at Barnwell Priory was advised always to have 'ginger, cinnamon, peony and the like ready in his cupboard, so as to be able to render prompt assistance to the sick' (*The Observances in Use at the Augustinian Priory of S. Giles and S. Andrew at Barnwell, Cambridgeshire*, ed. J. Willis Clark (Cambridge, 1897), p. 203).
57. G.J. Aungier, *The History and Antiquities of Syon Monastery* (London, 1840), pp. 395–6.
58. *Visitation of Religious Houses in the Diocese of Lincoln*, ed. A.H. Thompson (Canterbury and York Soc., XXIV, 1919), pp. 121, 123.

CONCLUSION

In a sermon preached at St Paul's Cross, London, in about 1388, Thomas Wimbledon addressed the topic of Christian accountability in a sinful world. His text, which is preserved in several copies and seems to have made a lasting impression on the congregation, is notable not only for a discussion of the ways in which illness might be used by God to inspire fear, humility, patience and obedience, but also for a novel view of the day of reckoning. He compares 'the sekenesse of the world' before doomsday with the condition of a patient on his or her deathbed. Whereas the latter would experience either a sharp decline in the body's natural heat or a dangerous rise in temperature, the former was destined to suffer simultaneously from the fires of promiscuity and a cooling of religious zeal.[1] In each case the humoral balance had been irretrievably disturbed, with only one possible outcome. This was a powerful simile to which Wimbledon's listeners could easily respond: all would be familiar, to a greater or lesser extent, with the medical theory involved; and most would themselves have experienced at first hand the various ways in which physicians, surgeons or empirics put these ideas into practice.

A few years later, at the beginning of the fifteenth century, the author of a withering attack on standards of morality in public life, known to historians as *Mum and the Sothsegger*, likewise felt that his argument could be most forcefully expressed through recourse to humoral imagery. Just as it was essential for the boils, apostumes and swellings of the sick to be lanced and dressed before the evil matter turned inward, with fatal consequences, so too the shire knights in parliament should 'berste oute alle the boicches and blayens of the hert and lete the rancune renne oute a-russhe al at oones, leste the fals felon festre with-ynne'.[2] Men and women who had recently witnessed the fall of Richard II and the outbreak of protracted civil unrest under his successor did not need reminding that 'venym' trapped within the body politic would rapidly corrupt the entire organism, and the open sore of disaffection turn to gangrene.

This book contains many examples of the ways in which contemporary ideas about the human body and medicine came to enjoy a general currency throughout late medieval English society. Churchmen, preoccupied with the disease of sin, seized upon a vocabulary which was graphic, immediate and, above all, appropriate to those entrusted with the cure of souls. Quite sophisticated concepts from the pages of the *regimen sanitatis* were, moreover, deployed alongside predictable allusions to cautery, purgation and the phlebotomist's knife. The spiritual benefits of fasting could be explained in medical terms, since there were clear parallels to be drawn between the positive effects of careful diet on the body and of penance on the soul. Indeed, given the holistic approach adopted by medieval priests and physicians alike, treatment of one was assumed to exert a direct influence upon the other. A Lenten fast, undertaken as 'phlegmatic' winter was giving way to 'sanguine' spring, would 'drye the erthe' of the body in the same way as the sun caused moisture to evaporate from the soil, burning off the lethal fumes of lust: 'Fastyng hit clansyth a mannys flesch of evyll steryng and lyst to syn of gloteny and of lechery; for thes byn synnys of the flesch.'[3]

Although they leave the reader in no doubt as to the discomfort of treatment, such references rarely betray much in the way of contempt or hostility towards trained practitioners. On the contrary, the reassuring figure of Christ the Physician, so frequently invoked in medieval homiletic literature, suggests that the upper reaches of the medical profession, if not the rank and file, may have commanded rather more respect and admiration than contemporary satirists would have us believe. Significantly, although the leech and the lawyer were often classed together as mercenary parasites preying upon their victims, the contrasting metaphor of Christ the serjeant-at-law pleading for the souls of men in a celestial court of King's bench never exercised much hold over the popular imagination. This was in part because the lives of ordinary people were more immediately touched by illness and pain than they were by litigation, but the symbolic potential of the learned *medicus* with his profusion of cures was obviously far greater.

The idea of professional rivalry at the patient's bedside could, for instance, be elaborated to illustrate the superiority of the Christian faith. As one preacher noted when expounding upon the medicinal qualities of the Eucharist and the purpose of the Crucifixion:

> Frendis, Crist dois this as the grett fesicions and leches don when that thei com owte of a farre contrey: thei aspie where that othur leches have fayled, and thethur thei goy and geven here medecyns for to shewe here connynge [skill]. Ryght so Crist Ihesu, when all prophetis be the lawe of Moyses fayles for to save mans sowle, for that was the lawe of vengeaunce, than com Crist, and with is preciouse blode he made man hole.[4]

Others dwelt upon the remedies offered by Christ to those who had to endure misery on earth, drawing as they did so upon widespread knowledge of surgical practice and the *regimen* of health:

> And I maintain that the blows of this world are like a strong corrosive powder which these masters [of surgery] apply to these wounds when they perceive that there is any dead flesh, or that there is too much raw flesh. They apply a concentration of corrosive powder which eats away the flesh very aggressively. But however much the patient must suffer, it does him great good afterwards, and as a result of this pain he will escape a far worse fate which would otherwise overtake him, or perhaps even death. And so it is when a man is sick: the master does all manner of things to him, and prescribes for him syrups to drink and electuaries to take, which may perchance be both bitter and evil smelling to swallow. Nevertheless, unless the master recognizes the great urgency of internal and external treatment, I would neither undertake nor submit to it. . . .[5]

Nor should we forget the comparison made between the Virgin Mary and a quiet, competent nurse, adept in her care of the patient but always obedient to the wishes of her superior, the physician. If contemporary medical theory tended to support the ambivalent, sometimes overtly hostile views of the female sex adopted by many theologians, in practice most of the treatment available in medieval England was, none the less, undertaken by women, either on a commercial basis, as midwives, herbalists, empirics and even surgeons, or as an important part of routine domestic duties. In the countryside, where trained practitioners were few and far between, women would be expected to fill the gap, acquiring at least a rudimentary knowledge of academic medicine as well as mastering the herbal lore customarily passed on by word of mouth and practical demonstration from one generation to the next. Literature abounds with examples of their skill, which drew upon both traditions. Since there is no local apothecary to prescribe for her ailing husband, Chaucer's Dame Pretelote takes it upon herself to diagnose and treat his condition, recommending heavy purgation to rid his body of excessive choler, and warning him that sunshine will intensify the humoral imbalance, perhaps to the point of death. Just like the best physician, she is careful to suggest a 'digestive' before embarking upon the more aggressive aspects of therapy, with laxatives made of hellebore, ground ivy and other plants to be found at home in their barnyard. For although she is only a hen, she knows well enough that dreams provide a sure indication of the 'greet superfluytee' of melancholic, phlegmatic or choleric vapours, usually caused by overeating.[6]

The professional medical establishment, which comprised a small élite of university-educated physicians lacking any formal collegiate or organizational structure, and a far larger group of master surgeons and barbers whose practice was strictly controlled by urban craft guilds, feared the threat to their incomes and status posed by 'unskilled' or 'unlearned' rivals of either sex, and were also anxious about competition from the apothecaries whom they employed to make up (but not prescribe) drugs. Attempts, especially by barbers, to corner the urban market in the fifteenth century, were, however, bound to achieve only limited success: besides the factor of cost, which placed their services beyond the reach of the poor, the uncertain, painful nature of so many of the 'cures' on offer meant that most people wanted to postpone the ordeal for as long as possible. Having exhausted the range of readily available domestic remedies, many would turn next to the charms, potions and salves which constituted the stock in trade of wise-women and herbalists, while at the same time considering the state of their immortal souls. Pilgrimage to the shrine of a saint or holy relic notable for miraculous cures might well be left as a final resort, when all else had failed, but was, on the other hand, regularly undertaken as a kind of insurance policy against future sickness.

Even for those lucky enough to possess a robust constitution, good health must have seemed a fragile, ephemeral gift, to be fostered at all costs. Only the very rich could afford to employ their own personal physicians, whose mastery of theological, medical and astrological texts enabled them to advise their patrons on almost every aspect of life and death. But a growing corpus of literature was obtainable in English for the guidance of men and women with an interest in

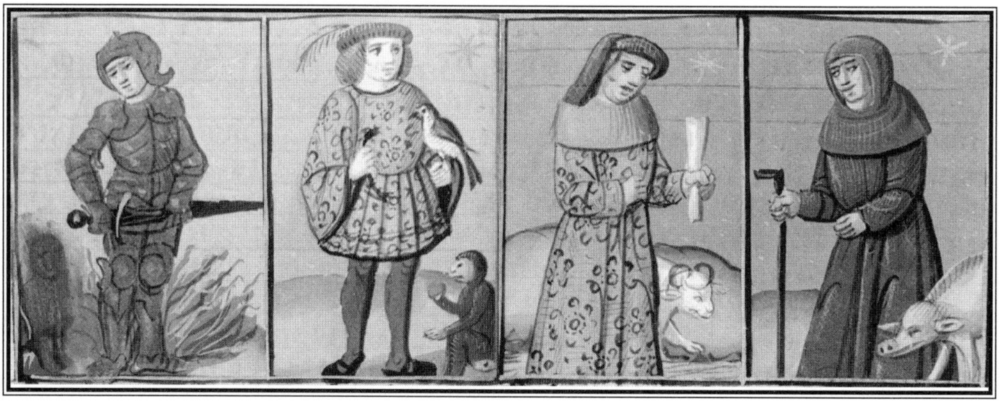

A late fifteenth-century depiction of the four humours with their salient characteristics. The choleric man of war, the sanguine courtier, the phlegmatic merchant and the melancholic clerk have by this date acquired symbolic animals, being accompanied, respectively, by a lion, an ape, a goat and a pig, which represent degrees of drunkenness.

medicine; and the ubiquity of references to such concepts as the influence of the heavens on the human body or the hierarchy of bodily parts testifies to its popularity. Clearly, during a period when master surgeons commonly had recourse to charms and prayers when attempting difficult operations, and herbalists were well versed in humoral theory it is important to recognize the strength of these common beliefs and shared assumptions. However much differences of gender, class or training may have set practitioners apart from one another, the patient was rarely disposed to maintain rigid distinctions: for him or her the rich diversity of physical or spiritual treatment offered a continued hope, desperately sought, of relief from suffering.

NOTES

1. *Wimbledon's Sermon Redde Rationem Villicationis Tue*, ed. I.K. Knight (Duquesne Studies, Philological Series, IX, 1967), p. 110.
2. *Mum and the Sothsegger*, ed. M. Day and R. Steele (Early English Text Soc., CIC, 1936), pp. 59–60.
3. John Mirk, *Mirk's Festial: A Collection of Homilies,* ed. T. Erbe (Early English Text Soc., XCVI, 1905), pp. 253–4.
4. *Middle English Sermons* ed. W.O. Ross (Early English Text Soc., CCIX, 1940, reprinted 1960), p. 126.
5. Henry of Lancaster, *Le Livre de Seyntz Médicines*, ed. E.J. Arnould (Oxford, 1940), p. 196.
6. Geoffrey Chaucer, *Works*, ed. F.N. Robinson (Oxford, 1970), pp. 200–1.

FURTHER READING

Readers wishing to explore the subject of medieval medicine in greater depth are urged to begin with K. Park's authoritative survey, 'Medicine and Society in Medieval Europe, 500–1500', in *Medicine in Society*, ed. A. Wear (Cambridge, 1992). This essay describes the wide variety of treatment on offer and the interconnection between different types of practice, as well as discussing major developments in public and private health care over a period of one thousand years. C.H. Talbot, *Medicine in Medieval England* (London, 1967), and S. Rubin, *Medieval English Medicine* (Newton Abbot, 1974), remain standard works, and are extremely readable, setting the English experience in the wider European context. Both rely largely upon printed sources, and are neither as original nor as scholarly as N.G. Siraisi, whose *Medieval and Early Renaissance Medicine* (Chicago, 1990) is warmly recommended, especially to those with an interest in medical education. However, this book reflects the author's own specialization in Italian and academic medicine, and has comparatively little to say about England, which lagged far behind the Continent in many respects.

Detailed information about health care in England during the earlier Middle Ages may be found in E.J. Kealey, *Medieval Medicus* (Johns Hopkins, 1981), which concentrates upon the first half of the twelfth century. Kealey paints a rather optimistic picture of the availability and effectiveness of medical resources, but at least this counteracts the relentlessly gloomy and often anachronistic approach to medieval medical history adopted by nineteenth- and early twentieth-century writers, who tended to be physicians or surgeons themselves and were thus preoccupied with the idea of 'progress'. R. Gottfried, *Doctors and Medicine in Medieval England* (Princeton, 1986), is marred by errors on almost every page, and should be used with great caution.

Our understanding of the theory and practice of medieval medicine is greatly enhanced by the survival of many illuminated manuscripts. The best introduction to this important visual source is P. Murray Jones, *Medieval Medical Miniatures* (London, 1984), which contains a clear and comprehensive account of contemporary ideas and their application. Although their commentary is less informative, A.S. Lyons and R.J. Petrucelli cover most aspects of medical iconography from ancient times to the present day in the lavishly produced *Medicine: An Illustrated History* (New York, 1976). For practical, consultative purposes, L. Mackinney's catalogue and finding aid, *Medical Illustrations in Medieval Manuscripts* (London, 1965) remains an invaluable reference work. Some writing on humoral theory makes a new and potentially difficult subject virtually unintelligible, but F.M. Getz's introduction to her edition of the pharmaceutical writings of Gilbertus Anglicus, *Healing and Society in Medieval England* (University of Wisconsin Publications in the History of Science and Medicine, VIII, 1991), is a model of clarity. The essays collected by S. Campbell, B. Hall and D. Klausner in *Health, Disease and Healing in Medieval Culture* (Toronto, 1992) cover a wide range of topics and source materials, reflecting the rich diversity of treatment, from diet to cautery, available to the patient. A more specialized book of papers, *Practical Medicine from Salerno to the Black Death*, edited by L. Garcia-Ballester and others (Cambridge, 1994), examines a variety of medical texts and their academic background.

Although they are principally concerned with two French practitioners and their work, both L. Demaitre, *Doctor Bernard Gordon: Professor and Practitioner* (Toronto, 1980), and M.C. Pouchelle, *The Body and Surgery in the Middle Ages* (Polity Press, 1990), have much to say which is of general interest. Further insights into continental practice may also be found in K. Park, *Doctors and Medicine in Early Renaissance Florence* (Princeton, 1985), and M.R. McVaugh, *Medicine before the Plague: Practitioners and their Patients in the Crown of Aragon 1285–1345* (Cambridge, 1993). No comparable study has yet been produced for England, partly because the sources are so very different and the material available far more limited. F.M. Getz's chapter on 'The Faculty of Medicine before 1500', in *The History of the University of Oxford, Volume II, Late Medieval Oxford,* ed. J.I. Catto and R. Evans (Oxford, 1992), is essential reading for those who want to learn more about the education of physicians, as, to a lesser degree, is D.R. Leader's briefer investigation of medical training in his *History of the University of Cambridge, Volume I, the University to 1546* (Cambridge, 1988). The papers presented in *Essays on the Life and Work of Thomas Linacre* c. *1460–1524*, ed. F. Maddison, M. Pelling and C. Webster (Oxford, 1977), most notably that by C. Webster on 'Thomas Linacre and the Foundation of the Royal College of Physicians', constitute a useful starting-point for readers wishing to explore the sixteenth century, and also tell us more about the problems facing England's two faculties of medicine in the later medieval period.

English surgeons and barbers are less well served, although T. Beck provides useful extracts from original documents in his otherwise rather variable monograph, *The Cutting Edge: Early History of the Surgeons of London* (London, 1974). The biographical register of *Medical Practitioners in Medieval England* compiled by C.H. Talbot and E.A. Hammond (Wellcome Historical Medical Library, London, new series, vol. VIII, 1965) presents a mass of evidence about more than 1,200 specific individuals, but is marred by a number of misidentifications and other errors, as well as by the omission of apothecaries and barbers. It should be used in conjunction with F.M. Getz's additions and revisions which appear in *Social History of Medicine*, III (1990), pp. 245–83. The question of medical incomes is addressed in C. Rawcliffe, 'The Profits of Practice: the Wealth and Status of Medical Men in Later Medieval England', *Social History of Medicine,* I (1988).

As will have become clear from this book, religion and magic played an important part in the healing process. R.C. Finucane examines one area of ecclesiastical influence in *Miracles and Pilgrims: Popular Beliefs in Medieval England* (London, 1977); and J.R. Guy reveals another in 'The Episcopal Licensing of Physicians, Surgeons and Midwives', *Bulletin of the History of Medicine*, LVI (1982). Essays by M. Carlin, M. Rubin and J. Henderson in *The Hospital in History*, ed. L. Granshaw and R. Porter (London, 1990), assess the relative importance of spiritual, as opposed to physical, medication in English and Italian hospitals. The highly ambivalent attitude of the Church and society towards lepers is eloquently described by S.N. Brody, *The Disease of the Soul: Leprosy in Medieval Literature* (Cornell, 1974), while P.B.R. Doob, *Nebuchadnezzar's Children: Conventions of Madness in Middle English Literature* (Yale, 1974), looks at the fate of the insane. It should be stressed, however, that neither writer has consulted the kind of legal or administrative source material which casts a more favourable light upon contemporary practice. A lucid account of the use of charms and magic in medicine may be found in R. Kieckhefer, *Magic in the Middle Ages* (Cambridge, 1990). K. Thomas's classic study, *Religion and the Decline of Magic* (London, 1984), also contains valuable material for the medievalist.

The subject of ecclesiastical prejudice towards the female body is explored by U. Ranke-Heinemann, in a polemical study, *Eunuchs for Heaven: The Catholic Church and Sexuality* (London,

1990). Her views are somewhat less measured than those of D. Jacquart and C. Thomasset, whose *Sexuality and Medicine in the Middle Ages* (Cambridge, 1988) presupposes a degree of historical and medical knowledge on the part of the reader, but manages, even so, to entertain as well as inform. Medical ideas about male and female bodies are also investigated in T.W. Laqueur's thought-provoking book, *Making Sex: Body and Gender from the Greeks to Freud* (Harvard, 1990).

Although the care of the sick in medieval and early modern England was largely undertaken by women in the home or local community, and university-trained or otherwise licensed practitioners were in fact responsible for only a limited clientele, historians have devoted a disproportionate amount of attention to the emergent medical profession at the expense of other healers. It has, moreover, generally been assumed that members of this profession showed little interest in 'female problems', a belief which explains the relative paucity of books about practical obstetrics and gynaecology. A stimulating article by M. Green on 'Women's Medical Practice and Health Care in Medieval Europe' (*Signs*, XIV (1989)) challenges such preconceptions, and shows how much is still to be learned about this neglected field.

Unfortunately, B. Rowland's edition of a vernacular gynaecological text, *Medieval Woman's Guide to Health* (Kent, Ohio, 1981), is misleading in some respects, not least with regard to the identity of the now legendary female practitioner, Trotula of Salerno. Readers are advised to consult J.F. Benton, 'Trotula, Women's Problems, and the Professionalization of Medicine in the Middle Ages', *Bulletin of the History of Medicine*, LIX (1985), which dispels for good some hoary myths about 'Dame Trot'. A more rigorous examination of the dissemination of medical knowledge among laymen and -women than that offered by Rowland may be found in L.E. Voigts's contribution to *Book Production and Publishing in Britain, 1375–1475*, ed. J. Griffiths and D. Pearsall (Cambridge, 1984).

M.E. Wiesner's chapter on midwives in her *Working Women in Renaissance Germany* (Rutgers, 1986), and her discussion of 'Early Modern Midwifery', in *Women and Work in Pre-Industrial Europe*, ed. B.A. Hanawalt (Indiana, 1986), show, once again, how different English practice was from that in other parts of Europe. J. Donnison's *Midwives and Medical Men* (London, 1988) briefly explores the medieval period, and P.P.A. Biller, 'Childbirth in the Middle Ages', *History Today*, XXXVI (1986), provides some useful illustrations and an accessible overview of the subject. The topic of nursing in general has attracted little attention from medievalists, and material about the contribution made by women to the running of English hospitals is widely scattered. M. Wade Labarge, *Women in Medieval Life* (London, 1986), describes the regime at the Hôtel Dieu in Paris, while R.M. Clay's classic study, *The Mediaeval Hospitals of England* (London, 1909), remains a standard, if not always well-documented, source.

BIBLIOGRAPHY

UNPUBLISHED PRIMARY SOURCES

British Library, Dept of Mss, Add. Mss 27582, 35115; Arundel 42; Egerton 2572; Harley 1736; Sloane 4, 5, 6, 96, 468, 775, 983

Borthwick Institute, York, York Registry Wills, vols I–V

Clywyd RO, Ruthin, DD/WY/6642

Canterbury Cathedral, City and Diocesan RO, Consistory Court Wills, Register VII

Eton College Records, vol. XLVII

Longleat House (Mss of the Marquess of Bath), Ms. 6415

New College, Oxford, Archives, Ms. 3691

Norfolk County RO, DCN1/10/1–38 (infirmarers' rolls of Norwich Cathedral Priory); press G, case 24, shelf A, general accounts of the Great Hospital, 1465–1501, 1485–1508, 1509–1527

PRO, C1/42/108, 64/154, 68/44, 111/11–12, 113/52, 131/8, 230/53, 252/13–16, 309/43–44; C88/128/34; C260/20/9, 25/2; C270/22; DL28/3/2; E36/220; E101/45/5, 48/3, 69/4/409, 402/18, 20, 404/21, 24, 410/14, 518/5; E135/8/48; E153/1066/1–2; E159/282; E179/242/25; E404/16/399, 31/420, 34/101, 46/299, 59/126, 60/73, 64/199, 72/2/27, 72/4/5, 54, 74/1/110, 75/1/20, 76/1/21; E405/70; Probate Court of Canterbury, Logge 2, 5; SC8/231/11510, 304/15189; SP1/19, 22

Trinity College Library, Cambridge, Mss R.14.32, 52

Wellcome Library, Western Mss 290, 537, 564, 626, 784

York Minster Library, Ms. XVI. E. 32

PUBLISHED PRIMARY SOURCES

Abélard, Peter, *The Letters of Peter Abélard*, ed. B. Radice (pbk, London, 1974)

Albucasis, *Albucasis on Surgery and Instruments*, ed. M.S. Spink and G.L. Lewis (London, 1973)

An Alphabet of Tales, A–H, ed. M.M. Banks (Early English Text Soc., CXXVI, 1904)

Ane Addicioun of Scottis Croniklis and Deidis, ed. T. Thomson (Edinburgh, 1819)

Anglicus, Bartholomaeus, *On the Properties of Things: John Trevisa's Translation of Bartholomaeus Anglicus' De Proprietatibus Rerum*, ed. M.C. Seymour and others (3 vols, Oxford, 1975–88)

Anglicus, Gilbertus, *Healing and Society in Medieval England: A Middle English Translation of the Pharmaceutical Writings of Gilbertus Anglicus*, ed. F.M. Getz (Wisconsin Publications in the History of Science and Medicine, VIII, 1991)

Anglicus, Johannes, *Rosa Anglica, sev Rosa Medicinae Johannis Anglici*, ed. W. Wulff (Irish Text Soc., XXV, 1929)

Anjou, René of, *Oeuvres Complètes du Roi René*, ed. Le Comte de Quatrebarbes (4 vols, Angers, 1845–6)

Annals of the Barber Surgeons of London, ed. S. Young (London, 1890)

Arderne, John of, *Treatises of Fistula in Ano*, ed. D. Power (Early English Text Soc., CXXXIX, 1910)

Augustine, St, *Concerning the City of God against the Pagans*, trans. H. Bettenson (pbk, London, 1984)

Bale, John, *The Complete Plays*, ed. P. Happe (2 vols, Woodbridge, 1985–6)

Beverley Town Documents, ed. A.F. Leach (Selden Soc., XIV, 1900)

The Book of the Knight of La Tour-Landry ed. T. Wright (Early English Text Soc., XXXIII, 1868)

The Book of Vices and Virtues, ed. W.N. Francis (Early English Text Soc., CCXVII, 1942, reprinted 1968)

Brakelond, Jocelin of, *Chronicle of the Abbey of Bury St Edmunds*, ed. D. Greenway and J. Sayers (pbk, Oxford, 1989)

Brunne, Robert of, *Robert of Brunne's Handlyng Synne*, ed. F.J. Furnivall (Early English Text Soc., CXIX, 1901)

Burton, Robert, *The Anatomy of Melancholy*, ed. T.C. Faulkener and others (2 vols, Oxford, 1989–90)

Calendar of Close Rolls

Calendar of Coroners' Rolls of the City of London 1300–1378, ed. R.R. Sharpe (London, 1913)

Calendar of Early Mayor's Court Rolls of the City of London, 1298–1307, ed. A.H. Thomas (Cambridge, 1925)

Calendar of Fine Rolls

Calendar of the Freemen of Norwich, 1317–1603, ed. W. Rye (London, 1888)

Calendar of Inquisitions Miscellaneous

Calendar of the Letter Books of the City of London

Calendar of Papal Letters

Calendar of Papal Petitions

Calendar of Patent Rolls

Calendar of Plea and Memoranda Rolls of London

Calendar of State Papers Venetian, 1202–1509, ed. R. Brown (London, 1864)

Calendar of Wills Proved and Enrolled in the Court of Hustings, ed. R.R. Sharpe (2 vols, London, 1889–90)

Calendars of the Proceedings in Chancery in the Reign of Queen Elizabeth

Catalogue des Manuscrits de Médecine Médiévale de la Bibliothèque de Bruges, ed. A. de Pooter (Paris, 1924)

Catalogue of Western Manuscripts on Medicine and Science in the Wellcome Historical Medical Library, ed. S.A.J. Moorat, vol. I, *Mss. Written before 1650 A.D.* (London, 1962)

Catherine of Siena, *The Letters of St Catherine of Siena*, ed. S. Noffke (4 vols in progress, Medieval and Renaissance Texts and Studies, Binghampton, New York, 1988 onwards)

Caxton, William, *Dialogues in French and English*, ed. H. Bradley (Early English Text Soc., extra series, LXXIX, 1900)

——, *The Game and Playe of the Chesse*, ed. W.E.A. Axon (London, 1883)

Chartularium Universitatis Parisiensis, ed. H. Denifle and A. Chatelain (4 vols, Paris, 1897–9)

Chaucer, Geoffrey, *Works*, ed. F.N. Robinson (Oxford, 1970)

Chauliac, Guy de, *The Cyrurgie of Guy de Chauliac*, ed. M.S. Ogden (Early English Text Soc., CCLXV, 1971)

Chronicon Angliae 1328–1388, ed. E.M. Thompson (Rolls Series, 1874)

Collection de Documents pour Servir a l'Histoire des Hôpitaux de Paris, ed. M. Briele and others (4 vols, Paris, 1881–7)

A Common-Place Book of the Fifteenth Century, ed. L.T. Smith, (London, 1886)

Commynes, Philippe de, *Mémoires*, ed. J. Calmette (3 vols, Paris, 1924–5)

A Contemporary Narrative of the Proceedings Against Dame Alice Kyteler, ed. T. Wright (Camden Soc., XXIV, 1843)

Councils and Synods, 1205–1313, ed. F.M. Powicke and C.R. Cheney (2 vols, Oxford, 1964)

The Dance of Death, ed. F. Warren (Early English Text Soc., CLXXXI, 1931)

Daniel, Walter, *The Life of Ailred of Rievaulx*, ed. F.M. Powicke (London, 1950)

Dante Alighieri, *Hell*, trans. S. Ellis (London, 1994)

Dives and Pauper, ed. P. Heath Barnum (Early English Text Soc., CCLXXV, 1976, and CCLXXX, 1980)

Documentazioni Cronologiche per la Storia della Medicina, Chirurgia e Farmacia in Venezia 1258–1382, ed. V. Stefanutti (Venice, 1961)

Dunbar, William, *The Poems of William Dunbar*, ed. J. Kinsley (Oxford, 1979)

Early English Meals and Manners, ed. F.J. Furnivall (Early English Text Soc., XXXII, 1868)

The Early English Versions of the Gesta Romanorum, ed. S.J.H. Heritage (Early English Text Soc., extra series, XXXIII, 1879)

The English and Scottish Popular Ballads, ed. F.J. Child (5 vols, Folklore Press, New York, 1957)

English Gilds, ed. T. Smith, L.T. Smith and L. Brentano (Early English Text Soc., XL, 1890)

English Medieval Handwriting, comp. A. Rycraft, Borthwick Wallet, III (York, 1973)

English Metrical Homilies, ed. J. Small (Edinburgh, 1862)

The English Text of the Ancrene Riwle, ed. A. Zettersten (Early English Text Soc., CCLXXIV, 1976)

English Wycliffite Sermons, ed. A. Hudson (3 vols, Oxford 1983–90)

Erasmus of Rotterdam, *The Correspondence of Erasmus, Letters 1523–24*, trans. R.A.B. Mynors and A. Dalzell (*The Collected Works of Erasmus*, Toronto, X, 1992)

——, *In Praise of Folly*, ed. H. Hopewell Hudson (Princeton, 1970)

The Exchequer Rolls of Scotland

Expeditions to Prussia and the Holy Land Made by Henry, Earl of Derby, ed. L. Toulmin Smith (Camden Soc., new series, LII, 1894)

Extracts from the Records of the Burgh of Edinburgh, 1403–1528 (Scottish Burgh Records Soc., 1869)

Fabric Rolls of York Minster, ed. J. Raine (Surtees Soc., XXXV, 1858)

Fasciculus Morum: A Fourteenth-Century Preachers' Handbook, ed. S. Wenzel (Pennsylvania, 1989)

Fisher, John, *English Works of John Fisher*, ed. J.E. Mayor (Early English Text Soc., extra series, XXVII, 1876)

Foedera, Conventiones, Litterae et cuiuscunque Generis Acta Publica, ed. T. Rymer (20 vols, The Hague, 1704–35)

Fortescue, John, *De Laudibus Legem Anglie*, ed. and trans. S.B. Chrimes (Cambridge, 1949)

Foxe, John, *Acts and Monuments of John Foxe*, ed. G. Townsend and S.R. Cattley (8 vols, London, 1837–41)

Freemen of the City of York, 1272–1558, ed. F. Collins (Surtees Soc., XCVI, 1896)

Froissart, Sir John, *Sir John Froissart's Chronicles*, ed. and trans. T. Jones (4 vols, Haford, 1803–5)

Galen, *Galen on the Usefulness of the Parts of the Body*, ed. M.T. May (2 vols, Cornell, 1968)

The Goodman of Paris, ed. G.G. Coulton and E. Power (London, 1928)

Gower, John, *The Complete Works*, ed. G.C. Macaulay (4 vols, Oxford, 1899–1902)

——, *The English Works*, ed. G.C. Macaulay (Early English Text Soc., LXXXI, LXXXII, 1900)

Hall, Edward, *Hall's Chronicle Containing the History of England During the Reign of Henry the Fourth and the Succeeding Monarchs* (London, 1809)

Henryson, Robert, *The Poems and Fables of Robert Henryson*, ed. H.H. Wood (Edinburgh and London, 1958)

Hippocratic Writings, ed. G.E.R. Lloyd (pbk, London, 1983)

The Historical Collections of a Citizen of London, ed. J. Gairdner (Camden Soc., new series, XVII, 1876)

Historical Manuscripts Commission, Sixth Report

Hoccleve, Thomas, *Hoccleve's Works: The Minor Poems*, ed. F.J. Furnivall and I. Gollancz (Early English Text Soc., extra series, LXI, 1892, LXXIII, 1925, reprinted in one vol. 1970)

——, *Hoccleve's Works: The Regiment of Princes and Fourteen Minor Poems*, ed. F.J. Furnivall (Early English Text Soc., LXXII, 1897)

Horae Beatae Mariae Virginis, ed. E. Hoskins (London, 1901)

Household Accounts from Medieval England, ed. C.M. Woolgar (Records of Social and Economic History, new series, XVII, 1992)

The Household Books of John Howard, Duke of Norfolk, 1462–1471, 1481–1483 (1 vol. in 2 parts, Stroud, 1992)

Illustrations from The Life of Bertrand Duguesclin by Jean Cuvelier, ed. H.Y. Thompson (London, 1909)

Intrates: A List of Persons Admitted to Live and Trade within the City of Canterbury 1392–1592, ed. J. Meadows Cowper (Canterbury, 1904)

Inventaires Mobiliers et Extraits des Comptes des Ducs de Bourgogne, 1363–1471, ed. B. and H. Prost (2 vols, Paris, 1902–13)

Issues of the Exchequer, ed. F. Devon (London, 1847)

John of Gaunt's Register, Part I, 1371–75, ed. S. Armitage-Smith (Camden Soc., third series, XX, 1911)

John of Gaunt's Register, 1379–83, ed. E.C. Lodge and R.S. Somerville (Camden Soc., third series, LVI, 1937)

Kempe, Margery, *The Book of Margery Kempe*, ed. W. Butler-Bowdon (Oxford, 1954)

——, *The Book of Margery Kempe*, ed. S.B. Meeche (Early English Text Soc., CCXII, 1940)

Lancaster, Henry of, *Le Livre de Seyntz Médicines*, ed. E.J. Arnould (Oxford, 1940)

Lanfrank, *Lanfrank's 'Science of Cirurgie'*, ed. R. von Fleischhacker (Early English Text Soc., CII, 1894)

Langland, William, *The Vision of Piers Plowman*, ed. A.V.C. Schmidt (London, 1978)

——, *Piers the Plowman*, ed. W.W. Skeat (2 vols, Oxford, third impression, 1961)

A Leechbook or Collection of Medical Recipes of the Fifteenth Century, ed. W.R. Dawson (London, 1934)

Letters and Papers of Henry VIII

The Libelle of Englyshe Polycye, ed. G. Warner (Oxford, 1926)

The Liber de Diversis Medicinis, ed. M.S. Ogden (Early English Text Soc., CCVII, reprinted 1969)

The Life of St Hugh of Lincoln, ed. D.L. Douie and H. Farmer (2 vols, London, 1961–2)

The Lisle Letters, ed. M. St Clare Byrne (5 vols, Chicago, 1981)

A Litil Boke the Whiche Trayted and Reherced Many Gode Thinges Necessaries for the . . . Pestilence (John Rylands Facsimiles, III, 1910)

The Little Red Book of Bristol, ed. F.B. Bickley (2 vols, Bristol, 1900)

Loris, Guillaume de, and Jean de Meun, *The Romance of the Rose*, ed. and trans. C. Dahlberg (New England, 1983)

Lydgate, John, *The Minor Poems: Secular Poems*, ed. H.N. MacCracken (Early English Text Soc., CXCII, 1939)

——, *The Minor Poems: Religious Poems*, ed. H.N. MacCracken (Early English Text Soc., CVII, 1911, reprinted 1961)

Malory, Thomas, *Le Morte d'Arthur*, ed. J. Cowen (pbk, 2 vols, London, 1986)

Mandeville, John, *Mandeville's Travels*, ed. P. Hamelius (Early English Text Soc., CLIII, 1919)

Manuscript Archives of the Worshipful Company of Grocers of the City of London 1345–1463, ed. J.A. Kingdon (2 vols, London, 1886)

Medieval Woman's Guide to Health, ed. B. Rowland (Kent, Ohio, 1981)

Memorials of London and London Life in the Thirteenth, Fourteenth and Fifteenth Centuries, ed. H.T. Riley (London, 1868)

Le Ménagier de Paris, ed. G.E. Brereton and J.M. Ferrier (Oxford, 1981)

Metham, John, *The Works of John Metham*, ed. H. Craig (Early English Text Soc., CXXXII, 1916)

Les Métiers et Corporations de la Ville de Paris, ed. R. de Lespinasse (3 vols, Paris, 1886–97)

Middle English Sermons, ed. W.O. Ross (Early English Text Soc., CCIX, 1940, reprinted 1960)

Milton, John, *Paradise Lost*, ed. M.Y. Hughes (New York, 1935)

The Miracles of King Henry VI, ed. R. Knox and S. Leslie (London, 1923)

Mirfeld, Johannes de, *Johannes de Mirfeld: His Life and Works*, ed. P. Horton-Smith-Hartley and H.R. Aldridge (Cambridge, 1936)

Missale ad Usum Insignis Ecclesiae Eboracensis, ed. W.G. Henderson (Surtees Soc., LXIX and LX, 1872)

Monmouth, Thomas of, *The Life and Miracles of St William of Norwich*, ed. A. Jessopp and M.R. James (Cambridge, 1896)

More, Thomas, *The Workes of Sir Thomas More, Knyght* (London, 1557)

——, *The Apology*, ed. J.B. Trapp (*The Complete Works of St Thomas More*, New Haven, IX, 1979)

——, *A Dialogue Concerning Heresies*, ed. T.M.C. Lawler and others (*The Complete Works of St Thomas More*, New Haven, VI, 1981)

Moryson, Fynes, *An Itinerary* (4 vols, Glasgow, 1907–8)

Mum and the Sothsegger, ed. M. Day and R. Steele (Early English Text Soc., CIC, 1936)

Myrc, John, *Instructions for Parish Priests*, ed. E. Peacock (Early English Text Soc., XXXI, 1868, revised 1902)

—— [Mirk], *Mirk's Festial: A Collection of Homilies*, ed. T. Erbe (Early English Text Soc., XCVI, 1905)

Norton, Thomas, *Thomas Norton's Ordinal of Alchemy*, ed. J. Reidy (Oxford, 1975)

The Observances in Use at the Augustinian Priory of S. Giles and S. Andrew at Barnwell, Cambridgeshire, ed. J. Willis Clark (Cambridge, 1897)

Original Letters Illustrative of English History, ed. H. Ellis (3 series in 11 vols, London, 1824–46)

The Oxford Dictionary of Saints, ed. D.H. Farmer (Oxford, 1978)

Paris, Matthew, *Chronica Majora*, ed. H.R. Luard (7 vols, London, 1872–84)

Parish Fraternity Register: Fraternity of the Holy Trinity and SS Fabian and Sebastian in the Parish of St Botolph without Aldersgate, ed. P. Basing (London Record Soc., XVIII, 1982)

Paston Letters and Papers of the Fifteenth Century, ed. N. Davis (2 vols, Oxford, 1971–6)

Pecock, Reginald, *The Reule of Crysten Religioun,* ed. W.C. Greet (Early English Text Soc., CLXXI, 1927)

Phares, Symon de, *Receuil des Plus Célèbres Astrologues et Quelques Hommes Doctes*, ed. E. Wickersheimer (Paris, 1929)

Pisan, Christine de, *The Treasure of the City of Ladies*, trans. S. Lawson (pbk, London, 1985)

The Political Songs of England, ed. T. Wright (Camden Soc., VI, 1839)

Polydore Vergil's English History, ed. H. Ellis (Camden Soc., XXIX, 1845)

Privy Purse Expenses of Elizabeth of York, ed. N.H. Nicolas (London, 1830)

Procès de Condamnation de Jeanne d'Arc, ed. P. Tisset (3 vols, Paris, 1960–71)

The Prymer off Salysburye Use (John Growle, London, 1533)

Rabelais, François, *The Histories of Gargantua and Pantagruel*, trans. J.M. Cohen (pbk, London, 1969)

Records of the Borough of Nottingham, ed. W.H. Stevenson (3 vols, Nottingham, 1882)

Records of the City of Norwich, ed. W. Hudson and J.C. Tingey (2 vols, Norwich, 1906–19)

Records of the Wardrobe and Household 1285–1286, ed. B.F. Byerly and C.R. Byerly (London, 1977)

Records of the Wardrobe and Household 1286–1289, ed. B.F. Byerly and C.R. Byerly (London, 1986)

The Register of Edward the Black Prince, ed. M.C.B. Dawes (4 vols, London, 1930–3)

The Register of Henry Chichele, ed. E.F. Jacob (Canterbury and York Soc., XLII, 1937)

The Register of John Stafford, ed. T.S. Holmes (Somerset Record Soc., XXXI–XXXII, 1915–16)

Religious Lyrics of the Fifteenth Century, ed. C. Brown (Oxford, 1962)

Reports of the Deputy Keepers of the Public Records

Reynes, Robert, *The Common Place Book of Robert Reynes of Acle, an Edition of Tanner Ms. 407*, ed. C. Louis (Garland, New York, 1980)

The Roll of the Freemen of the City of Canterbury, 1392–1800, ed. J. Meadows Cowper (Canterbury, 1903)

Rolle, Richard, *Yorkshire Writers: Richard Rolle of Hampole*, ed. C. Horstman (2 vols, London, 1895–6)

Rolls of the Justices in Eyre for Yorkshire, ed. D.M. Stenton (Selden Soc., LVI, 1937)

Rotuli Parliamentorum

Rutebeuf, *Oeuvres Complètes*, ed. M. Zink (2 vols, Paris, 1989–90)

Scripta Leonis, Rufini et Angeli Sociorum S. Francisci, ed. R.B. Brooke (Oxford, 1990)

Secretum Secretorum, ed. M.A. Manzalaoui (Early English Text Soc., CCLXXVI, 1977)

Secular Lyrics of the Fourteenth and Fifteenth Centuries, ed. R.H. Robbins (Oxford, 1952)

The 'Sekenesse of Wymmen', ed. M.R. Hallaert (Brussels, 1982)

Select Cases in the Court of King's Bench under Richard II, Henry IV and Henry V, ed. G.O. Sales (Selden Soc., LXXXVIII, 1971)

Shillingford, John, *Letters and Papers of John Shillingford*, ed. S.A. Moore (Camden Soc., new series, II, 1871)

The Siege of Jerusalem, ed. E. Kolbing and M. Day (Early English Text Soc., CLXXXVIII, 1932)

Sir Gawain and the Green Knight, ed. B. Stone (pbk, London, 1974)

Skelton, John, *The Complete English Poems*, ed. J. Scattergood (Yale, 1983)

Society at War, ed. C.T. Allmand (Edinburgh, 1973)

Songs, Carols and Other Miscellaneous Poems, ed. R. Dyboski (Early English Text Soc., extra series, CI, 1907)

Soranus, *Soranus' Gynaecology*, ed. O. Temkin (Johns Hopkins, 1956)

Starkey, Thomas, *A Dialogue Between Cardinal Pole and Thomas Lupset, in England in the Reign of King Henry the Eighth*, ed. J.M. Cowper (Early English Text Soc., extra series, XII, 1871, and XXXII, 1878, reprinted 1971)

Statutes of the Realm

Les Statuts et Règlements des Apothicaires, ed. F. Prevet (15 vols, Paris, 1950)

Stonor Letters and Papers, ed. C.L. Kingsford (Camden Soc., third series, XXIX and XXX, 1919)

Strassburg, Gottfried von, *Tristan*, ed. A.T. Hatto (pbk, London, 1967)

The Thornton Manuscript (Scolar Press, 1975)

Three Prose Versions of the Secreta Secretorum, ed. R. Steele (Early English Text Soc., extra series, LXXIV, 1898)

Twenty-Six Political and Other Poems, ed. J. Kail (Early English Text Soc., CXXIV, 1904)

Valor Ecclesiasticus, ed. J. Caley and J. Hunter (6 vols, London, 1810–34)

Villanova, Arnald de, *De Dosi Tyriacalium Medicinarum*, in *Opera Medica Omnia*, vol. III, ed. M.R. McVaugh (Barcelona, 1985)

Villon, François, *Le Testament Villon*, ed. J. Rychner and A. Henry (2 vols, Geneva, 1974)

Visitation Articles and Injunctions, ed. W.H. Frere (Alcuin Club Collections, XIV–XVI, 1910)

Visitation of Religious Houses in the Diocese of Lincoln, ed. A.H. Thompson (Canterbury and York Soc., XXIV, 1919)

Visitations of the Diocese of Norwich, 1492–1532, ed. A. Jessopp (Camden Soc., new series, XLIII, 1888)

Voragine, Jacobus de, *The Golden Legend of Jacobus de Voragine*, ed. and trans. G. Ryan and H. Ripperger (New York, 1969)

Walsingham, Thomas, *Historia Anglicana*, ed. H.T. Riley (2 vols, Rolls Series, 1863–4)

Webb, J., 'Translation of a French Metrical History of the Deposition of Richard II', *Archaeologia*, XX (1824)

Wills and Inventories from the Registers of the Commissary of Bury St Edmunds, ed. S. Tymms (Camden Soc., XLIX, 1850)

Wimbledon, Thomas, *Wimbledon's Sermon Redde Rationem Villicationis Tue*, ed. I.K. Knight (Duquesne Studies, Philological Series, IX, 1967)

Woman Defamed and Woman Defended, ed. A. Blamires (Oxford, 1992)

Wyclif, John, *Select English Works of John Wyclif*, ed. T. Arnold (3 vols, Oxford, 1869–71)

York City Chamberlains' Account Rolls 1396–1500, ed. R.B. Dobson (Surtees Soc., CXCII, 1978–9)

York Civic Ordinances 1301, ed. M. Prestwich (University of York, Borthwick Paper, XLIX, 1976)

York Memorandum Book 1376–1419, ed. M. Sellars (Surtees Soc., CXX, 1911)

York Memorandum Book 1388–1493, ed. M. Sellars (Surtees Soc., CXXV, 1914)

SECONDARY SOURCES

Alston, M., 'The Attitude of the Church towards Dissection before 1500', *Bulletin of the History of Medicine*, XVI (1944)

Amundsen, D.W., 'Medical Deontology and Pestilential Disease in the Later Middle Ages', *Journal of the History of Medicine*, XXXII (1977)

——, 'Medieval Canon Law on Medical and Surgical Practice by the Clergy', *Bulletin of the History of Medicine*, LII (1978)

——, 'Medicine and Faith in Early Christianity, *Bulletin of the History of Medicine,* LVI (1982)

—— and Ferngren, G.B., 'Philanthropy in Medicine: Some Historical Perspectives', in *Beneficence and Health Care*, ed. E.E. Shelp (*Philosophy and Medicine*, XI, 1982)

Arbesmann, R., 'The Concept of *Christus Medicus* in St Augustine', *Traditio*, X (1954)

Aries, P., *The Hour of Our Death*, trans. H. Weaver (pbk, London, 1987)

Arnould, E.J., *Étude sur le Livre des Saintes Médécines du Duc Henri de Lancastre* (Paris, 1948)

Aungier, G.J., *The History and Antiquities of Syon Monastery* (London, 1840)

Baildon, W.P., 'Notes on the Religious and Secular Houses of Yorkshire', *Yorkshire Archaeological Soc.* (Record Series, XVII, 1894)

Barkai, R., 'A Medieval Hebrew Treatise on Obstetrics', *Medical History*, XXXIII (1989)

Beauvoir, S. de, *The Second Sex*, trans. H.M. Parshley (pbk, London, 1988)

Beck, T., *The Cutting Edge: Early History of the Surgeons of London* (London, 1974)

Benedek, T.G., 'The Changing Relationship between Midwives and Physicians during the Renaissance', *Bulletin of the History of Medicine*, LI (1977)

Benton, J.F., 'Trotula, Women's Problems, and the Professionalization of Medicine in the Middle Ages', *Bulletin of the History of Medicine*, LIX (1985)

Biller, P.P.A., 'Birth Control in the West in the Thirteenth and Early Fourteenth Centuries', *Past and Present*, XCIV (1982)

——, 'Childbirth in the Middle Ages', *History Today*, XXXVI (1986)

——, 'Marriage Patterns and Women's Lives: A Sketch of a Pastoral Geography', in *Woman Is a Worthy Wight: Women in English Society* c. *1200–1500*, ed. P.J.P. Goldberg (Stroud, 1992)

Bloch, M., *The Royal Touch: Sacred Monarchy and Scrofula in England and France*, trans. J.E. Anderson (London, 1973)

Bober, H., 'The Zodiacal Miniature of the *Très Riches Heures* of the Duke of Berry', *Journal of the Warburg and Courtauld Institutes*, XI (1948)

Bolton, J., *The Medieval English Economy 1150–1500* (pbk, London, 1980)

Bond, E.A., 'Notices of the Last Days of Isabella, Queen of Edward II', *Archaeologia*, XXXV (1853)

Bradford, C.A., *Heart Burial* (London, 1933)

Brody, S.N., *The Disease of the Soul: Leprosy in Medieval Literature* (Cornell, 1974)

Brown, E.A.R., 'Death and the Human Body in the Later Middle Ages', *Viator*, XII (1981)

Brown, P., and Butcher, A., *The Age of Saturn* (Oxford, 1991)

Brundage, J.A., *Law, Sex and Christian Society in Medieval Europe* (Chicago, 1987)

Buhler, C.F., 'Prayers and Charms in Certain Middle English Scrolls', *Speculum*, XXXIX (1964)

Bullough, V.L., 'Medical Study at Medieval Oxford', *Speculum*, XXXVI (1961)

——, 'Medieval Medical and Scientific Views of Woman', *Viator*, IV (1973)

—— and Voght, M., 'Women, Menstruation and Nineteenth-Century Medicine', *Bulletin of the History of Medicine*, XLVII (1973)

Bynum, C.W., *Holy Feast and Holy Fast: The Religious Significance of Food to Medieval Women* (University of California Press, 1987)

Cadden, J., *Meanings of Sex Difference in the Middle Ages* (Cambridge, 1993)

Campbell, A.M., *The Black Death and Men of Learning* (New York, 1931)

Carey, H.M., 'Astrology at the English Court in the Later Middle Ages', in *Astrology, Science and Society*, ed. P. Curry (Woodbridge, 1987)

——, *Courting Disaster: Astrology at the English Court and University in the Later Middle Ages* (London, 1992)

Carlin, M., 'Medieval English Hospitals' in *The Hospital in History*, ed. L. Granshaw and R. Porter (pbk, London, 1990)

Charmasson, T., *Recherches sur une Technique Divinatoire: La Géomancie dans l'Occident Médiéval* (Paris, Geneva, 1980)

Cholmeley, H.P., *John of Gaddesden and The Rosa Medicinae* (Oxford, 1912)

Chrimes, S.B., *English Constitutional Ideas in the Fifteenth Century* (Cambridge, 1936)

Clark, C., 'The Zodiac Man in Medieval Astrology', *Journal of the Rocky Mountain Assoc.*, III (1982)

Clark, G.N., *A History of the Royal College of Physicians of London* (2 vols, Oxford, 1964)

Clay, R.M., *The Medieval Hospitals of England* (London, 1909)

Comrie, J.D., *History of Scottish Medicine* (2 vols, London, 1932)

Connor, R.D., *The Weights and Measures of England* (London, 1987)

Coopland, G.W., *Nicole Oresme and the Astrologers* (Harvard, 1952)

Coyecque, E., *L'Hôtel Dieu de Paris au Moyen Age* (2 vols, Paris, 1889–91)

Cullum, P.H., *Cremetts and Corrodies: Care of the Poor and Sick at St. Leonard's Hospital, York, in the Middle Ages* (University of York, Borthwick Paper, LXXIX, 1991)

——, 'Poverty and Charity in Early Fourteenth-Century England', in *England in the Fourteenth Century*, ed. N. Rogers (Stamford, 1993)

Demaitre, L., 'The Idea of Childhood and Child Care in Medical Writings of the Middle Ages', *Journal of Psychohistory*, IV (1977)

——, *Doctor Bernard de Gordon: Professor and Practitioner* (Toronto, 1980)

——, 'The Description and Diagnosis of Leprosy by Fourteenth-Century Physicians', *Bulletin of the History of Medicine*, LIX (1985)

Donnison, J., *Midwives and Medical Men* (London, 1988)

Doob, P.B.R., *Nebuchadnezzar's Children: Conventions of Madness in Middle English Literature* (Yale, 1974)

Duby, G., *The Three Orders: Feudal Society Imagined*, trans. A. Goldhammer (Chicago, 1980)

Duffy, E., *The Stripping of the Altars: Traditional Religion in England* c. *1400*–c. *1580* (Yale, 1992)

Duke Humphrey's Library and the Divinity School 1488–1988 (Bodleian Library, Oxford, 1988)

Dyer, C., *Standards of Living in the Later Middle Ages* (pbk, Cambridge, 1989)

Ell, S.R., 'The Two Medicines: Some Ecclesiastical Concepts of Disease and the Physician in the High Middle Ages', *Janus*, LXVIII (1981)

Emden, A.B., *Biographical Register of the University of Oxford to 1500* (3 vols, Oxford, 1957–9)

——, *Biographical Register of the University of Cambridge* (Cambridge, 1963)

Finucane, R.C., *Miracles and Pilgrims: Popular Beliefs in Medieval England* (London, 1977)

Flanagan, S., *Hildegard of Bingen, A Visionary Life* (pbk, London, 1990)

Fletcher, J.M., 'Linacre's Lands and Lectureships', in *Essays on the Life and Work of Thomas Linacre* c. *1460–1524*, ed. F. Maddison, M. Pelling and C. Webster (Oxford, 1977)

Flint, V.J., 'The Transmission of Astrology in the Early Middle Ages', *Viator*, XXI (1990)

——, *The Rise of Magic in Early Medieval Europe* (Princeton, 1991)

Forbes, T.R., 'Verbal Charms in British Folk Medicine', *Proceedings of the American Philosophical Soc.,* CXV (1971)

Garcia-Ballester, L., 'Changes in the *Regimina Sanitatis*: The Role of the Jewish Physicians' in *Health, Disease and Healing in Medieval Culture*, ed. S. Campbell, B. Hall and D. Klausner (Toronto, 1992)

Gask, G.E., 'The Medical Services of Henry the Fifth's Campaign of the Somme in 1415', in his *Essays on the History of Medicine* (London, 1950)

Geoghegan, D., 'A Licence of Henry VI to Practise Alchemy', *Ambix*, VI (1957/8)

Getz, F.M., 'Charity, Translation and the Language of Medical Learning in Medieval England', *Bulletin of the History of Medicine*, LXIV (1990)

——, 'To Prolong Life and Promote Health: Baconian Alchemy and Pharmacy in the English Learned Tradition', in *Health, Disease and Healing in Medieval Culture*, ed. S. Campbell, B. Hall and D. Klausner (Toronto, 1992)

——, 'The Faculty of Medicine before 1500', in *The History of the University of Oxford, Volume II, Late Medieval Oxford*, ed. J.I. Catto and R. Evans (Oxford, 1992)

Gilchrist, R., 'Christian Bodies and Souls: The Archaeology of Life and Death in English Hospitals', in *Death in Towns: Urban Responses to the Dying and the Dead, 100–1600*, ed. S. Bassett (Leicester, 1992)

Gilson, J.P., 'A Defence of the Proscription of the Yorkists in 1459', *English Historical Review*, XXVI (1911)

Goff, J. Le, *The Birth of Purgatory*, trans. A. Goldhammer (London, 1984)

Grafton, A.J., and Swerdlow, N.M., 'Calendar Days in Ancient Historiography', *Journal of the Warburg and Courtauld Institutes*, LI (1988)

Gransden, A., *Historical Writing in England II:* c. *1307 to the Early Sixteenth Century* (London, 1982)

Green, M., 'Women's Medical Practice and Health Care in Medieval Europe', *Signs*, XIV (1989)

Griffiths, R.A., 'The Trial of Eleanor Cobham: An Episode in the Fall of Duke Humphrey of Gloucester', *Bulletin of the John Rylands Library*, LI (1968/9)

——, *The Reign of King Henry VI* (London, 1981)

Gunther, R.T., *Early Science in Oxford* (14 vols, Oxford, 1925–45)

Guy, J.R., 'The Episcopal Licensing of Physicians, Surgeons and Midwives', *Bulletin of the History of Medicine*, LVI (1982)

Hall, D.J., *English Medieval Pilgrimage* (London, 1965)

Hammond, E.A., 'The Westminster Abbey Infirmarers' Rolls as a Source for Medical History', *Bulletin of the History of Medicine*, XXXIX (1965)

Hanawalt, B., 'Childrearing among the Lower Classes in Late Medieval England', *Journal of Interdisciplinary History*, VIII (1977/8)

Harvey, B., *Living and Dying in England 1100–1540: The Monastic Experience* (Oxford, 1993)

Harvey, J., 'Henry Daniel: A Scientific Gardener of the Fourteenth Century', *Garden History*, XV (1987)

Harvey, J., *Medieval Gardens* (pbk, London, 1990)

Hatcher, J., 'Mortality in the Fifteenth Century: Some New Evidence', *Economic History Review*, second series, XXXIX (1986)

Hayum, A., *The Isenheim Altarpiece: God's Medicine and the Painter's Vision* (Princeton, 1989)

Hébert, M., 'L'Armée Provençale en 1374', *Annales du Midi*, XCI (1979)

Henderson, J., 'The Hospitals of Late Medieval and Renaissance Florence', in *The Hospital in History*, ed. L. Granshaw and R. Porter (pbk, London, 1990)

——, 'The Black Death in Florence: Medical and Communal Responses', in *Death in Towns: Urban Responses to the Dying and the Dead, 100–1600*, ed. S. Bassett (Leicester, 1992)

—— and Park, K., '"The First Hospital Among Christians": The Ospedale di Santa Maria Nuova in Early Sixteenth-Century Florence', *Medical History*, XXXV (1991)

Herlihy, D., 'Life Expectancies for Women in Medieval Society', in *The Role of Women in the Middle Ages*, ed. R.T. Morewedge (London, 1975)

The History of Parliament: The House of Commons 1386–1421, ed. J.S. Roskell, L. Clark and C. Rawcliffe (4 vols, Stroud, 1993)

Holmes, G., *Augustan England, Professions, State and Society 1680–1730* (London, 1982)

Holmes, G.A., *The Good Parliament* (Oxford, 1975)

Honeybourne, M.B., 'The Leper Hospitals of the London Area', *Transactions of the London and Middlesex Archaeological Soc.*, XXI (1967)

Hooper, B., and others, 'The Grave of Sir Hugh de Hastyngs, Elsing', *Norfolk Archaeology*, XXXIX (1984)

Houlbrooke, R.A., *The English Family 1450–1700* (pbk, London, 1984)

Hughes, M.J., *Women Healers in Medieval Literature* (New York, 1943, reprinted 1968)

Huizinga, J., *The Waning of the Middle Ages*, trans. F. Hopman (pbk, London, 1976)

Hunt, T., *Popular Medicine in Thirteenth-Century England* (Woodbridge, 1990)

Jackson, R., *Doctors and Diseases in the Roman Empire* (London, 1988)

Jacquart, D., *Dictionnaire Biographique des Médecins en France au Moyen Age* (Hautes Études Médiévales et Modernes, series 5, XXXV, 1979)

——, *Le Milieu Médical en France du XIIe au XVe Siècle* (Hautes Études Médiévales et Modernes, series 5, XLVI, 1981)

——, and Thomasset, C., *Sexuality and Medicine in the Middle Ages* (Cambridge, 1988)

James, M., 'Ritual, Drama and Social Body in the Late Medieval English Town', *Past and Present*, XCVIII (1983)

Jamison, C., *The History of the Royal Hospital of St Katherine* (Oxford, 1952)

Jarcho, S., 'Guide for Physicians (Musar Harofim) by Isaac Judaeus', *Bulletin of the History of Medicine*, XV (1944)

Jewson, C.B., *History of the Great Hospital Norwich* (Norwich, 1980)

Johnstone, H., 'Poor Relief in the Royal Households of Thirteenth-Century England', *Speculum*, IV (1929)

Jones, M.K., and Underwood, M.G., *The King's Mother* (Cambridge, 1992)

Jones, P.M., *Medieval Medical Miniatures* (London, 1984)

——, 'Four Middle English Translations of John of Arderne', in *Latin and Vernacular: Studies in Late Medieval Texts and Manuscripts*, ed. A.J. Minnis (Woodbridge, 1989)

Kealey, E.J., 'England's Earliest Women Doctors', *Journal of the History of Medicine*, XL (1985)

Kelly, H.A., 'English Kings and the Fear of Sorcery', *Mediaeval Studies*, XXXIX (1977)

Kennedy, V.I., 'Robert Courson on Penance', *Mediaeval Studies*, VII (1945)

Kibre, P., 'Lewis of Caerleon, Doctor of Medicine, Astronomer and Mathematician', *Isis*, XLIII (1952)

Kibre, P., 'Arts and Medicine in the Universities of the Later Middle Ages', *Mediaevalia Louaniensia*, series one, VI (1978)

——, *Studies in Medieval Science: Alchemy, Astrology, Mathematics and Medicine* (London, 1984)

Kieckhefer, R., *Magic in the Middle Ages* (pbk, Cambridge, 1990)

Kittredge, G.L., *Witchcraft in Old and New England* (Cambridge, Mass., 1928)

Knowles, D., and Hadcock, R.N., *Medieval Religious Houses of England and Wales* (London, 1971)

Krivatsky, P., 'Erasmus' Medical Milieu', *Bulletin of the History of Medicine*, XLVIII (1973)

Labarge, M. Wade, *Women in Medieval Life* (London, 1986)

Lang, S.J., 'John Bradmore and His Book Philomena', *Social History of Medicine*, V (1992)

Laqueur, T.W., *Making Sex: Body and Gender from the Greeks to Freud* (Harvard, 1990)

Leader, D.R., *A History of the University of Cambridge, Volume I, The University to 1546* (Cambridge, 1988)

Lecat, J.P., *Le Siècle de la Toison d'Or* (Paris, 1986)

Lemay, H.R., 'Anthonius Guainerius and Medieval Gynecology', in *Women of the Medieval World*, ed. J. Kirshner and S.F. Wemple (Oxford, 1985)

Levey, M., *Early Arab Pharmacology* (Leiden, 1973)

Lindberg, D.C., 'The Transmission of Greek and Arab Learning to the West', in *Science in the Middle Ages*, ed. D.C. Lindberg (Chicago, 1978)

Lyons, A.S., and Petrucelli, R.J., *Medicine: An Illustrated History* (New York, 1978)

McDougall, I., 'The Third Instrument of Medicine: Some Accounts of Surgery in Medieval Iceland', in *Health, Disease and Healing in Medieval Culture*, ed. S. Campbell, B. Hall and D. Klausner (Toronto, 1992)

Macfarlane, A., 'Illegitimacy and Illegitimates in English History' in *Bastardy and Its Comparative History*, ed. P. Laslett and others (London, 1980)

McFarlane, K.B., *England in the Fifteenth Century* (pbk, London, 1981)

Mackinney, L.C., 'Medical Ethics and Etiquette in the Early Middle Ages', *Bulletin of the History of Medicine*, XXXVI (1952)

McMurray Gibson, G., 'Saint Anne and the Religion of Childbed: Some East Anglian Texts and Talismans', in *Interpreting Cultural Symbols: Saint Anne in Late Medieval Society*, ed. K. Ashley and P. Sheingorn (Athens, Georgia, 1990)

McNiven, P., 'The Problem of Henry IV's Health, 1405–1413', *English Historical Review*, C (1985)

McVaugh, M.R., and Voigts, L.E., 'A Latin Technical Phlebotomy and Its Middle English Translation', *Transactions of the American Philosophical Society*, LXXIV (1984)

Maddicott, J.R., 'Parliament and the Constituencies' in *The English Parliament in the Middle Ages*, ed. R.G. Davies and J.H. Denton (Manchester, 1981)

Martin, C.T., 'Clerical Life in the Fifteenth Century', *Archaeologia*, LX (1907)

Matthews, L.G., 'King John of France and the English Spicers', *Medical History*, V (1961)

——, The Spicers and Apothecaries of Norwich', *Pharmaceutical Journal*, CXCVIII (1967)

——, *The Royal Apothecaries* (London, 1967)

Mayer, C.F., 'A Medieval English Leechbook and its Fourteenth-Century Poem on Bloodletting', *Bulletin of the History of Medicine*, VII (1939)

Miller, B.D.H., 'She Who Hath Drunk Any Potion', *Medium Aevum*, XXXI (1962)

Mooney, L.R., 'A Middle English Verse Compendium of Astrological Medicine', *Medical History*, XXVIII (1984)

Moore, R.I., 'Heresy as Disease', in *The Concept of Heresy in the Middle Ages*, ed. W. Lordaux and V. Verhelst (*Mediaevalia Louaniensia*, series one, IV, 1976)

——, *The Formation of a Persecuting Society* (Oxford, 1987)

Mustain, J.K., 'A Rural Medical Practitioner in Fifteenth-Century England', *Bulletin of the History of Medicine*, XLVI (1972)

Myers, A.R., *The Household of Edward IV* (Manchester, 1959)

——, 'The Jewels of Queen Margaret of Anjou', *Bulletin of the John Rylands Library*, XLII (1959–60)

——, *Crown, Household and Parliament in the Fifteenth Century* (London, 1985)

Noorda, S.J., 'Illness and Sin, Forgiving and Healing' in *Studies in Hellenistic Religions*, ed. M.J. Vermaseren (Leiden, 1979)

North, J.D., *Horoscopes and History* (Warburg Institute Surveys and Texts, XIII, 1986)

Opsomer-Halleux, C., 'The Medieval Garden and its Role in Medicine' in *Medieval Gardens*, ed. E.B. MacDougall (Dumbarton Oaks, 1986)

Origo, I., *The Merchant of Prato* (pbk, London, 1986)

Otway-Ruthven, J., *The King's Secretary and the Signet Office in the Fifteenth Century* (Cambridge, 1939)

Owst, G.R., *Literature and the Pulpit in Medieval England* (Oxford, 1961)

Pagels, E., *Adam, Eve, and the Serpent* (pbk, London, 1990)

Palmer, K., 'The Church, Leprosy and Plague in Medieval and Early Modern Europe', *Studies in Church History*, XIX (1982)

Park, K., *Doctors and Medicine in Early Renaissance Florence* (Princeton, 1985)

—— and Henderson, J., '"The First Hospital Among Christians": The Ospedale di Santa Maria Nuova in Early Sixteenth-Century Florence', *Medical History*, XXXV (1991)

Phillips, E.D., *Greek Medicine* (London, 1973)

Porter, R., *A Social History of Madness* (pbk, London, 1989)

——, *Mind Forg'd Manacles: A History of Madness in England from the Restoration to the Regency* (pbk, London, 1990)

Post, J.B., 'Doctor Versus Patient: Two Fourteenth Century Law Suits', *Medical History*, XVI (1972)

Pouchelle, M.C., *The Body and Surgery in the Middle Ages*, trans. R. Morris (Oxford, 1990)

Poulle, E., 'Horoscopes Princiers des XIVe et XVe Siècles', *Bulletin de la Société Nationale de Antiquaires de France* (Feb. 1969)

Power, E., 'Some Women Practitioners of Medicine in the Middle Ages', *Proceedings of the Royal Soc. of Medicine*, XV (1922)

Radford, U.M., 'The Wax Images Found in Exeter Cathedral', *Antiquaries Journal*, XXIX (1949)

Ranke-Heinemann, U., *Eunuchs for Heaven: The Catholic Church and Sexuality*, trans. J. Brownjohn (London, 1990)

Rawcliffe, C., *The Staffords, Earls of Stafford and Dukes of Buckingham, 1394–1521* (Cambridge, 1978)

——, 'The Hospitals of Later Medieval London', *Medical History*, XXVIII (1984)

——, 'Richard, Duke of York, the King's "Obeisant Liegeman", a New Source for the Protectorates of 1454 and 1455', *Historical Research*, LX (1987)

——, 'The Profits of Practice: the Wealth and Status of Medical Men in Later Medieval England', *Social History of Medicine*, I (1988)

——, 'Consultants, Careerists and Conspirators: Royal Doctors in the Time of Richard III', *The Ricardian*, no. 106 (1989)

Reutter de Rosemont, L., *Histoire de la Pharmacie à travers les Ages* (2 vols, Paris, 1931)

Richards, P., *The Medieval Leper and his Northern Heirs* (Cambridge, 1977)

Richardson, R., *Death, Dissection and the Destitute* (pbk, London, 1988)

Riddle, J.M., 'Theory and Practice in Medieval Medicine', *Viator*, V (1974)

Robbins, R.H., 'Medical Manuscripts in Middle English', *Speculum*, XLV (1970)

Roberts, K.B., and Tomlinson, J.D.W., *The Fabric of the Body: European Traditions of Anatomical Illustration* (Oxford, 1992)

Ross, C.D., *Edward IV* (London, 1975)

Rubin, M., *Charity and Community in Medieval Cambridge* (Cambridge, 1987)

——, 'Development and Change in English Hospitals, 1100–1500', in *The Hospital in History*, ed. L. Granshaw and R. Porter (pbk, London, 1990)

——, *Corpus Christi: The Eucharist in Late Medieval Culture* (pbk, Cambridge, 1992)

Rubin, S., *Medieval English Medicine* (New York, 1974)

Sabine, E.L., 'Butchering in Mediaeval London', *Speculum,* VIII (1933)

——, 'The Latrines and Cesspools of Mediaeval London', *Speculum,* IX (1934)

——, 'City Cleaning in Mediaeval London', *Speculum,* XII (1937)

Schmitt, C.B., 'Thomas Linacre and Italy', in *Essays on the Life and Work of Thomas Linacre c. 1460–1524,* ed. F. Maddison, M. Pelling and C. Webster (Oxford, 1977)

Scully, T., 'The Sickdish in Early English Recipe Collections', in *Health, Disease and Healing in Medieval Culture,* ed. S. Campbell, B. Hall and D. Klausner (Toronto, 1992)

Shinners, J.R., 'The Veneration of the Saints at Norwich Cathedral in the Fourteenth Century', *Norfolk Archaeology,* XL (1987)

Shorter, E., *A History of Women's Bodies* (London, 1983)

Siegel, R.E., *Galen's System of Physiology and Medicine* (New York, 1968)

Siraisi, N.G., *Medieval and Early Renaissance Medicine* (pbk, Chicago, 1990)

Skinner, S., *Terrestrial Astrology: Divination by Geomancy* (London, 1980)

Somerville, R., *The Savoy* (London, 1960)

South, D., and Power, J.F., *Memorials of the Craft of Surgery* (London, 1886)

Stratford, J., 'The Manuscripts of John Duke of Bedford: Library and Chapel' in *England in the Fifteenth Century,* ed. D. Williams (Woodbridge, 1987)

Talbot, C.H., and Hammond, E.A., *The Medical Practitioners in Medieval England* (London, 1965)

——, *Medicine in Medieval England* (London, 1967)

——, 'Medical Education in the Middle Ages', in *The History of Medical Education,* ed. C.D. O'Malley (Berkeley, California, 1970)

——, 'Medicine' in *Science in the Middle Ages,* ed. D.C. Lindberg (Chicago, 1978)

Tester, J., *A History of Western Astrology* (Woodbridge, 1987)

Thomas, K., *Religion and the Decline of Magic* (pbk, London, 1984)

Thompson, A.H., *The History of the Hospital and the New College of the Annunciation of St Mary in the Newarke, Leicester* (Leicestershire Archaeological Soc., 1937)

Thorndike, L., *A History of Magic and Experimental Science* (8 vols, London and Columbia, 1923–58)

——, *Science and Thought in the Fifteenth Century* (New York, 1929)

Thrupp, S.L., *The Merchant Class of Medieval London* (pbk, Ann Arbor, 1962)

Tout, T.F., *Chapters in the Administrative History of Medieval England* (6 vols, Manchester, 1920–33)

Townend, B.R., 'The Story of the Tooth Worm', *Bulletin of the History of Medicine,* XV (1944)

Trease, G.E., 'The Spicers and Apothecaries of the Royal Household in the Reigns of Henry III, Edward I and Edward II', *Nottingham Medieval Studies,* III (1959)

——, *Pharmacy in History* (London, 1964)

Ussery, H.E., *Chaucer's Physician: Medicine and Literature in Fourteenth Century England* (Tulane, 1971)

Vale, M., 'Cardinal Henry Beaufort and the "Albergati" Portrait', *English Historical Review,* CV (1990)

The Victoria County History of the County of York, ed. W. Page (3 vols, 1907–13, reprinted 1974)

The Victoria County History of London, ed. W. Page (London, 1909)

Voigts, L.E., 'Scientific and Medical Books', in *Book Production and Publishing in Britain, 1375–1475*, ed. J. Griffiths and D. Pearsall (Cambridge, 1984)

——, and McVaugh, M.R., 'A Latin Technical Phlebotomy and its Middle English Translation', *Transactions of the American Philosophical Soc.*, LXXIV (1984)

——, 'The Latin Verse and Middle English Prose Texts on the Sphere of Life and Death in Harley 3719', *The Chaucer Review*, XXI (1986)

——, and Hudson, R.P., 'A Surgical Anesthetic from Late Medieval England', in *Health, Disease and Healing in Medieval Culture*, ed. S. Campbell, B. Hall and D. Klausner (Toronto, 1992)

Warner, M., *Alone of All Her Sex: The Myth and Cult of the Virgin Mary* (pbk, London, 1976)

Webb, E.A., *The Records of St. Bartholomew's Priory* (2 vols, Oxford, 1921)

Webster, C., 'Thomas Linacre and the Foundation of the College of Physicians', in *Essays on the Life and Work of Thomas Linacre c. 1460–1524*, ed. F. Maddison, M. Pelling and C. Webster (Oxford, 1977)

Wenzel, S., 'Pestilence and Middle English Literature: Friar John Grimestone's Poems on Death', in *The Black Death: The Impact of the Fourteenth-Century Plague*, ed. D. Williman (New York, 1982)

White, L., 'Medical Astrologers and Late Medieval Technology', *Viator*, VI (1975)

Wickersheimer, E., *Dictionnaire Biographique des Médecins en France au Moyen Age* (Paris, 1936)

Wiesner, M.E., 'Early Modern Midwifery', in *Women and Work in Pre-Industrial Europe*, ed. B.A. Hanawalt (Indiana, 1986)

——, *Working Women in Renaissance Germany* (Rutgers, 1986)

Wilken, R.L., *The Christians as the Romans Saw Them* (Yale, 1984)

Wilson, G., *Theriac and Mithridatum, A Study in Therapeutics* (London, 1966)

Wormald, F., 'The Rood of Bromholm', *Journal of the Warburg Institute*, I (1937/8)

Wylie, J.H., *History of England under Henry IV* (4 vols, London, 1898)

Wyman, A.L., 'The Surgeoness: The Female Practitioner of Surgery 1400–1800', *Medical History*, XXVIII (1984)

Yates, F.A., *The Art of Memory* (pbk, London, 1969)

INDEX

The indexing of medieval names poses many problems. In the interests of consistency, saints and persons whose names include prefixes (de, of, von) are entered under their christian names. For the benefit of readers interested in the medical profession, the abbreviations (a)pothecary, (b)arber, (m)idwife, (p)hysician or leech and (s)urgeon denote late medieval practitioners.